Adverse Events,
Stress,
and Litigation

Adverse Events, Stress, and Litigation

A Physician's Guide

SARA C. CHARLES, M.D.
Professor of Psychiatry (Emerita)
University of Illinois School of Medicine at Chicago

PAUL R. FRISCH, J.D.
General Counsel
Oregon Medical Association

Illustrations by Ronald Bailey

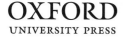

OXFORD
UNIVERSITY PRESS

2005

OXFORD
UNIVERSITY PRESS

Oxford University Press, Inc., publishes works that further
Oxford University's objective of excellence
in research, scholarship, and education.

Oxford   New York
Auckland   Cape Town   Dar es Salaam   Hong Kong   Karachi
Kuala Lumpur   Madrid   Melbourne   Mexico City   Nairobi
New Delhi   Shanghai   Taipei   Toronto

With offices in
Argentina   Austria   Brazil   Chile   Czech Republic   France   Greece
Guatemala   Hungary   Italy   Japan   Poland   Portugal   Singapore
South Korea   Switzerland   Thailand   Turkey   Ukraine   Vietnam

Copyright © 2005 by Sara C. Charles and Paul R. Frisch

Published by Oxford University Press, Inc.
198 Madison Avenue, New York, New York 10016

www.oup.com

Oxford is a registered trademark of Oxford University Press

Library of Congress Cataloging-in-Publication Data
Charles, Sara C.
Adverse events, stress, and litigation : a physician's guide / Sara C. Charles,
Paul R. Frisch ; illustrations by Ronald Bailey.
p. ; cm.
Includes bibliographical references and index.
ISBN-13 978-0-19-517148-8
ISBN 0-19-517148-9
1. Physicians—Malpractice.   2. Defensive medicine.   3. Medical errors—Psychological
aspects.   4. Physicians—Psychology.   5. Physicians—Job stress.   I. Frisch, Paul R.   II. Title.
[DNLM: 1. Malpractice.   2. Adaptation, Psychological.   3. Physicians—psychology.   4. Stress,
Psychological. W 44.1 C477a 2005]
RA1056.5.C437 2005
344.04'121—dc22   2004054790

9 8 7 6 5 4 3 2 1

Printed in the United States of America
on acid-free paper

Dedicated to America's Physicians

Bad outcomes occur with some frequency in medical practice, even though they infrequently lead to litigation. However, in the lifetime of a physician, as in anyone's lifetime, one lawsuit is enough. According to a 2003 survey of the members of the American College of Obstetricians and Gynecologists, an average of 2.64 suits had been filed against the typical member and 76.3 percent of the respondents have been sued at least once.

The characteristic bright confidence of, and bold reassurances by, good lawyers do not necessarily allay the anxiety and shaken self-assurance that physicians feel when they are sued for malpractice. Lawyers avoid taking personally what physicians cannot help taking personally. Lawyers dwell both within the case and outside of it, disengaging at the end of the day from the experience that not only rides home with sued physicians but burrows deeply into their dreams as well. Lawyers view litigation from a very different angle than do physicians. Lawyers have traveled on this ship many times, lifeboat drills are second nature to them, and when storms strike, they order fresh drinks and go on playing cards. The voyage is all new to physicians, or similar litigants, who easily lose their footing and feel that they may be swept overboard at any moment.

Abundant evidence attests that the health of physicians affects the kind of care they deliver and that prolonged stress leads to impairment. Physicians in possession of the knowledge and skills that enable them to recognize and deal rapidly with practice-associated stressors are better able to moderate the impact of these stressors and to meet their professional obligations without interruption and without suffering any illness themselves. In this book, defendants tell their own stories in their own voices, explaining the steps they found helpful. They describe the emotional ebb and flow of the process and the potential snags and tell how, in the midst of busy lives, they navigated through the rapids.

Knowledge of what others went through can help us keep our psychological balance and control our reactions to stress. Our hope is that this book will help readers acquire such composure so that as defendants they will be better able to partner with their legal counsel and so participate more actively and effectively in their defense.

Chicago, Illinois   S. C. C.
Portland, Oregon   P. R. F.

Acknowledgments

We are grateful for the contributions of many extraordinary citizens as well as the many dedicated and anonymous physicians who gave generously of their time and shared their experiences of litigation so that others might find some understanding and support in facing one of life's greatest challenges.

We thank in particular our consultants, associates, and friends—many who remain unnamed—for their willingness to be interviewed and for their contributions to this book, including those who painstakingly reviewed its drafts: Richard Allen, MD, Maureen Anderson, Proctor Anderson, MD, Laurie Arnold, MD, Cynthia Baines, Mike Barnicle, Lori Bartholomew, Beverly M. Brazauskas, Saul Bellow, Leonard Cerullo, MD, Thomas E. Cooney Esq., Philip H. Corboy Esq., Joseph Daley, MD, Cynthia Davis, PhD, Linda Esser, Anne Finucane, Bob Fields, Steve Fountain, MD, Tom Fox, Maurice Garvey Esq., Norman Mailer, Maureen Mondor, David Myers, Eli Newberger, MD, Roni Pressler, Barbara Rockett, MD, Tim Saunders, Mary Santos, MD, John Schmidt, MD, Ruth Shea, Albert Strunk, MD, JD, Darryl Thomas, Mike Wallace, Laura West, MD, Thomas White, Audrey Vanagunas, Ron Ziarko, and Deborah Zarin, MD. We are also grateful to members of the Physician Insurers Association of America, the ISMIE Mutual Insurance Company, and the Council of Medical Specialty Societies for their help.

Special thanks go to the Helen Brach Foundation and its president, Raymond Simon, Esq., without whose support this book could not have been completed. We are grateful to our editor, Jeff House, who shepherded along the project. Last, we owe a special debt of gratitude to our spouses and families, Eugene Kennedy and Nancy, Alexis, and Jesse Frisch, whose contributions are immeasurable.

Contents

Adverse Events,
Stress,
and Litigation

Prologue

Four Days in the Nineties:
The Making of a Defendant

August 13, 1993

Dr. Richard Allen was finishing up his last day of work before leaving for a long-awaited 10-day vacation. He had just completed a preoperative evaluation of a 60-year-old woman that had been requested by a local orthopedic surgeon. Although aware of the woman's history of chronic back pain and disability, Dr. Allen remained concerned about whether she was really suitable for elective surgery. In examining her, he had noted her marked obesity, poorly controlled hypertension, and an anemia that had been neither definitively diagnosed nor treated. He recommended that she be evaluated for this latter condition before surgery. The last thing he did before leaving town was to sign out, as usual, to his partner, who would cover for him.

August 23, 1993

The evening Dr. Allen returned, refreshed and eager to get back to work, he notified his partner that he was back. As was their custom, his partner signed Dr. Allen's patients back to his care, mentioning no particular problems that should concern him. He did say that the woman Dr. Allen had seen earlier in consultation had, in the interim, undergone back surgery, had some postoperative complications, and was still in the hospital. Dr. Allen learned that the orthopedist had decided, given her serious and unremitting back pain, that the potential relief

1

offered by surgery outweighed the continuing discomfort she would experience during any delay for further examination.

On his rounds the next morning, Dr. Allen noted a flurry of activity at the room of this patient and was told that she had just died. He was "totally confused about what had happened" and requested an autopsy, which eventually revealed a large retroperitoneal bleed, apparently associated with oozing from the operative site, further complicated by the use of anticoagulants prescribed for a pulmonary embolus she had sustained postoperatively. The cause of death was attributed to shock secondary to irreversible blood loss.

March 24, 1995

This Friday was like any other Friday: rounds, a mid-day teaching conference, patients scheduled until 4:00 PM, and then a few patients who needed attention at the hospital before finishing the day. Sitting alone in his office, Dr. Allen opened an envelope that had been left earlier by the local sheriff. He unfolded a complaint telling an unfamiliar story that he was about to enter as a leading character.

Shortly after the patient's death, Dr. Allen was informed that the hospital chart had been subpoenaed. Even though he had been out of town at the time of the patient's hospitalization, he learned that his name was "splashed all over the chart." The nurses had continued to call his office and his partner had responded for him. He felt certain that, along with his partner and other physicians, he was going to be named in the malpractice suit that was bound to come. Having had no contact with the issue for 19 months, Dr. Allen felt "like someone who has a malignancy in remission. . . . you know it's there and you try to suppress it. You put it in the back part of your mind, in your subconscious but it always creeps back. . . . You *know* that it's going to show up."

Dr. Allen was overwhelmed as he read the complaint. Along with his partner and the radiologist, he was charged with negligent care. The name of the orthopedic surgeon was, he noticed immediately, nowhere in the complaint. The events flashed through his mind; he had recommended that the surgery be delayed; he was not even in town when the patient was in the hospital. He looked up from the few pages that changed his life, depressed, a rage building within him. Even though he had known that this moment would come, Dr. Allen was stunned.

March 25, 1995

He spent the evening trying to keep his balance in a buffeting whirlwind of disturbing emotions. He was being charged with the death of a patient when he had not even been on the scene. Some of those who were, including the orthopedic surgeon, had escaped being named in the complaint. He felt trapped, consumed by uncharacteristic rage, furious at what had happened. After many restless hours, he finally fell asleep.

Early Saturday morning Dr. Allen awoke with what he instinctively knew, even though he had never experienced it before, was atrial fibrillation. He went to the emergency department, where one of his associates was called in to assess his medical history, complete the appropriate physical examination, order the diagnostic tests to confirm the diagnosis, and prescribe the appropriate medication. It is ironic, he thought, that this cardiologist did not inquire about any recent stressors. He decided not to tell him what had happened unless asked. His cardiologist did not try to lift the curtain on the previous day but Dr. Allen knew that his sudden illness was intimately connected with his newly acquired designation. As of Friday, he had become, for the first time in his life, a *defendant*.

1

Adverse Events: A Basis for Litigation

Physicians usually become defendants through their involvement, sometimes centrally, sometimes peripherally, in an adverse event. An *adverse event* is defined in the 1999 Institute of Medicine (IOM) report *To Err Is Human* as "an injury resulting from medical intervention . . . not due to the underlying condition of the patient."[1] Such an event can throw physicians into what one describes as "the most stressful experience of my entire life."[2] Even if the untoward event never explodes into a malpractice claim, its impact is often so serious that it trips off powerful feelings in the patient as well as in all of the health professionals involved in the incident.

Consider the story of the surgeon in a well-publicized Florida case in which a 7-year-old boy was admitted for a third surgery for the removal of scar tissue and a benign tumor from his left ear.[3] Before surgery, two doses of epinephrine were prepared. A small dose (lidocaine 1 percent with epinephrine 1:100,000) was to be injected to constrict blood vessels and to limit bleeding; a larger topical adrenaline dose (1:1,000) was prepared for external application around the ear to decrease surface bleeding. Approximately twenty minutes into anesthesia, the patient was injected with what was thought to be 3 ml of lidocaine 1 percent with epinephrine 1:100,000. The patient's heart rate and blood pressure rose dramatically, necessitating treatment with propanolol, labetalol, and lidocaine to stabilize him. The surgical team concluded that he had had a transient response to the medication and the surgery resumed. Within a few minutes, his blood pressure and heart rate suddenly dropped and he began to exude frothy pink pulmonary edema. Within twenty-four hours he was dead.

Here was a healthy 7-year-old whom the surgeon had known since he was 18 months old. Had he killed him? Was he responsible for the death of a child who was the same age as one of his own? How was he to explain to the father and mother of a 7-year-old that their basically healthy child was now comatose and on life support? The surgeon was devastated, perplexed, and overwhelmed. What could possibly have happened to cause such an outcome? He had never experienced anything like this before.

Who was responsible: the surgeon, the anesthesiologist, the surgical nurse, or the pharmacist? Because the source of the problem was unknown and the hospital was committed to the systems approach to investigating adverse events, blame was not laid at anyone's door. The hospital immediately began a thorough investigation of the death that was widely publicized in the local media. To forestall litigation, the hospital quickly moved to reach a financial settlement with the child's family. Three months later, repeated and independent laboratory analyses revealed that the syringe thought to contain lidocaine 1 percent with 1:100,000 epinephrine actually contained topical adrenaline 1:1,000. Clearly a mistake had occurred: the wrong medication had been injected into the patient. Everyone involved, however, was emotionally traumatized by this tragic event. The three-month lag in discovering the source of the problem cast a further shadow over all participants, so chilling their relationships and wounded feelings that they could not be easily restored.

The Dilemma: The Human Element

Health-care professionals face a searing dilemma. In everyday practice they are constantly trying to balance their sense of being in control—even in certain circumstances, feeling omnipotent—with the nagging opposite of feeling vulnerable, uncertain, and limited. An adverse event confronts physicians with an intense psychological conflict about the possibility that they may have failed to meet their self-imposed ideals as well as the expectations of the profession. On an intellectual plane, physicians may realize that error-free medicine is unattainable. Still, trying the best they can to achieve near-perfect performance remains their psychological and ethical imperative.

The culture in which we live and in which physicians must practice reinforces the dilemma of this classic double bind. The 1999 IOM report advocates "a shift from blaming individuals for their past behavior to a focus on preventing future errors by designing safety into the system."[4] At the same time, it moves the responsibility back to physicians by placing the burden for improving safety on "the intrinsic motivation of health care providers, shaped by professional ethics, norms, and expectations."[4] As if unaware of the conflict, the Robert Wood Johnson Foundation began in early 2001 to fund a new initiative entitled "Pursuing Perfection: Raising the Bar for Health Care Perfection."[5] Such approaches reinforce the expectation that error-free medicine could be attained if only practitioners would work harder to achieve it.

A recent survey of practicing physicians and the public on the subject of medical errors further reveals the American expectation of perfection in health care. Both physicians and lay persons believe that medical error comes more from the failure of *individuals* than from that of institutional systems.[6] A basic principle of the IOM report, however, is the opposite—that medical error more often arises from the failure of institutions than from the misdeeds of individual practitioners. If, in fact, institutional problems rather than individual failures contribute to most medical errors, a significant gap exists between perception and reality.

Technological advances and the ready availability of sophisticated tests and drugs encourage both the physician and patient to expect something close to perfection. Patients want physicians to be sensitive and caring as only humans can be, but they also want physicians to perform in the consistent and controlled manner of machines. If a bad outcome occurs, the onus is immediately placed on the physician, who "should" have known or done something to prevent the event from happening. Thus, the dilemma is created to which most physicians are ill prepared to respond. Recognizing that medical practice, like every other human endeavor, is necessarily fraught with uncertainty and altered by ever-expanding knowledge, most training programs focus on improving abstract knowledge and practical skills while giving less attention to the human, interpersonal aspect of being a physician. House officers who make mistakes in institutional medicine, for example, are discouraged by supervisors and the institution itself from discussion of these events, thereby losing the opportunity to learn from and deal with such events.[7]

In his thoughtful memoir, David Hilfiker[8] captures the dilemma:

> The medical profession seems to have no place for its mistakes. Indeed, one would almost think that mistakes were sins. And if the medical profession has no room for doctor's mistakes, neither does society. . . . The drastic consequences of our mistakes, the repeated opportunities to make them, the uncertainty about our culpability, and the professional denial that mistakes happen all work together to create an intolerable dilemma for the physician. We see the horror of our mistakes, yet we cannot deal with their enormous emotional impact. Perhaps the only way to face our guilt is through confession, restitution, and absolution. Yet within the structure of modern medicine there is no place for such spiritual healing.

Views on Adverse Events: Are They Errors?

The IOM report suggests that errors refer only to adverse events that could be anticipated and therefore prevented.[9]

The Clinician's Perspective

The Florida surgeon knew instinctively that something had gone wrong and immediately began to experience a wide range of bad feelings. Completely at a loss to explain what had happened, his first question was, Did *I* make a mistake? As trained scientists, physicians are prepared to learn from their mistakes and lapses.

In the past, health-care professionals denied the emotional impact of such events and, in accord with the general cultural expectation, they generally hid their feelings. When physicians cannot acknowledge their feelings, their ability to explore what actually happened is seriously compromised. Only in recent years have physicians begun to reveal their personal encounters with bad outcomes, that is, those undesirable outcomes that may arise from complications, an error, or the underlying nature of the illness or injury. These physicians commonly acknowledge feelings of guilt and self-accusation about failing to provide adequate care to the patient.[10] Physicians are also understandably fearful about the short- and long-term repercussions of such events on their personal and professional lives. In addition to feelings of devastation, shock, and shame, they commonly obsess over the details of the event, their possible role in it, and whether the event was preventable. As one physician described this obsessing that may continue for many years, "I hold court in my mind, replaying events. . . ."[11]

The Human Factors Psychology Perspective

Psychologist James Reason, who has researched human error for more than a generation, suggests that error occurs when "a planned sequence of mental or physical activities fails to achieve its intended outcome, and when these failures cannot be attributed to the interventions of some chance agency."[12] He expands on Danish researcher Jens Rasmussen's previously described classification of human performance. The first type, *skill-based* errors, includes slips and lapses. *Slips* are errors committed at a skill-based level of performance when, for example, the neurosurgeon operates at the wrong level of the vertebrae. *Lapses* are memory failures or omissions that also occur at a skill-based level. An example would be neglecting to follow up on a questionable laboratory report.

Reason calls the second type of error a *rule-based* mistake. A *rule* is a pattern of behavior used to achieve a particular goal. The rule may be misapplied or a bad rule may be chosen to achieve a given goal, resulting in a mistake. This happens when the health-care professional, who should follow a specific procedure for administering medication, places the wrong drug in a designated syringe. Reason terms the third type of error a *knowledge-based* mistake. This occurs when a decision for action is based on insufficient knowledge or a biased interpretation of relevant knowledge. The psychiatrist commits this error when he or she fails to test for agranulocytosis in a psychotic patient on clozapine. Slips or lapses are sometimes immediately evident to us and therefore are often easier to identify than are mistakes.

Errors as a Function of a System

The traditional approach to assessing responsibility for adverse events focuses on the individual at the *sharp* end of the event chain, that is, the person in direct contact with the patient, such as the physician, nurse, or pharmacist. If the erring person can be identified, he or she can be blamed and punished and the problem is seemingly addressed.

James Reason emphasizes *latent* errors within the *organization* or *system* in which skilled individuals work.[13] Given human fallibility, Reason maintains that if a system creates conditions that lessen the possibility for error, fewer errors will occur. Systems cannot change human nature but they can change the conditions in which humans work. When bad outcomes occur, the *systems approach* evaluates how resources and constraints imposed by the overall system influence the behavior of those at its *sharp end*.

Error, according to this approach, is not a function of one isolated cause but rather of many systemic and, at first, seemingly unrelated factors. Reason illustrates his approach to highly technical or high-reliability organizations with the Swiss cheese model of accidents (Fig. 1–1).[14] Virtually all organizations have layers of defenses and safeguards, including physical barriers, automatic shut downs or alarms, established procedures, and operator behaviors (for surgeons, pilots, and others), to prevent errors or negative outcomes. Reason envisions these layered safeguards as slices of cheese whose natural weaknesses, or holes, are plugged by effective defenses. A failure, or hole, in one layer does not necessarily lead to a final outcome because firewalls intervene in the deck of layers. When, however, a series of independent failures become aligned, as shown in Figure 1–1,

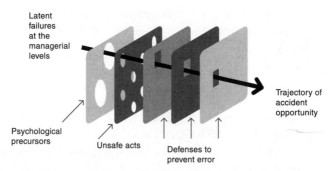

Figure 1–1. The "Swiss cheese" model illustrates how multiple, usually small, failures in an organization align simultaneously to contribute to an error. Latent failures that permit inadequate staffing or poorly maintained technology align with active failures or unsafe acts by persons at the "sharp end" to penetrate the organization's usual defenses against error. Adapted from James Reason, *Human Error* (Cambridge, England: Cambridge University Press, 1990), 208.

they open a "trajectory of accident opportunity" that can serve as a conduit for this now conjoined series of incidents and become the pathway to an error or a bad outcome. Such an outcome, as illustrated by a multistate blackout, occurs only when a series of almost random occurrences align, making a passageway for a particular failure that was unpredictable beforehand. According to this model, if any of the firewalls had been effective, the event would not have occurred.

The investigation of error in high-reliability organizations such as hospitals do not focus on finding *someone to blame* but rather on *discovering ways to limit the recurrence of this and similar events*. In the Florida incident, the hospital administrators, after studying the system and analyzing the factors associated with the problem, isolated a faulty medication delivery system that did not sufficiently distinguish closely related drugs. It subsequently changed the operating room policy for the administration of medications onto a sterile field to prevent such events from recurring.

The Patient Safety Movement's Perspective

Adherents of the Patient Safety Movement espouse the systems approach to error and view adverse events as public health problems that need identification, tracking, and appropriate interventions to prevent their reoccurrence. Frequently cited studies, one from New York and one from Colorado and Utah, estimate the incidence of adverse events at 3.7 percent and 2.8 percent of hospitalizations, respectively.[15–17] Death occurred in 13.6 percent of the New York cases and in 6.6 percent of the Western states' cases. Both studies estimated that between almost one third and one half of these adverse events were due to negligence or were preventable. These widely circulated results estimated the number of deaths due to errors as between 44,000 and perhaps 98,000 and became the foundation for the IOM report's call to action. Some researchers disagree about the conclusions of these studies, suggesting that they do not establish a correlation between the adverse events and the patients' deaths.[18,19] Both physicians and the public, however, believe that the number of deaths in hospitals due each year to error is fewer than 5,000, far lower than IOM estimates.[20]

We may view an error that occurs within an institution from two perspectives. It may be the result of an *active failure*, defined as an unsafe act committed by the people in direct contact with the patient.[21] It may also be attributed to a *latent condition* that inheres in the health-care system as a result of decisions made by designers, builders, procedure writers, and management.[21] These latter decisions can lead to under-staffing, staff fatigue, inadequate equipment, untrustworthy alarms, poor procedures, or other system weaknesses that may burgeon into latent errors. The full explanation of the event may identify a complex interaction between the system and the health-care professionals in which the physician is only one link in a complicated chain.

The Institution Perspective

Hospital and clinic administrators do not like adverse publicity or financial risk. An adverse event, its gravity magnified by media attention, compromises and may derail the primary mission of an institution. Ideally, the institution has policies that protect and inform patients about adverse events as well as programs to minimize adverse publicity and financial loss and support the medical and nursing staff involved. However, when such events arise, hospitals may have a greater interest in protecting their reputation and financial status than in protecting the personnel, such as the physicians who were involved in the adverse event.

When the Florida case is presented nationally as a model for improving patient safety, administrators, rather than the nurses and physicians most intimately involved in the case, generally lead the discussion. Does this mean that the hospital and its staff have different perspectives in perceiving and resolving such events? Does it mean that the clinical staff is outside the resolution process and that its input is either not solicited or ignored, so that as outsiders they feel no "ownership" of the settlement? In this and similar situations, the interests of the institution can supercede those of the individual staff members, who may feel they have been "hung out to dry." This in turn can generate unhealthy tensions and intolerable work conditions. Institutions whose leaders include all parties in discussions of difficult situations work in concert with the clinical staff to resolve the consequences of an adverse event. Whether an error or not, a catastrophic event can stimulate an institution to examine and change its culture or, unhealed and unattended, to infect the environment with dissension and disruption for many years.

The Insurer's Perspective

The ideal insurance company pools the risk for a large number of homogeneous, but independent, random events, to maintain its financial stability and make a profit for its shareholders.[22] Professional liability insurers specifically protect the physician against the legal expense of defending against, or paying for, claims that arise from the risks associated with medical practice and, in exchange, charge a premium to assure their financial stability. Medical malpractice insurance is not regarded as an easy or guaranteed business because the pool of potential policyholders is relatively small, the pool of claims is even smaller, the time period for processing a claim is lengthy, and a broad range of variables make the final payouts difficult to predict. As businesses abandon unprofitable endeavors, so did for-profit malpractice insurers in the mid-1970s and mid-1980s. In 2002 and 2003, both the St. Paul Companies and Farmers Insurance Group withdrew entirely from the medical malpractice market. Responding to escalating premiums and the unavailability of insurance in the mid-1970s, physicians, often in association with state medical societies, formed independent physician-owned mutual insurance companies. These companies sought to provide affordable coverage by changing from *occurrence* to *claims made* policies, that is, from issuing policies that cover physicians for any incident that arises during the policy period regardless of when the claim is filed to policies that cover incidents that occur *and* are reported while the policy is in force. They also introduced a number of physician-friendly but financially responsible innovations. Although such companies now insure over 40% of American physicians, they have, because of recent losses, diminished investment income, and a variety of other factors, raised their premiums significantly.

The company must make some decisions that are good for them but costly to physicians' pockets and pride. In the event of a claim, and despite protestations one way or another, the likelihood of a physician settling or going to trial is determined primarily by the financial repercussions of the decision on the insurance company. The salient issue is not whether an error occurred but whether the claim can be defended successfully without threatening the assets of the insurance company. Failing to make tradeoff decisions in its own interest, the insurer diminishes the likelihood that physicians will have the insurance necessary for their work.

Tort Law Perspective

In tort law, errors are judged as significant if they violate the *prevailing standard of care*, which is defined as a standard of practice adhered to by reasonably competent physicians in the same or similar circumstances, either in their own locality, termed the *community standard*; or in their medical specialty, termed the *national standard*. The latter is commonly applied. Because the function of tort law is to assign blame or exonerate some person or entity and to award compensation accordingly, it is necessary to determine whether the standard of care has been breached. Judges and juries rely on the opinions of peers, the expert witnesses. In a jury trial, the judge rules on the law applicable to the case and the jury is known as the finder of fact, that is, it judges what the facts are in a particular case. Little, however, prevents the finders of fact from basing their decision on such nonobjective matters as emotion, theatrics, or their perception of the plaintiff's injuries.

The Medical Expert's Perspective

The medical expert, as an agent of the legal process, is called on to decide objectively whether an adverse event was preventable. This is a difficult task because it may take years to identify and analyze all of the elements in such complex events. Medical experts must testify (*1*) that the care failed to comply, or complied, with the applicable standards and (*2*) that this failure more likely than not caused the injuries or damages claimed by the plaintiff or, from the defendant's expert testimony, that the physician's care met the standard and did not cause the injuries. Credible experts, who make most of their judgments in retrospect, can differ as to whether an error occurred. This process can invoke either *explicit criteria*, or some specific, predetermined criteria against which to measure care, or *implicit criteria*, or a subjective, independent review of the care based on reasonable and prudent professional practice.[23] Professional clinical venues and the courts usually follow the latter procedure to reach judgments about reasonable and prudent practice. Shortcomings, such as bias, are inherent, however, in such retrospective analyses. The more serious the outcome, Caplan found, the more likely that care is judged as inappropriate.[24] In his study, reviewers were presented with identical matched cases, differing only in the severity of outcome. Those who knew that a permanent, adverse outcome occurred were more likely to judge the involved physician as failing to provide appropriate care. Those who knew that a temporary, adverse outcome occurred were less likely to come to such conclusions. This study illustrates the ambiguities of viewpoint, judgment, and experience associated with expert medical testimony about adverse events.

Putting the Varied Viewpoints into Perspective

For physicians, such differing perspectives on adverse events are often a source of intense confusion, frustration, and anger. Physicians need to recognize and attempt to understand that each participant views the incident from a different perspective and that they themselves cannot change the script of the drama seen from such varying viewpoints. Physicians must accept that the truth of every incident depends on the viewer's angle of vision and that they must adapt to this reality as positively as they can.

The tort law model still dominates the field as a way to settle disputes. If physicians cannot change the way tort law works, they can learn about how it functions and prepare themselves to work with, rather than rage against, it. We will examine how the ordinary physician can do this in subsequent chapters.

An Adverse Event: The Real World and the Systems Approach

American health-care organizations, sensitized to the public's interest in discovering the roots of medical error and in improving patient safety, increasingly advocate the systems approach as a model for addressing such issues. This requires changing the "blaming" bias of the larger culture to one that emphasizes safety and accountability. The American regulatory environment and the tort system, however, continue to focus first on identifying those responsible for the event and therefore constitute a significant barrier to educating people to a new perspective on bad outcomes. Harvard University researcher Troyen Brennan[25] captures the conflict:

> Any effort to prevent injury due to medical care is complicated by the dead weight of a litigation system that induces secrecy and silence. No matter how much we might insist physicians have an ethical duty to report injuries resulting from medical care

or to work on their prevention, fear of malpractice litigation drags us back to the status quo.

Physicians find themselves at that hazardous intersection between the institutional need to prevent negative events and the inevitable search for someone to blame. They want to respond to patients openly and ethically and, as scientists, to explore and learn from such events. But they also recognize that doing either naively could result in a lawsuit or licensure action. Physicians may value the opportunity to learn from mistakes while also experiencing a natural urge to shelter the incident from examination to protect both their sense of themselves as persons and as professionals and their financial security.

Recommendations for Dealing with Adverse Events

When a bad outcome occurs, physicians are concerned for the patient but they are quickly pressed by demands to participate immediately in an investigation to help the patient, the institution, and themselves to understand exactly what happened. This process is of indeterminate length because it switches physicians to the timetable of a retrospective clinical and legal analysis of all of the factors that may have contributed to the bad outcome. During this period, physicians are doubly vulnerable: they lack knowledge about practical responses to what may be going on in the legal arena and they lack awareness of what is going on inside themselves. Unless they are knowledgeable about their legal vulnerabilities and how they can understand, accept, and strengthen themselves against them, their lives and careers fall rapidly under the shadow of legal jeopardy. Unless they understand their own feelings and how they can influence their actions, they may behave in ways that help neither their patients nor themselves.

Before the Event

ESTABLISH GOOD COMMUNICATION WITH PATIENTS. Physicians can take many practical steps to enhance their work with patients. Some experts recommend that patients, while waiting, complete a short form that prepares them for the current visit. It may include such questions as the following. What are the key things that you want to discuss today? What are the key symptoms that you want your doctor to know about? Do you have specific questions about tests, procedures, forms, and prescriptions, etc., that need to be discussed today? This form should also include a family history for patients seen in consultation or for their first visit. When patients focus on an agenda, aided by written notes, both physician and patient work together better.

On meeting the patient, physicians should communicate a clear message: "I am interested only in you at this moment." Physicians can greet patients warmly and shake hands and then sit down with them and ask what they would like to talk about. If patients compile lists with too many items, physicians have the opportunity to help them rank their concerns, from the most to the least urgent. Finally, physicians should assess how much patients understand what is discussed with them, perhaps by simply asking them what they have heard in their discussion. If the physician has an accent or the patient has limited English proficiency, an extra effort, including the use of an interpreter, must be made to ensure that physician and patient understand each other. Factors such as ethnicity, educational level, and age, according to research on "health literacy," contribute to patients misunderstanding advice on how to use their medication.[26] When physicians are better attuned to patients and their perception of such issues, they are more successful in caring for them.

WHEN RECOMMENDING TREATMENT, MAKE SURE PATIENTS UNDERSTAND INFORMED CONSENT. Establishing a good understanding of the risks and benefits of a procedure or treatment before it begins prepares patients and physicians for the range of possible outcomes. Many physicians think that informed consent is just a legal hurdle that has little clinical value. While the possibility of different outcomes, including harmful ones, is not inconceivable for physicians, even their patients with some intellectual appreciation of "unexpected outcomes" generally do not anticipate them and, as a result, regard them as mistakes or as necessarily harmful when they occur. Physicians help patients by explaining that complications are not usually caused by mistakes, that different outcomes occur because of patients' biological differences, and that undesired outcomes are often not permanent.

Physicians should cover four areas in any informed consent session: (1) describe the proposed procedure or treatment in clear, lay terms; (2) describe the likely benefits of the procedure or treatment; (3) explain the alternatives to, and risks of, the procedure or treatment, including the risks of doing nothing; and (4) answer any questions the patient may have as fully and professionally as possible. Discussion of these issues equips patients and their families psychologically to face the inevitable uncertainty of any procedure. Such discussions will also better prepare them for the contingencies that may occur in the emergency department or other locations when, in our absence, they see other health-care professionals. Anecdotal evidence indicates that the way in which physicians deal with informed consent may be a factor in the desire of patients or their families to pursue a lawsuit should a bad outcome occur. Many risk managers believe physicians enhance the informed consent process by providing patients with written explanatory information, if possible, even before the informed consent discussion takes place.

The state medical society, liability insurer, or private attorney can provide physicians with information about the specific informed consent laws in their locality. Some state laws are relatively inclusive, addressing consent from minor children and physically or mentally handicapped individuals, the need for consent during emergencies, and documentation of informed consent, as well as listing circumstances in which informed consent is mandated.

PREPARE FOR DEALING WITH ADVERSE EVENTS BY PARTICIPATION IN AVAILABLE TRAINING SESSIONS. Trained to respond to clinical emergencies, physicians can also train themselves to deal with the emotional exigencies of an unexpected bad outcome in the same way. Local risk managers can be useful resources about available training programs. Some institutions have produced simulations of a variety of emergencies and critical events.[27-30] Videotapes have been developed that illustrate how to respond to crises and how to conduct effective disclosure sessions.[31,32] Anticipation and practice are not only useful ways to prepare for these difficult clinical events, but they may also assist physicians in their daily practice.

BE FAMILIAR WITH ANY GUIDELINES THAT YOUR INSTITUTION HAS ESTABLISHED FOR HANDLING ADVERSE EVENTS. In July 2001, the Joint Commission on Accreditation of Healthcare Organizations (JCAHO) mandated standards for the reduction in and management of adverse patient outcomes.[33] The hospital's risk manager or medical staff coordinator can explain whether the institution has such mandated guidelines in place or if they are under development. It is in the interest of physicians to participate in the development of these guidelines by their hospitals, not the least of all because the hospital's legal interests may diverge dramatically from those of the medical staff. Collaborating in the development of the guidelines not only familiarizes physicians with them but also makes it more likely that they will operate effectively in concert with the institution and with a clear understanding of their own responsibilities when unintended patient outcomes occur.

BE FAMILIAR WITH YOUR MALPRACTICE INSURANCE COMPANY'S GUIDELINES FOR HANDLING ADVERSE EVENTS. Most malpractice insurers provide their insureds with specific guidelines for handling adverse events. It is essential to review these materials each time one renews a policy. Insurers deal with bad outcomes every day. Their goal is to protect physicians from experiencing a lawsuit and to obtain a successful resolution if one is initiated. Their staff members are trained to respond calmly and objectively to insured physicians to protect them both professionally and financially and to help physicians deepen their understanding of the process.

During the Immediate Postevent Period

TAKE ADVANTAGE OF INSTITUTIONAL AND OTHER AVAILABLE SUPPORT SYSTEMS. The Dana Farber Cancer Institute, for example, has a policy for handling adverse events that outlines the processes for notification of relevant staff throughout the system, documentation, and disclosure to the patient.[34] Also in place is a rapid response multidisciplinary team that can provide emotional support to physicians and other members of the health-care team who are responding clinically to patients who are in crisis.

NOTIFY THE INSTITUTION'S RISK MANAGER AS SOON AS POSSIBLE AFTER AN INCIDENT. When an adverse event occurs, physicians should follow the written recommendations of their health-care institution and contact the risk manager as soon as possible. These persons are experienced in handling adverse events and should be able to provide appropriate and timely advice and counsel. They can also help physicians view the event objectively, pierce the fog of confusion that sits thickly on it, and anticipate their reactions to the process that will seek the cause of the problem. Experienced professionals can also provide advice and support as physicians plan the next steps they must take to deal effectively with the impact of the event.

NOTIFY THE PROFESSIONAL LIABILITY CARRIER AS SOON AS POSSIBLE AFTER THE INCIDENT. Physicians are often afraid to contact their insurer about an adverse event out of anxiety about being "punished" with higher premiums or denial of coverage in the next renewal period. Some may wonder if they should act unilaterally to make it "right" directly with the patient. This is understandable but neither prudent nor useful. Physicians should always contact their insurance carrier and seek their advice on how to proceed. In some instances, they authorize the forgiveness of a patient charge or suggest that the physician offer a subsequent surgery without charge as a response that may ward off either a claim or a malpractice suit. In most instances, an early consultation giving the insurance personnel the details of an adverse event enables them to obtain information about the event, set a defense in motion, and so minimize the immediate impact of a claim as well as its later impact on the physician's insurability.

AFTER AN ADVERSE EVENT, SOME PHYSICIANS FEEL MORE COMFORTABLE NOTIFYING THEIR PERSONAL LAWYER FOR ADVICE. This is often a natural response even though personal attorneys, as a rule, do not practice as defense attorneys. Physicians, more commonly, perhaps, talk in a general way to a family member or friend who is either a lawyer or physician. Although such persons can be extremely supportive, they should not provide legal or medical advice but instead guide physicians to contact the insurer, who will, if necessary, appoint an attorney with whom they may consult. It is not unusual for a physician's personal attorney to have a relationship with the defense law firm affiliated with the physician's malpractice insurance company. Personal attorneys may then play a role in facilitating contact with a specific attorney in the firm.

WHEN INDICATED, SEEK FURTHER CONSULTATION WITH RISK MANAGERS, HOSPITAL ADMINISTRATORS, ETHICS COMMITTEES, AND OTHERS. Individual circumstances always determine their response, but sometimes this is necessary even before the physician talks with the family. Dr. Richard Allen, whose experience is detailed in the prologue, on arriving on the unit immediately after the patient's death, met with the orthopedist who, although he was not the treating physician but was covering for his own partner, had managed the resuscitation. These physicians shared their view of what might have caused the patient's death. Dr. Allen suggested that they request an autopsy to find out what happened. Because he had met them once before and Dr. Allen, as a consultant, had not, the orthopedist agreed to meet with the family and the risk manager was contacted only after this initial session. In other circumstances, as we have noted, the risk manager may serve as the initial and key resource when a bad outcome occurs.

SEEK IMMEDIATE CONSULTATION IF THE MEDIA BECOME INVOLVED. Institutions generally have an established relationship with the media, whereas physicians ordinarily do not. The institution wants to put its best face forward regarding the event and to calm and reassure the public. The hospital administrators' view of the outcome and its antecedents may not always agree with that of the physician. Physicians may be tempted to tell their side of the story publicly for "truth's sake," a temptation they are well advised to resist. Physicians should remember that the media are keenly interested in conflict and negative information and allow contact with the media to be the province of the malpractice carrier or defense lawyer. Ideally, the lawyers and other representatives craft a message together that will serve fairly all of the various interests involved.

As SOON AS POSSIBLE, DICTATE OR WRITE DOWN A DESCRIPTION OF THE CLINI-CAL EVENTS FOR INCLUSION IN THE MEDICAL RECORD. This should be done according to the usual protocol and should be a complete and accurate rendering of the event.

As SOON AS POSSIBLE, REVIEW THE MEDICAL RECORD FOR ACCURACY. Resist at all costs the impulse to modify what is already in the medical record to clarify ambiguous remarks or to remove apparently damaging information. These efforts, although understandable, never succeed and, should a claim arise, can compromise its defense. Almost always, the alteration of records severely undermines the defense of one's case and, even if the physician was not negligent, can lead to nonrenewal of coverage and possible licensure sanctions. If something in the record needs clarification or correction, physicians should consult their insurance carrier or hospital protocol and write a note that includes the time and date of the addition under their signature or initials.

WRITE A NARRATIVE OF THE CASE AS SOON AS POSSIBLE. This should be done promptly, as described later in Chapter 6, while the events are fresh in one's mind.

When a physician reports a claim to his or her insurer, most malpractice insurers recommend that a case narrative be written as a letter and addressed to a named attorney. The latter may or may not eventually serve as the physician's defense attorney. This places the narrative under the protection of an *attorney work product*, shielding it against any effort by the patient's attorney to subpoena it and to force its disclosure. As a separate document prepared only for the use of the defense attorney, it is legally protected and, because it is written for personal reasons, is not part of the clinical record. As an account of the facts, impressions, perceptions, and feelings associated with the event, it is essentially a timely and complete rendering of what occurred and should be kept in a safe place separate from the patient's chart until the carrier-assigned attorney requests it.

During the Postevent Period

Physicians experience a bad outcome or a medical error as a significant, and usually traumatic, life event. Despite the trauma, physicians need to respond effectively to patients and their families, who carry the burden of the outcome, and participate fully with the associated legal and regulatory sequelae. When the institution focuses on understanding the nature of the mistake and provides support rather than a search for someone to blame, physicians learn much that will benefit them in the future. The ideal response and the demands of the current climate of health care, however, remain in conflict. The formidable deterrents to a quick resolution to a bad outcome contribute to a range of conflicted feelings that physicians need to identify correctly, accept, and address calmly. Doing so will lessen the likelihood of similar occurrences in the future. It will also help physicians communicate effectively with their patients during this time of heightened emotion and gain some measure of hard-won peace for themselves.

2

Adverse Events: What We Feel and Why

Dr. Laura West, the youngest full-time member of an obstetric-gynecology university faculty, was under the additional pressure of preparing for her specialty board examinations. Faced with a very complex case involving a young woman at risk for a life-threatening bleed from a placental abnormality, Dr. West prepared for every contingency. She had been trained in a high-density litigation environment and anticipated lawsuits with every difficult case regardless of the outcome. Before the patient's delivery, she planned for the necessary backup and conducted and recorded a detailed informed consent session that included a list of relevant references. "It was the perfect chart. And what could happen, happened."[1]

The patient became an obstetric emergency and probably, in retrospect, had an amniotic fluid embolus. She did well initially but spent a long time in the intensive care unit (ICU) recovering from the complication of adult respiratory distress syndrome. For months after the patient's delivery, Dr. West visited the patient daily in the ICU, treating her complications and monitoring her slow recovery. She described herself and her patient as feeling "miserable." After an extended hospital stay, a fatty emulsion feeding that should have been administered via stomach tube was administered through the patient's intravenous line instead, leading to a cardiac arrest secondary to a fatty pulmonary embolus and sudden death. Dr. West felt both freed from the burden of caring for her patient and guilty for welcoming the relief. Even though Dr. West had done "everything right," she was devastated by the outcome and was certain that she would eventually be sued.[1]

> I was a young doctor, ... people didn't know me ... I had this catastrophic event ... and every day I questioned myself. ... I had graduated first in my class, I had been the chief resident and I was as well prepared as I could be but [after the event] I doubted myself every day. ... It was just agony.

One sequela was particularly distressing. She began to have difficulty in closing abdomens and was obsessed with the possibility that every patient would bleed to death. After each surgery, before falling asleep that night, she would lie awake wrestling with concerns about how the patient was doing and obsessing about whether the patient was seeping blood. Almost 2 years passed before she had regained some overall feeling of equilibrium. It was during that period that she was sued.

Adverse Events as Traumatic Life Events

Patients and their families are obviously the primary victims of adverse events. Physicians who also suffer emotionally whether or not these incidents are due to errors are now understood to be victims, too.[2–5] Physicians report experiencing feelings of anger, remorse, disappointment, panic, and shame that are disruptive and painful and that they feel they must bear in silence. Studies reveal that not all physicians stand with the majority of their colleagues who tend to be self-accusatory. Some physicians who feel they have less influence or control over their work appear to be less disturbed than do those who tend to hold themselves responsible for everything that happens.[3]

A study of the "perceived" past mistakes made by fifty-three family physicians helps us understand why they have these feelings.[6] Physicians generally attribute the mistake to their own behavior, most commonly to (1) feeling hurried or distracted by an awareness that other patients needed their attention; (2) premature closure of the diagnostic process; (3) misleading normal findings in the patient; and (4) a lack of knowledge about the issue confronting them. In this study, 47 percent of the patients died. The patients sustained no adverse outcome after 26 percent of the mistakes, and only four of the fifty-three incidents (7.5 percent) generated malpractice suits. Another study identifies misplaced optimism, a drive for perfection, and acting with insufficient restraint or deliberation, excessive haste, impatience, overconfidence, or inadequate peer group consultation as causal factors.[7] Although such self-accusatory reactions are not unusual in highly trained obsessive persons, they can still have serious consequences.

A slight shift in attitude toward the causes of error in health care is appearing among physicians and the public that may slightly alter physicians' emotional reactions to them. In a recent survey, 53 percent of physicians identified under-staffing of nurses in hospitals as a cause of error, whereas 50 percent cited their own overwork, stress, or fatigue.[8] Patients, by contrast, attribute errors to physicians who do not take sufficient time with them (72 percent); to overwork, stress, or fatigue among health-care professionals (70 percent); to the failure of health-care professionals to work and communicate with one another (67 percent); and to the understaffing of nurses (65 percent). We may interpret many of these as failures of the institution to create a proper work environment for its health-care professionals rather than as any failure of the professionals themselves.

Although errors are a normal and expected aspect of human behavior,[9] they are always undesirable, especially in health care. The depth of error's emotional impact on physicians is a measure of how strongly they repudiate error when it does occur. That physicians are conscientious, caring, and competent practitioners is an image deeply ingrained in them on many levels and they are loath to accept any deviation from this high ideal.

Traumatic Life Events Defined

A *traumatic life event* may be defined as the direct personal experience or the witnessing of "an event that involves actual or threatened death or serious injury or other threat to one's physical integrity . . . or learning about unexpected or violent death, serious harm, or threat of death or injury experienced by a family member or other close associate."[10] In most circumstances, physicians feel closely related to their patients. Exposure to their serious injury or death generates feelings of fear, helplessness, or horror that are especially severe when the stressor is "of human design" rather than a natural phenomenon.[11]

When we participate in, or oversee, a serious adverse event in our practice, we witness not only an often totally unexpected tragedy but also one that may plague us with speculative or direct concerns about whether we played some role in, or contributed to, the design of its occurrence. This acutely poignant reality of being personally involved or seemingly responsible for its occurrence may stir deep and unsettling emotions within physicians.[12]

A traumatic event is not a discrete event that is over and done with immediately. It generally triggers a process that inflicts other losses to which we must adapt. A recent widow not only lost her husband but also experiences changes in her social and financial status. For those of us in health care, a traumatic event may generate the additional trauma of legal action with its threat of serious personal, financial, and professional losses.

The Impact of Traumatic Events

As more people are exposed to terrorism, researchers are learning more about how traumatic events affect individuals, what personal characteristics render them either more vulnerable to difficulties or more likely to develop symptoms, and how they may better cope in such circumstances. The initial response to trauma, often termed *distress*, is common to all people and considered normal and adaptive. Subsequent responses, both short and long term, differ considerably among individuals. They may range from the most common response of complete recovery to the chronically debilitating posttraumatic stress disorder (PTSD). These findings on stress responses can help physicians, who have close contact with tragedy on a daily basis, to anticipate and cope with the predictable reactions to such traumatic events.

A Framework for Understanding Reactions to Traumatic Life Events

Emotional turmoil and confusion are most common when an adverse outcome is unanticipated and severe. The surgeon whose story is told in Chapter 1 had a gentle and encouraging conversation before surgery with the 7-year-old child he had known for some years. Within a few hours, the physician was confronted with the failing heart of a limp, anesthetized boy. Faced with this situation, he experienced fear, dread, and a rush of stress hormones that shifted him to highest alert. He had decisions to make and directions to give. He had to calm the anxiety of his team and assert control over the event. He was faced with a catastrophe and did not know why it had occurred. If it was the result of a mistake, what was its nature and who played a role in it?

Exposure to stress affects the total person and our reactions to traumatic events are rooted in our personalities, biology, and basic instincts for self-preservation. Our emotions flow from the complex changes that occur within us in our neuroendocrine, neurochemical, and neuroanatomical systems as they respond to stress. The literature on the biology of stress, especially in the psychological and psychiatric literature, may be of interest to some readers.[13-16] Our discussion, however, focuses on the common subjective experience of stress that we describe when we talk about our reactions to traumatic events.

Our attention is so intensely focused in a crisis that, for a brief period, our behavior becomes almost automatic, especially if we are well trained to respond to emergencies. The sensations and human emotions generated by the event generally remain outside of our conscious awareness. We are running, we often say, on adrenaline.

The emotions that accompany traumatic events are initially so overwhelming, immobilizing, and frightening that we cannot easily name them or fully absorb them into our consciousness. The psychological power of such traumas flows from the way the original event is etched into our memory and merged inextricably with intense emotions. Shock and heightened anxiety protect us from a full awareness of this utterly devastating emotional overload.

In Figure 2–1 the psychoanalyst Mardi Horowitz conceptualizes the normal process that follows such serious life events as divorce, the death of a close friend

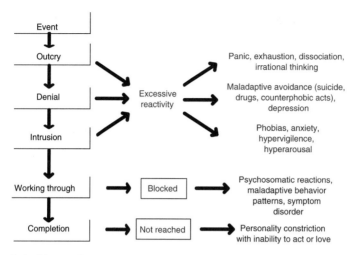

Figure 2–1. Phases of response to stressor events. From Mardi J. Horowitz, *Treatment of Stress Response Syndromes* (Washington, DC: American Psychiatric Press, 2003), with permission.

or relative, financial reverses, exposure to some natural disaster, or a serious adverse event and subsequent litigation.[17] When the normal process is interrupted or blocked, pathological reactions and symptoms develop.

We cannot initially believe that any of these events have happened. Its impact is too powerful for us to absorb, and our first response is to deny it through an outcry, any of many variations of, "Oh, no, this has not happened."

We have already entered the gloomy tunnel in which we alternate between denial, in which we cannot face the reality of the event, and *intrusion*, in which uninvited thoughts about the event invade us with a bombardment of distractions. We draw down great stores of psychological energy just keeping these aggressor notions from overrunning us.

As we begin to calm down, we may still feel anxious and jumpy and experience waves of reminders as well as memories, called *intrusions*, that cause us to feel dread, fear, and panic. Placed suddenly into a situation that seems beyond our control, we may feel overwhelmed, impotent and vulnerable. We may experience confusion and later have problems remembering exactly how we behaved and what we said. We may feel in a daze and have difficulty grasping the full significance of the event. Some people describe feeling out of it, disconnected, remote, and lacking in emotion. Those who are ordinarily close to us may feel distant. In addition, restlessness, hypersensitivity, and sleep disturbances contribute to a state of generalized physiological arousal. We may also experience intense anger, depression, irritable mood, and nightmares, all of which can disrupt our personal relationships.

Against this background, we keep working through, consciously and unconsciously, this disordering experience, carrying out the psychological labor we must do for ourselves so that we can accept the reality of what has happened to us.

Many clinicians believe that because these symptoms of distress are temporary, they will dissipate gradually, often in a matter of days.[18] Instead of being incorrectly labeled as "pathological," these symptoms should be recognized as healthy and normal responses to a significant threat to our persons.

It should not be surprising that we may be reminded of the event, quite unexpectedly, even many years later, by some seemingly innocuous situation or sensation. Returning to the operating room where the critical event took place, for example, or seeing the face of that dying child in our mind's eye can overwhelm us with a barrage of unanticipated and uncomfortable emotions. We may be surprised at the intensity of the feelings that seem as fresh as if the event had happened yesterday. Researchers know that emotionally intense events are remembered for longer periods than neutral events, but why this is so and what role psychological and neurobiological forces play in consolidating memories remain unknown.[19,20]

Longer-Term Reactions

Initial reactions at times do not dissipate as quickly as we hoped, and we may become aware of symptoms that remain and interfere with our everyday life. According to the *DSM-IV*, the PTSD that may follow exposure to trauma encompasses three groups of symptoms that must be present for at least one month to warrant the diagnosis: (*1*) persistent intrusive and involuntary thoughts about the event that may be triggered by seemingly innocuous stimuli; (*2*) avoidance of stimuli that are associated with the event that may be accompanied by feelings of numbness as well as constriction of interpersonal relationships; and (*3*) symptoms associated with increased arousal such as sleep disturbances, irritability, hypersensitivity, and an exaggerated startle response.[21]

After careful evaluation, an alternative diagnosis, acute stress disorder, may be assigned to some individuals who have symptoms within the first month after exposure to a trauma.[21] These individuals have similar and slightly overlapping symptoms with PTSD but are affected for a shorter period of time and exhibit what are known as dissociative symptoms, such as feeling psychologically detached and a subjective sense of numbing. They are often encouraged to engage in interpersonal and cognitive therapies that enable them to gain perspective and psychological distance from the event. In addition, individuals who develop this disorder appear to be more vulnerable to the later development of PTSD.

Studies consistently find that female gender, a history of previous sexual or physical abuse, and psychiatric illness are well-established predictors of posttraumatic symptomatology.[22] If we are aware of these factors in our own life and we are exposed to a major trauma in our work, we may usefully seek psychiatric consultation to diminish or monitor the emergence of significant symptoms and, if indicated, to initiate rapid treatment.

In addition to, and often accompanying, the conditions just described, we may experience symptoms associated with a range of psychiatric disorders. After trauma, women are at greater risk of PTSD and clinical depression than are men, who are more vulnerable to substance abuse.[23] Those who have experienced major depression in the past are vulnerable to a recurrence. Symptoms of other diagnoses that may develop among trauma-exposed individuals include those of adjustment disorders, mood disorders, anxiety disorders, and a range of medically unexplained physical complaints.

Beginning to Heal the Wound

Exposure to trauma generates expected reactions that may be called normal responses to abnormal events. Although these reactions dissipate within a few days or weeks, individuals may continue to experience periodic waves of intrusive thoughts about the event or impulses to avoid places or people that remind them of the event. Many persons, however, are resilient, that is, able to withstand exposure to extreme stress without developing serious symptoms. They are more likely to possess this characteristic if they have a well-developed capacity for, and availability of, stable and supportive relationships, a pattern of active problem-solving coping, an adaptive personality, and a lack of previous psychiatric illness.[24]

Physicians who think that the traumatic event may have been foreseeable and under their control and that they could have prevented it from happening may complicate an already horrible event with feelings of failure, regret, guilt, and shame. Focusing on these feelings and endlessly obsessing about them make it difficult to gain the distance and perspective necessary to heal and return to effective work. Discussing these situations with trustworthy and empathic colleagues or family members is one way of achieving some degree of comfort and putting an end to these wearying preoccupations.

It is helpful but generally not enough to be reassured that these distressing feelings will rapidly dissipate. The peculiarly human need to talk to others about a significant stressor is a natural coping mechanism that hastens recovery.[25] Talking about the accident or tragedy that a physician has just witnessed is part of finding a safe place away from the enormity of the event. In its shelter, physicians can put an end to their wearying preoccupations and find soothing the presence of other persons who understand, support, and live with them as they emerge from the fear and terror that trail off such an event.

The specter of the law looms large for physicians after any adverse event in medicine. Can physicians take advantage of sharing their reactions with others without feeling constrained by the law? Although we discuss this in greater detail in Chapter 4, physicians should generally behave like everyone else. There is no lawsuit at the moment. By confiding in a trustworthy and understanding person, without disclosing any confidential health information, a physician may reclaim emotional calm.

Debriefing After the Event

Debriefing is a common but controversial approach to posttraumatic reactions. Originally developed in the military, it is frequently used to help emergency responders to disasters and multiple trauma events. *Debriefing* after a traumatic event, as Watson and her group[26] suggest, means different things to different people. They note that although the term is popularly used to describe any intervention that encourages talking through the experience, a recent consensus conference on psychological reactions after mass tragedies suggests limitations: Debriefing should refer only to routine individual or group sessions that review the details of the event from a factual perspective to provide the opportunity for ventilation, support, and education. The military and emergency personnel who use debriefing on a regular basis generally understand and support this carefully defined use of the process.

Some researchers, however, find that, even defined in this way, debriefing can be unhelpful to recently traumatized individuals. They contend that for many people the traumatic event is so overwhelming and their instinct to avoid any reminders of it is so intense that the mandatory exposure to, or urging of, a detailed review exacerbates rather than relieves the impact of the trauma.[27] Some observers suggest that such interventions serve to re-traumatize already traumatized individuals.

As parties to a traumatic event in the clinical setting, physicians are immediately involved in the numerous reviews that follow. A detailed debriefing is now institutionalized in health care and, although physicians may dislike it, they cannot avoid being involved. The investigation of the event, although limited in time and confined to the institutional setting, may also become an extensive, far-reaching, and public lawsuit that can be contested for many years.

Some evidence suggests that if a fact-finding debriefing is convened in close proximity to the traumatic event, it may be less effective and more threatening to the participants than if it is delayed until a reasonable amount of time passes. A forced, detailed, and premature debriefing may distort recollection of the event and interfere with the resolution of distress. A case can be made for delaying any in-house debriefing or investigation for at least two or three days, and perhaps for as long as a month, after the event to allow everybody involved to regain some measure of psychological equilibrium. During that time, however, physicians should refrain from developing a game plan with other participants as a way of defending themselves.

Recommendations for Helping Physicians
Help Themselves

RECOGNIZE AND ACKNOWLEDGE EMERGING FEELINGS. Many physicians deny or try to cover up their emotions to avoid feeling out of control. Although understandable in the short run, such denial inhibits effective resolution of the feelings. Conscientious physicians find that even considering the possibility of error is emotionally painful. Time and patience are our allies in getting ourselves into focus so that we can eventually identify and acknowledge our true feelings about the event.

BE UNDERSTANDING OF OTHERS WHO ARE INVOLVED IN THE EVENT AS WELL AS OF ONESELF. Resist any rush to judgment about what caused the event. The good that physicians do for patients outweighs the bad by any measure. In a long-range perspective in which physicians treat thousands of patients over the span of many years, error occurs infrequently. Accustomed to self-scrutiny, when an adverse event happens, physicians must guard against excessive self-criticism and ward off immobilizing feelings of guilt and shame. They should see their colleagues in this same true light. Finger-pointing is among the most destructive of post-bad outcome behaviors. Physicians must remember that they usually are not the most objective judges of what really happened in events that may take days or weeks to untangle. A lack of restraint only benefits the plaintiff lawyers.

DO NOT BE SURPRISED WHEN REPEATED AND PREOCCUPYING THOUGHTS OF THE EVENT PERSIST. The central psychological dynamic at work in physicians after a mistake or bad outcome is the question, "Was it my fault?" and its variant, "Could I have controlled or prevented this event from happening?" Physicians tend to examine every event from every angle. Time is needed to sort out with others the specifics of what actually happened. Third-party evaluations from people outside the event can help to settle obsessions that are second nature to physicians.

PARTICIPATION IN DEBRIEFING AND SUBSEQUENT INVESTIGATIONS MAY HELP US GAIN SOME OBJECTIVITY ABOUT THE EVENT. Like it or not, when bad things happen, physicians must begin to learn how to live with them. Sometimes the apparent facts speak in a way that urges them to acknowledge a measure of guilt. Difficult as it is, acknowledging and accepting this possibility will help disperse the obsessive and preoccupying gloom that may settle on us after a bad outcome.

TALK WITH ONE'S SPOUSE, A TRUSTED COLLEAGUE, OR A CLOSE FRIEND ABOUT ONE'S REACTIONS. Because physicians are often conflicted about doing this, this is discussed in more detail in Chapter 4.

3

Disclosure After an Adverse Event

Common sense tells us that when something bad happens, physicians should talk about it with the patient and family. The American Medical Association (AMA) Code of Medical Ethics states that "it is a fundamental requirement that a physician should at all times deal honestly and openly with patients."[1] In situations that result from a mistake or poor judgment, "the physician is ethically required to inform the patient of all the facts necessary to ensure understanding of what has occurred." Most physicians believe that the obligation to disclose is a basic function of open communication with the patient and that any outcome—good or bad— should be discussed. Remaining silent is not an option and attempting a cover-up is not only unethical but, in today's world, probably impossible.

It is much easier to advise disclosure than it is to disclose, especially after a truly adverse outcome. The impact of these large events is directly related to their gravity. Physicians view events of death or irreversible injury as failures that traumatize everybody involved. Effective discussion about these events with patients is filled with challenges.

Why Physicians Hesitate to Disclose

Many physicians believe that straightforward honesty about their role in a bad outcome increases their chances of being sued. They are also wary that, if a claim is made against them, any expression of regret or sympathy may be translated into a legally binding admission of fault. The logic goes something like this: (*1*) an expression of regret equals an apology; (*2*) an apology equals an admission of negligence; (*3*) an admission of negligence equals a lawsuit; and therefore, (*4*) an expression of regret equals a lawsuit.

Disclosure means different things to different people. Technically, to disclose means to "expose to view; to make known or public."[2] For many physicians, disclosure carries the connotation of an *acknowledgment* that "implies the disclosing of something that has been or might be concealed."[3] Will acknowledging that "a mistake has occurred and I'm truly sorry this has happened" imply something physicians do not intend, that is, "I also am responsible for this event?" Can empathy be expressed without a possibly ambiguous apology?

An *apology* is defined as "an admission of error or discourtesy accompanied by an expression of regret."[4] Some risk managers, patients, policy experts, and others, in contrast to defense lawyers, argue that an empathic acknowledgment is insufficient and that an explicit apology, including an acceptance of responsibility, is an essential component of any disclosure. If physicians apologize, do they thereby admit fault? The cloud of meaning that hovers around "apology" in our culture explains why expressions of regret are often easily misinterpreted.

If physicians acknowledge that a mistake has been made but make no reference to "fault," does the patient see them as being honest and truthful? If they explicitly apologize and acknowledge fault, are they not turning themselves over to the courts by confessing negligence, a charge against which there then may be no defense? These are not minor matters. The above distinction underscores the protections under the law in current disclosure legislation in many states in which expressions of beneficence are often protected while the acknowledgment of fault is not.[5]

Recent Developments Regarding Disclosure

Theoretically, any adverse event, or even one perceived to be adverse, can become the subject of litigation. For many years, malpractice insurers have warned physicians not to acknowledge fault for such events. In 1994, the St. Paul Fire and Marine Insurance Company, which was until 2002 one of the nation's largest medical malpractice insurers, stated in its guidelines: "Do not be apologetic. Do not in any way imply that the bad outcome is the fault of you or another health provider. For most bad outcomes, an unusual result is at least as likely as malpractice. If there is fault, that can be determined later when everyone can be more objective."[6] The following year, an AMA/Specialty Society Medical Liability Project (AMA/SSMLP) publication advised: "When a complication or iatrogenic injury occurs, the patient should be informed, preferably by his or her primary physician, in a timely manner that accurately presents the facts of the situation, but does not draw conclusions of liability or fault."[7] For many physicians, this approach to dealing with adverse events reflects a deeply held conviction: State the facts, be empathic, but do not use words that could be interpreted as an apology.

In 2000, the National Patient Safety Foundation, a not-for-profit research and education group, circulated a policy that has since been implemented by many hospitals. It encourages a "truthful and compassionate explanation about the error and the remedies available to the patient."[8] One year later, the Joint Commission on the Accreditation of Healthcare Organizations (JCAHO) published a revised standard stating that, "Patients and, when appropriate, their families are informed about the outcomes of care, including unanticipated outcomes."[9] This standard requires that responsible practitioners, or their designee, explain not only the outcome of any treatment or procedure to patients and their families but also any outcomes that differ significantly from those that had been anticipated.[9] Although neither organization requires an explicit apology for such events, they do set an institutional standard and, quite possibly, a standard of care. Many proponents of this position assume that an apology is included in these disclosures. Some, in fact, term an expression of regret without an explicit apology and assignment of fault as non-disclosure.[10] Physicians fear, quite correctly, that these demands are the equivalent of crying "Fire" in a crowded movie. Physicians live and practice in a highly combustible legal environment, and any seeming admission of fault or error may set it ablaze.

Such standards about disclosure seem workable and track the AMA's Code of Medical Ethics that requires full disclosure of errors.[11] They differ, however, from the opinion of some malpractice insurers and defense attorneys who continue to discourage any full disclosure, especially any use of the term "mistake," for fear it will be construed as an admission of fault. These differing views therefore put physicians into conflict because if they do the right thing, they make themselves targets for lawsuits. Although surgeon Lucian Leape is a strong proponent for disclosure, he acknowledges that, "The realities of the malpractice threat provide strong incentives against disclosure or investigation of mistakes. Even a minor error can place the physician's entire career in jeopardy. . . . It is hardly surprising that a physician might hesitate to reveal an error to either the patient or hospital authorities. . . ."[12] A terrible irony of this "make-everything-right" environment is that being honest, forthright, and empathic about a physician's proximity to the event turns such forth-comings into admissions for which the physician may be legally punished.

This dilemma is illustrated by the case described by Chicago physician Dr. John Lantos. A patient with breast cancer experienced complications from a severe graft-versus-host response after a bone marrow transplant, renal failure, and multiple infections. After her death, the hospital discovered that during resuscitation, she received intravenous fluids that contained ten times the normal dose of potassium chloride. Uncertain about whether to notify the patient's family of the error, the physician consulted with the hospital ethics committee.[13]

The committee struggled with a range of questions. Did the mistake contribute to the patient's death? Would she have survived if she had not received the mistaken dose? If the staff knows about the mistake, shouldn't the patient's family also know? Because the patient had little hope of survival, isn't the information irrelevant? Hasn't the family experienced enough tragedy? But isn't telling the truth always best? If family members are not told and they find out later about the mistake, might they be upset and therefore initiate a malpractice action? If they are told about a clear mistake with attribution, however, might they not also file a malpractice suit? Lawyers on the ethics committee offered no opinion but suggested that the physician carefully document whatever steps he decided to take. Ultimately, the committee told the attending physician he could either tell or not tell the family about the error. Not surprisingly, he chose not to disclose it to the family.

According to the AMA's opinions on ethics and current regulations affecting hospitals, would this physician have had a choice? The question remains: What are the long-term consequences of telling the truth for both the patient's family and the physician?

Full Disclosure: A Two-edged Sword?

Physicians know that *anything* they say can be used against them in a court of law. They are also told that the failure to conduct a frank discussion, with an apology, contributes to the desire of patients and their families to pursue litigation. Little research exists to assess the validity of this largely anecdotally based assumption. Because only an estimated 1.53 percent of patients sue after a negligent adverse event,[14] prospective studies are practically unattainable. Because the subjects have already experienced an adverse event and are either planning for, or are already in litigation, retrospective studies, the only systematized data available, are subject to hindsight bias. Nonetheless, the available studies indicate that a major stimulus to a lawsuit is the perception that, after an injury, physicians fail to provide sufficient explanations about what has happened. Patients want to know what happened and why, and they want some assurance that it will not happen again.[15–16] More forthrightness and honesty, these studies posit, would make litigation less likely.

If we accept the premise that lack of disclosure is an alleged trigger for lawsuits, does disclosure prevent them? Although fully disclosing bad outcomes to patients would appear to defuse the reasons for litigation and so seem a common sense tactic, little research evidence supports the notion that disclosure immunizes against litigation. The Department of Veterans Affairs (VA) program in Lexington,

Kentucky, espouses "extreme honesty" in the event of a documented adverse outcome where legal fault is established through an in-house investigation. Patients and their families are told not only the specifics of the event but also what medical measures and additional steps are in place to diminish disability and financial loss to the family.[17] During 14 years of the program, "the total number of cases increased but the costs per case declined significantly."[18] By acknowledging an adverse event and legal fault, the hospital sustained more claims but also reached settlements more quickly, often without resorting to litigation, thereby reducing tort system costs.

Critics suggest that the VA system can sponsor a program that discloses and accepts liability because of the "deep pocket" of the U.S. government and because the VA system provides virtually free care to its patients and has a variety of remedial treatment and disability programs already in place. In addition, physicians within the VA system are protected from personal liability by law, so their professional reputations and financial security are not threatened. If, however, a payment is made on their behalf, they may, subject to a review panel's decision, be voluntarily reported to the National Practitioner Data Bank. Many question whether such a system could be effective in the private sector.

Current data suggest that although full disclosure appears to increase patient satisfaction, it may not decrease patients' desire to sue.[19] It appears that physicians and patients do not always agree about what constitutes an honest explanation. In one study, two-thirds of physicians thought they were honest in their discussion with the patient but only one third of the patients thought so.[20] One-fifth of these patients described their physicians as basically dishonest in telling them about what happened. Clearly, more research needs to be done on this subject.

Other Impediments to Disclosure

CERTAIN COMMON AND DEEPLY ROOTED PERSONALITY FEATURES HAVE THE POTENTIAL TO INHIBIT PHYSICIANS FROM DISCLOSING A BAD OUTCOME. When an adverse event occurs, their human instinct for self-preservation can be in direct conflict with physicians' deeply ingrained sense of professional responsibility for the well-being of the patient. Even in the healthiest of physicians, especially among those who have difficulties in admitting failure or apologizing, this clash is no small obstacle to overcome.

Physicians in practice and in training are consistently found to fear personal inadequacy and failure and to protect themselves strongly against criticism and uncertainty.[21,22] They use "hiding responses" when they experience intense shame at falling short of their ideals and at any suggestion of failure or the exposure of their shortcomings.[23] These responses include withdrawal from social contact, denial or avoidance of the facts of the situation, or behavior that distances them from the outcome. These normal responses diminish anxiety and preserve and restore psychological equilibrium by allowing persons to temporarily wall off reality to protect against psychological injury while they adjust. Hiding responses are not helpful, however, when a bad outcome occurs because walling off interferes directly with physicians' carrying out their ethical and legal responsibilities to talk with patients and their families as soon as possible after an adverse event. To withdraw from patients is to avoid duty, and this failure to fulfill obligations only intensifies the sense of shame and low self-esteem.

PHYSICIANS ARE INCREASINGLY PRESSURED TO REPORT BAD OUTCOMES DESPITE PERSONAL RISKS AND COSTS TO THEMSELVES. When confronted with an error or a bad outcome, physicians become subject to a range of reporting mandates. Regrettably, powerful disincentives to compliance with such regulations also exist. Only twenty-one states that require reports of adverse incidents also provide legal protections against disclosure of reported data. In other states that require reports, no similar protections exist and therefore reports may be subject to discovery in malpractice litigation.[24]

Adverse event reports are used in some states for a variety of other purposes. When Dr. Joseph Daley experienced an adverse event in his Massachusetts surgical practice, he met the requirement of his policy by notifying his insurer.[25] Shortly thereafter, in renewing his medical license, he checked "none" to the inquiry about "claims pending." Within a month or two, the Board of Registration notified Dr. Daley that he had improperly completed his license renewal form and that he was, as a result, subject to sanction. The board responded to the astounded physician's inquiry by alleging that by failing to acknowledge three claims against him, he had made a fraudulent response. Now flabbergasted, he said he knew of no such claims and asked for the details. The board listed: (*1*) the insurer's open file on the reported incident, which did not become a claim; (*2*) a failure to diagnose a wrist fracture, about which Dr. Daley had no knowledge, in a head injury patient whom he had treated and who had sued another physician; and (*3*) a case in which his insurer had asked him to testify on behalf of one of their insureds who had been sued by one of Dr. Daley's patients. Inquiring as to why he had been officially reprimanded, the Board of Registration told Dr. Daley that it was his obligation to monitor all information on events that involved him. Unfortunately for Dr. Daley, this incident occurred in the late 1980s soon after Massachusetts passed a tort reform bill. Part of the law transformed the Joint Underwriting Association (JUA) into a mutual insurance company. To set premium rates among the various specialties, the actuaries apparently reviewed all potential claims in each specialty. Without his knowledge, Dr. Daley's open files had been submitted, leaving him caught in the middle of a change that held extremely negative consequences for him personally.

In retrospect, it seems sensible that in such circumstances, the insurer should tell those it insures how it uses such data. Had Dr. Daley's insurer informed him about the technical nature of an open claim and that such information about him had been forwarded to the board, he would have approached his license renewal in a less naïve and better prepared fashion. The ironic outcome of this tale is that, unless served with legal papers, Dr. Daley no longer reports anything to the insurer.

Momentum is increasing at both the state and national levels to establish data banks, primarily in the hospital and freestanding surgical center settings, to record medical near-misses and errors. Managed care organizations often require reports of adverse events that may later become the basis for de-selection of reported physicians from clinician panels. JCAHO requires the reporting and analysis of *sentinel events*, defined as unexpected occurrences, or the risk of one, involving death or serious physical or psychological injury. The honest reporting and analysis of such an event, often in physician's own words, may be discoverable and made available to third parties, including the media.[26,27]

Physician-attorney Bryan Liang warns that the use of regulations to stimulate improvement in patient safety will fail because good plaintiff attorneys, with sub-poenas and other legal maneuvers, can easily penetrate existing peer review/quality assurance protections. When information designed to improve the system is dis-coverable, the potential negative impact on the individual clinician rises significantly.[28] Such regulations always bristle with the unintended consequences that are the side effect of legislative efforts to promote good: in this case, making physicians unwilling to admit mistakes. If such regulations are to bear fruit and dismantle the current system of blame, they must provide effective zones of pro-tection to support the legal and ethical practice of medicine.

PHYSICIANS ARE SUBJECT TO CHANGING LEGISLATION RELATIVE TO APOLOGIES AND MEDICAL ERROR. In the real world of catastrophic outcomes where the fine line between full disclosure and an admission of fault is often blurred, it is useful for physicians to know whether, and what, legal protections are in force in their jurisdiction. Such information, along with relevant new developments, should be made known to physicians by the legal counsel of their health care facility or state medical society. Physicians should also inform themselves specifically about the following.

- *Laws concerning voluntary and involuntary disclosure of adverse events in health care.* In states with mandatory error-reporting laws, the physician often has the legal duty to disclose adverse events to patients or their families. They may also be required to report the event to some state agency charged with counting and classifying these events. Such laws are more likely to affect physicians who have a hospital-based practice in which the institution's mandated reporting of incidents includes the name of the physician involved.
- *Laws regarding peer review and quality assurance protections.* Peer review statutes prohibiting disclosure of postevent deliberation activities, such as

morbidity and mortality (M&M) conferences, gained fashion in the late 1960s. Most courts had always been reluctant to grant such immunity. The courts upheld these protections to nondisclosure only because the legislation always stated in the policy preamble that, when information flows freely, these protections ensure improvement in quality of care. Trial lawyers have attacked this premise in cases and through the legislative process. No wholesale undoing of these privileges has yet occurred, although some states now have common law exceptions and limitations to nondisclosure.[29] It is therefore important to know not only the scope and substance but also the limitation of these protections in the physician's jurisdiction.

The game-like quality of legal maneuvers defeats good intentions every time. Despite reassurances that M&M conferences are protected as peer review activity, physicians are wary and uneasy about being fully forthcoming in such settings, turning such conferences into dried-out formal affairs that lack the easy exchange of information that would both further professional education and promote patient safety.

• *Laws preventing the admission into evidence of statements, writings, or benevolent gestures expressing sympathy or conveying a general sense of benevolence.* These fairly recent developments in tort law reflect a growing societal recognition and acceptance of apology as a tool to reduce unnecessary litigation and its associated costs. If saying one is sorry can modulate the motivation of an injured patient to sue, not only does society benefit but also the potential parties to the dispute are spared the agony and expense of litigation.

Increasingly, state legislatures are writing laws that protect physicians' statements of sympathy from being admitted as evidence of liability in a malpractice case. The devil is found, as usual, in the details. In California, for example, apologies are protected but specific admissions of fault are not.[30] The law (§1160.a)[31] states, "The portion of statements, writings, or benevolent gestures expressing sympathy of a general sense of benevolence relating to the pain, suffering, or death of a person involved in an accident and made to that person or to the family of that person shall be inadmissible as evidence of an admission of liability in a civil action. A statement of fault, however, which is part of, or in addition to, any of the above shall not be inadmissible pursuant to this section."

What does this actually mean for the clinician confronted with a catastrophic event or bad outcome? The law's protections apply to all actions to recover damages for accidental (nonwillful) injury to or death of a person. Clearly, a medical negligence action meets the definition of *accident*. Purely benevolent gestures made aloud or in writing to a patient or family member of a patient (*family* is broadly defined) are not admissible as evidence in a civil action. What can physicians say that will not be construed as a statement of fault? Most legal advisors suggest that it would be appropriate for a physician to say, "I am truly sorry this has happened to you" or "I'm so sorry that you are going through this." If a physician says, "I am so sorry that I did this to you," this statement could be used as an admission of fault.

Many physicians are unaware that such laws exist. Other physicians claim that these developments have done little to lessen the fear of litigation in these jurisdictions. Some risk managers applaud the distinctions offered by the legislation as a way of helping physicians learn the difference between expressing empathy and admitting fault. Insurers are concerned about the ambiguities in the law and are working to strengthen these legal protections to make them more predictable.

* *Laws limiting public access (especially newspapers and television reporters) to written materials submitted in connection with patient safety reporting and other oversight activities such as those of professional licensing boards and credentialing organizations.* The tension between the public's right to know and the privacy of the relationship between the patient and the physician has increased over the past decade under the media's demand that the public's right should open the doors on what goes on behind the closed doors of every state licensing board. The public interest is a function of the media coverage of such catastrophic events as that at Duke University in 2003, when a patient received improperly matched organs. Also, news is by its nature essentially negative and news organizations automatically swarm to any professional's fall from grace whether from incompetence, health problems, or emotional distress.

THE CONTEMPORARY APPLICATION OF LEGAL STANDARDS CAN APPEAR TO BE ARBITRARY AND FICKLE. Most physicians can tell at least one story, often their own, about reaching a settlement in a malpractice case for nonmedical reasons. A prime example is found in the horrendous settlements offered in breast implant cases, where charges were clearly based on flawed science. Physicians can also tell stories about errors that were followed by no litigation. Such variations in the rationale for lawsuits and in the unpredictability of outcomes and payouts reinforce physicians' beliefs that objectivity and the community standard of care as the measure of professional performance are not always honored in the courtroom. Whether juries award damages based on sympathy for the severity of injury rather than on evidence that the physician violated the standard of care is debated.[32-34] This suggests that the twin goals of medical malpractice law—to compensate patients injured through negligence and to deter substandard medical practice— are neither sought nor achieved.[35-37] Unpredictability in the application of the law not only demoralizes good practitioners but also fails to protect patients from substandard practitioners. It is understandable that, when honest disclosure propels physicians into the courtroom, physicians refer to themselves as "moving targets" and to the system as a "lottery."

THE FEELING THAT A LAWSUIT IS INEVITABLE IN THE EVENT OF A BAD OUTCOME. Physicians may overestimate the probability that a lawsuit will be filed. The evidence to date suggests that, compared with the actual number of medical errors, the risk of a claim is quite small.[38] Physicians may also lack sufficient information about, and overestimate, their risk for a claim[39] and know little about how the legal system relates to the issue of medical malpractice.[40] Physicians cannot, however, deny widely reported occurrences: claims that appear to be valid are not filed, whereas those seemingly not valid are filed. Also, they cannot deny that even though their medical care conforms to the standard of care, plaintiffs are at times awarded damages only because of the severity of their injuries. In addition, a nuisance case that everybody would expect to be dismissed may survive for years on legal life support before being dropped just before trial. In their need for certainty and their drive for perfection, physicians have good reason to view the legal system as an environment dominated by trial attorneys that is unfamiliar, adversarial, and unpredictable.

Scenarios for Disclosure

A Mistake That Results in No Harm

Sometimes physicians, or others on the health-care team, are aware of a mistake that brings no harm to the patient. Does the patient need to be told of the incident? Some will argue that it is unnecessary to reveal mistakes unless the result is significant harm to the patient that can be remedied or modified or for which financial compensation may be given. Others argue that even nonharmful mistakes should be shared with patients, a course reinforced by research findings that patients want to know about even minor mistakes, if only to have them acknowledged by their physician.[41]

> Dr. William King, a general surgeon, inadvertently nicked a vessel during surgery, recognized the problem, and repaired it immediately. He did not reveal the incident when talking with the family immediately after the surgery. After the patient awakened, however, he told her what had happened and how he dealt with it during the surgery. He also indicated what further steps, such as continued observation and regular blood studies, would be taken to prevent any potential complications.

Recalling their "most memorable error," fourteen of fifty-three family practitioners identified mistakes about which they felt guilty but which inflicted no harm on the patient.[42] Even when no harm comes to the patients, such incidents, like all near misses, affect physicians emotionally. As most clinicians know, there is no better reminder of how easily mistakes can occur and how vulnerable physicians are than when we experience a close call that could have led to serious consequences. Although they may not tell the patient or anyone else, physicians may question their competence, because they know that the patient "could have been" harmed.

As noted, how such events affect our emotions is a function of their nature and severity.[43] The more shaken physicians are by the event, the more likely they are to probe its causes and to explore their role in it. A known mistake is easy to dismiss if it is not serious or harmful to the patient. Failing to question a patient about allergies and prescribing a medication that causes a rash are, for example, easily remedied mistakes. Unless we tease out the roots of the problem and discuss them with the patient, however, we will neither learn from the incident nor be able to modify our professional habits.

Given the tendency of patients to misunderstand and that the mistake's very occurrence serves as an impetus for the physician to take steps to prevent its recurrence, some lawyers warn against any discussion of such mistakes. Nonharmful mistakes can be uniquely instructive. The decision to discuss the issue, however, is one of clinical judgment, and doing so has the potential to make such an experience more beneficial for both physician and patient. Taking the time to talk openly about the cause and the treatment of the allergic reaction alerts physicians so that they can mentor themselves. They reinforce good habits, and, through their disclosure, achieve a deeper level of trust with their patient. Reflective self-mentoring reduces pressure on physicians, enabling them to make major changes in their practice that both improve patient safety and lessen their risk of being sued in the future.

Complications: Harm but No Mistake

Sometimes a bad outcome is not due to a mistake but rather to a complication whose possibility was foreseen and was clearly explained to the patient during an informed consent session. Informed consent builds a collaborative relationship between physician and patient before treatment, but it is also valuable after such a complication actually occurs. Daniel O'Connell, Ph.D., of the Bayer Institute for Health Care Communication, emphasizes the importance of using the informed consent session to begin the discussion of potential complications to lay the groundwork, should complications occur, for the postevent discussion.[44] When a patient sustains "harm but no mistake" and the complication has been anticipated and discussed beforehand, physicians should have little anxiety about disclosing all the relevant facts of the outcome.

By instinct and by training, physicians do everything possible to avoid complications. Patients place both their trust and their hope in physicians, believing, as they must, that all will be well. Physician and patient are linked beforehand in

denying the possibility of a bad outcome, defending themselves against anticipating such an unhappy development.

In that interval after an adverse event and before talking with the patient, physicians must examine their own feelings about what has happened to gain control
over them and, by temporarily suppressing them, to make themselves emotionally available to the patient. Although a measured appreciation of the risk beforehand may lessen a physician's feelings of personal responsibility, even anticipated
complications can cause them great personal agony and self-criticism. A relatively
well-functioning 70-year-old man who is symptomatic before a well-executed
carotid endarterectomy and then does well postoperatively differs dramatically
from the same postsurgical 70-year-old man with a stroke. Despite the fact that
the procedure is performed appropriately and the patient is fully briefed about the
remote possibility of this complication, physicians still often feel personally responsible for any negative change in their patient's status. Physicians know as
well that even after an open, sincere, and inclusive discussion, some patients may
still pursue litigation to "find out what happened" and to seek compensation.

Mistakes and Questionable Mistakes

Ambiguity is not found in all instances. Although the mistake is sometimes clear,
at other times, it is truly questionable. When all of the potential defendants agree
that a mistake has been made, current tort system thinking looks for early disclosure, apology, and restitution, responses that may obviate the need for litigation.
Ambiguity nestles in questions about whether a mistake really has occurred, leaving
the physician uncertain about issues of disclosure, apology, and restitution and
the potential for eventual litigation.

"Questionable mistakes" set off the classic uncertainty that we feel when we
know that we are involved but are unclear about our precise role in a serious event.
We can establish perspective on the event only after an objective assessment is
made of all of the known facts. We do not settle down easily or find quick relief
while waiting in such a limbo.

Even when overwhelming evidence points to a mistake, physicians may obsess, reviewing it endlessly, hoping still to be freed of responsibility. Because
recognizing a serious or catastrophic mistake is painful and emotionally devastating, physicians first need time to absorb it. Like all professionals, they instinctively shield themselves from such feelings and shrink back from facing failure.
Aware that such occurrences trigger sentinel event reports and other quality assurance mechanisms, physicians may also be concerned about potential sanctions from
within the hospital. They may be tempted to withdraw from contact with others,
to avoid anything associated with the situation, to refuse to cooperate fully with
any investigation, or to blame others for what has happened. Physicians who have
never experienced such an event may be especially resentful about the seemingly

humiliating and unfair demands made on them. Their best selves recognize that they must eventually accede to the institution's requiring their cooperation and give their time to investigate the source of the outcome.

Investigating Bad Outcomes

As physicians go through the investigative process, they may find that long-buried feelings of low self-esteem begin to surface that they are unwilling to share with others. They tend to suffer these feelings in silence and attempt, in fact, to cover them up to avoid the shame that their revelation would cause them. Davidoff suggests that shame is particularly difficult for physicians because its moral implications challenge their core feelings of integrity, leaving them feeling personally exposed, inferior, and diminished as persons.[45] Although physicians care for their patients and work hard to act responsibly, mistakes signal their fallibility and the possibility that they have acted irresponsibly. This failure is directly related to a profound life change for patients and even their death. Regardless of the cause of the event, physicians may be suffused with feelings of disappointment in themselves and of devastation at the outcome. They wonder if they will ever enjoy going to work or feel good about themselves again. During this period, they may feel that they can control themselves, keep their own counsel, and preserve their feelings of invulnerability by working out these feelings on their own. By isolating themselves, they often experience unnecessary stress and pressure that they could modify by sharing their reactions with others.

The environment largely determines whether physicians feel comfortable with the investigation. As noted earlier, most state laws protect M&M conferences as a peer review activity.[46] Because the exchange is protected from use in any later legal case, participants, even though they may feel uncomfortable, should feel safe and free to discuss the full facts related to the case. Physicians emerge from such protected discussions better prepared to prevent similar events from recurring in the future.

Physicians experience additional threats from the actual and potential mistakes that occur within complex systems. Any one of the potential defendants, including the institution, may attempt to lay blame on the physician's doorstep. Improperly conducted investigations confront physicians with increased legal risk and its side effect of emotional turmoil. In the worst-case scenario, the investigation can be manipulated as smoothly as elections can be stolen, to unfairly deflect blame from the institution by shifting it to the physicians.

The importance of the tone of the investigation is revealed in a study of consultant psychiatrists in Scotland.[47] Participants clearly differentiated between the supportive and constructive team reviews of patient suicides that spurred learning and the formal reviews whose purpose was to identify a blameworthy individual. Physicians negatively viewed those proceedings—legal, regulatory, and disciplinary—that pursued the latter goal. Some suggested that the healing potential of any formal inquiry is a function of its allowing the emotional charge of the event to lessen before any discussion begins.

Participation in a properly conducted interrogation allows physicians to confront their wounded feelings and to begin the healing that restores their equilibrium. The long journey of investigation may find that the event could not have been anticipated or that some chain of events outside the physician's purview led to the outcome. The investigation may also decide that the physician may or may not have contributed to a clear mistake or series of mistakes that led directly to an adverse event.

Some Questions about Disclosure

When Should Disclosure Occur?
The rule of thumb is to inform patients or their families as soon as possible after discovery of the problem. Some institutional policies encourage discussion with patients within twenty-four hours.

As in any clinical situation, the potential benefits of any action should outweigh its risks. The patient's clinical status, psychological condition, or personal preferences may affect the timing and content of a physician's disclosure about an actual or a potential mistake. Although full disclosure is the ideal, physicians must, in all cases, respect the patient's wishes. At the same time, certain family members may need specific information if they are to act on the patient's behalf. If physicians have any questions about the appropriateness and focus of disclosure, they should consult with the risk manager, the ethics committee, or the hospital legal counsel.

Some physicians hold a very limited session with the patient and family to reveal the complication or error, give some indication of what has or is being done to deal with it, and schedule a second, fuller session as soon as they know enough to address the problem in greater detail. This allows the patient and family to take the first steps on the path of absorbing what has happened to prepare them to stay on course for its entire length.

Who Should Tell the Patient?
In general, the treating physician takes the lead in disclosing the outcome to patients. In hospitals or other health-care systems, such significant personnel as nurses, residents, risk managers, or administrative representatives may also participate in the session.

Growing acceptance is found in some hospitals and other facilities of conducting the official disclosure session without the presence of the treating physician.

At the previously described VA facility in Lexington, Kentucky, and in a model program described by Liang,[48-49] the disclosure process includes administrators and risk managers but not the treating physicians. This approach is rationalized by the belief that most errors are due to system rather than individual failures and that individuals directly involved in the care of injured patients may be so psychologically compromised immediately after the event that they are not as effective as others who are not as directly involved in making disclosures. Cantor[50] further argues that an institutionalized and predictable process is more helpful to patients and families than the haphazard approaches that are affected by the contingencies of the individual physician's training, experience, and psychological state.

As institutions play more prominent roles in maintaining contact with the patient, physicians may feel alienated and undermined if they are kept outside the process. Sometimes physicians feel not only that their input is ignored but also that they are the last ones to learn what actually happened and what the institution's plans are to resolve it. Traditional ethical obligations, however, seem to support the notion that physicians play a significant role in disclosure. Indeed, most physicians want to talk with patients after a bad outcome and participate in any continuing investigation of the incident.

Who Should Be Told?

Patients should be told directly about what has happened. They may want to have other family members or close associates with them for the session. When the discussion is expected to be complicated and to involve difficult decision making, the patient should be encouraged to choose at least one other person to be present. If the patient is a minor, has died, or is unable to appreciate the situation fully, the survivors or other designated persons representing the patient should be informed about the outcome.

How Can Physicians Prepare to Discuss Bad Outcomes With Patients?

Physicians must be in good emotional balance and possess all of the information needed to conduct a helpful meeting with the patient. Presenting information in a confused manner or conveying a defensive posture increases the difficulty involved in admitting a mistake. Even if not all of the facts are available—something patients can understand—it is better to have clear ideas beforehand about what can be communicated truthfully and empathically. It is understandable that physicians may try to include some hope in their first discussion with patients but, if none really exists, this tactic serves everybody—patient, family, and physician—poorly. When the event is the subject of further investigation, physicians may usefully suggest a plan, often with a specified timeline, to keep the patient informed about its progress. Patients can also understand that although some of these investigations impose confidentiality requirements on the institution, anything that can be communicated appropriately will be made available to them.

A physician might begin with such words as, "I'm afraid I have bad news." This is a small but significant opening for telling the patient what has happened.[51,52] Buckman[53] offers a model that presents a six-step process for breaking bad news by giving information in "small chunks." Bad outcomes generate emotional repercussions that are often so overwhelming for patients, their families, and the physician, that one may need to arrange for a series of sessions to complete these difficult discussions.

What Needs to Be Discussed?
Whether it covers a complication or a clearly established error or whether the cause of the problem is unknown, the information communicated about the bad outcome should be consistent. Physicians should tell the patient what they currently know about the incident and what they have done or plan to do to lessen the burden of any expected disability. The physician may also recall the discussion of such outcomes with the patient, using this as a foundation for this difficult conversation.

A physician should, of course, facilitate any warranted consultation. One study reveals that the number of patients who want to speak to another physician about the mistake increases as a function of the severity of the incident.[54]

What if the Patient and Family Express Anger Directly and Blame the Physician for the Outcome?
Physicians should not be surprised if the family feels angry and disappointed. When individuals lose something, they need to express their anger and rage and they often do so by displacing it, along with blame, onto others. Even if physicians are not at fault, they are so close to the event that they become available candidates for the displacement of these intense negative feelings. It is easy to withdraw from the patient and family, to blame others for the problem, or to "disappear" from the scene when confronted with such intense negative attacks. The physician's responsibility, however, is to understand these feelings as a function of their patient's loss even though they may feel it personally, and to remain available to patients and families to help them work through these feelings during this difficult transition.

Convey an Explicit Apology Only When It Has Been Cleared by the Insurer and Institution
Although most insurers support disclosure of mistakes, most of them also offer cautions about how candid this disclosure should be. Physicians should never speculate about fault. Most companies ask physicians to contact them before they assume any culpability for the outcome. A physician's defense can be compromised if, without first involving the malpractice insurer, he or she acknowledges fault in

a situation. Some insurance companies agree with defense attorneys who caution against using the word "sorry" because it can be interpreted by patients or juries as an admission of fault. Others permit the use of the word as an expression of concern or sympathy, but the best guide is the policy of the insurer. Dr. George Thomasson, formerly with the Colorado Physicians Insurance Company, notes that in such circumstances their insureds may use words like "mistake" and "sorry" and then let the courts decide liability.[55]

Recommendations: An Outline for Disclosure

The approach of physicians to disclosure is a function of the event itself, their role in the outcome, the suggestions offered by risk managers and consultants, the current state law, and the unique relationship between physician and his or her patient and family members. The following abbreviated outline of a disclosure session illustrates a series of helpful principles.

This illustration is based on Dr. Richard Allen's case. He is not the admitting physician and he has seen the patient in consultation on only one occasion. His partner, however, had followed the patient postoperatively. When Dr. Allen arrives on the unit, the patient is being resuscitated under the supervision of an orthopedic surgeon, Dr. Thomas, who is covering for his partner, the patient's primary physician. He has seen the patient a few times and met with the family on one occasion. Both Dr. Allen and Dr. Thomas have limited information on the patient and her course. They discuss what they know and what they think has happened, and they agree to request an autopsy. They decide that because Dr. Thomas has met them previously, he will talk with the family.

Setting the Stage

WORK TO ACHIEVE SOME EMOTIONAL EQUILIBRIUM ABOUT THE EVENT. Risk manager Deborah McBride describes how, immediately after such an event, in a ninety-minute telephone conversation with a physician, she gave him time to talk about the incident in great detail.[56] She discussed ways that he could explain the outcome to the family without resorting to medical jargon. Bolstered by her support, he felt that his emotional balance and objectivity had been restored and he was able to proceed. In Dr. Allen's case, he and Dr. Thomas compared views on what might have transpired. Often an associate, nurse, or risk manager is immediately available to help in such situations.

IDEALLY, BAD NEWS SHOULD BE COMMUNICATED IN PERSON. Circumstances may require telephone contact, but generally person-to-person contact is most helpful for conveying emotionally charged information.

TAKE THE TIME TO ARRANGE A PHYSICAL SETTING THAT IS PRIVATE AND CONVEYS A NONHARRIED ATMOSPHERE. The more serious the news, the more important is our management of the time and the circumstance of privacy. We should section off the room with a curtain if a separate, private room is not available and arrange for a place where everyone involved can sit down. This conveys our authority as well as our awareness of the seriousness of the session. It also conveys our sensitivity and our concern for others' feelings. Most of us feel more comfortable sitting with patients and families, close enough to offer our supporting hand or a needed tissue. Human touch conveys our concern well, and we should feel free to express our concern in this healthy manner.

ALLOCATE SUFFICIENT TIME FOR THE DISCLOSURE SESSION. Discussions about mistakes or bad outcomes that can have enormous long-term consequences for both patients and physicians cannot be hurried. To avoid feeling hurried, physicians may prudently schedule a minimum of one uninterrupted hour for these conferences. By giving patients a message that they are in a hurry and want to get the session over as quickly as possible, physicians can destroy their best intentions and waste everybody's time. We convey an effective and reassuring message to the patient by communicating clearly through our manner and behavior that "my time is your time."

Conducting the Session
Some of us have natural gifts to express sorrow about bad outcomes and to provide explanations to patients. Others achieve expertise slowly and may require training and significant practice before they can effectively express empathy. Few of us have ever had any explicit training in talking with patients in emotionally charged situations. To help physicians, The Bayer Institute publishes videos and books and holds sessions on communication that include special attention to dealing with bad outcomes.[57]

INTRODUCE YOURSELF AND ALL THOSE INVOLVED IN THE SESSION. It is essential that the patient's relationship to everyone involved in the session be clear. We should introduce those who accompany us and explain their role in the patient's care, identifying each team member appropriately as the nurse, resident, or risk manager. We might then ask the patient and those family members present if they are comfortable in their presence and, if for some reason they are not, we should excuse these associates from the session. If we have any doubts about the identity of an individual in the room, we should not hesitate to ask in a warm and concerned manner, "Are you a relative of Ms. Jones?"

EMPATHIZE WITH THE PATIENT AND THE FAMILY. Even though, for most of us, the situation is in and of itself anxiety provoking, we must try to be completely available emotionally so that we can respond to the person's immediate needs.

This may be as small a gesture as offering a tissue, holding the person's hand, or touching them in some sympathetic way.

OPEN THE SESSION IN A WAY THAT SETS THE STAGE BUT ALSO CONVEYS AN IN-TEREST IN THE PERSON'S CURRENT EMOTIONAL STATUS.

> PHYSICIAN: Well, Mr. Jones, I know that you have been called in suddenly by the nurse here and told that your wife was not doing very well. I'm sure this is very upsetting for you since you must suspect that something very serious is going on.
>
> MR. JONES: Yes, and then they stopped me at the nursing station and prevented me from going to her room. Why? What's going on? Has something happened?
>
> (In this scenario, the physician is both surprised that the patient's condition has deteriorated so rapidly and anxious that family members might not understand how things could change so completely within a period of twenty-four hours. The physician is aware that the patient's husband is anxious and irritated about being stopped in the corridor. This underscores the physician's need to control his own emotions in the face of varying circumstances so that he can be genuinely empathic in responding to Mr. Jones, who does not yet know that his wife has died. He may also express his own upset at this turn of events.)
>
> PHYSICAN: Yes. I came in this morning and I was really taken aback to find that your wife's condition had gotten so much worse so rapidly. I wanted to talk with you right away, so I had the nurse call you immediately. I feel very badly about all this, but I have to tell you that things have not gone well.

TELL THE TRUTH. Ideally, bad news is delivered in stages. In dire circumstances such as this, however, there is no good way to break the news gently so that the husband can gradually absorb the reality of the situation. The patient's husband must be told of the patient's death immediately and directly. Attempting to dissemble or delay only complicates an already difficult situation. A simple statement of fact is most respectful of the husband's situation and of his emotional maturity.

> PHYSICIAN: According to the nurses, your wife was fairly stable through the night, her blood pressure and pulse were good, but she suddenly went into shock and we were unable to bring her back. We really tried very hard to revive her, and, despite our best efforts, we could not save her and she died. I'm sure this is very difficult for you, when you thought you were going to see her alive and then be told she died.
>
> MR. JONES: What? She's died?
>
> PHYSICIAN: I'm afraid that she has. Our team worked very hard to save her, but it just was not possible. I'm very sorry to have to tell you in this way. I know this must be a great shock for you. (pause)

EXPRESS SORROW FOR THE PERSON'S LOSS. Because bad or catastrophic outcomes may happen so infrequently, we may not find it easy to talk with patients and their families and to maintain a sensible balance between expressing our sorrow and assigning any fault. Some of us may find that rehearsing such a session beforehand frees us up, making us more comfortable and more able to find the right words in an actual session. If the session is held before we feel ready and in control, we may communicate our own discomfort to the patient and family and nobody is well served. Some insurers and risk managers suggest that we should use the word "I" carefully. We may say, for example, "I'm sorry that this has happened to you," but not "I'm sorry that I did such and such. . . ." Our best approach in expressing sorrow is first to pause and think about what we mean to say and then to mean it when we say it in simple, direct words, "I'm sorry that this has happened." Speak it, as Spencer Tracy advised actors, "as truly as you can." The emotions that accompany sincere words will be clear to other persons and our meaning will be unmistakable.

(The physician should wait silently for a brief period of time to allow for the husband's initial reaction.)

> PHYSICIAN: I feel very badly because I know that it is such a surprise and such a painful loss to you and all your family. None of us can quite know how difficult this is for you.
>
> MR. JONES: I can't believe it. I saw her last night and she was talking and she told me she was feeling somewhat better. I can't believe it. What happened?

PUT ANY EXPLANATION IN CONTEXT. When serious injuries occur, as we have noted before, considerable pressure builds up for an explanation. What contributed to the final outcome is not always crystal clear, and most of us also have difficulty in absorbing the full impact of such shocking news. If the person expresses an interest in immediately knowing why the event happened, we should offer a short explanation of the known details and what has, or what might be, done. We may also suggest that they might be more comfortable if they waited to have a session later in that day or within a few days. This acknowledges that they may need time to pull themselves together after the initial shock and that we need some time to develop a better understanding of the outcome.

> PHYSICIAN: Well, as you know, your doctor is out of town but I talked with him before he left and he said he had talked with you and your wife yesterday. He told me about his concerns about her blood count and about the tests that were ordered. We simply don't know the whole story at this time about why she went into shock so suddenly. I feel very sorry that I have to tell you this news and sorry that this is all I can tell you right now.
>
> *One way for us to communicate true empathy in such situations is to wait and follow the pattern of the person's spontaneous associations or flow of ideas. These are clear indicators of what they are feeling. In this case, after a brief silence, the husband speaks about what is uppermost in his mind.*

MR. JONES: Where is she? Can I see her?

PHYSICIAN: Of course. She is still in her room. I'll call the nurse to arrange it. Is there anyone with you today that you might want to be with you?

MR. JONES: I called my son earlier and he should be on his way from his home. Maybe he's come by now. (pause) He's not going to believe this. (He begins to tear up.) I can't believe it.

PHYSICIAN: Let me have the nurse come and I'll check to see if your son has arrived. Do you mind if I leave for a minute? (Mr. Jones nods acceptance and the physician leaves. He shuts the door and returns shortly with the nurse and Mr. Jones' son. The physician has told the son on the way into the room that he is talking with his father about events that have occurred since the previous evening. The tearful father and son embrace.)

MR. JONES: (to his son) Did the doctor tell you what happened? (The son nods assent.)

PHYSICIAN: As I mentioned to you, things have gone very badly since last night. Your mother went into shock just a short time ago and although we tried very hard to save her, we were unable to do so. She died very quickly.

SON: What happened?

PHYSICIAN: As I was saying to your father earlier, my partner saw your mother yesterday and her blood pressure, pulse, and respiration were all normal so that what we call her vital signs all seemed to be in order. You know that she had a blood clot in the lung a few days ago that seemed to be responding to treatment. There was concern about her falling blood count, however, and we were starting to do some tests to find out why that was happening. Before they were completed, your mother's blood pressure began to fall very quickly early this morning and she went into shock. It doesn't seem likely that she had another blood clot but we would need to look into that. The nurses noticed her condition right away and despite all our efforts to save her, your mother died.

The physician has reiterated the news and given some initial hints about what the basic problem may be. He waits while the son and father talk gently with each other.

PHYSICIAN: We'll have to review all the tests and see if we can find out what was the source of her recent problems. I'll be talking to the other physicians as well who were working with her. (The father and son begin to get themselves ready to visit the patient's room.)

Perhaps, after you have a chance to see your wife, we can talk some more. I know that, like all families, you want to know what happened to cause her to die so suddenly. One of the most useful ways to do this is to have the pathologist conduct an autopsy. The results may give us a much better idea of what caused the shock. It can also help us identify the source of the problem. After you're finished with your visit, perhaps we can talk some more about this and we can have you sign the necessary papers.

The physician has now begun to set a pathway and propose processes that will help not only the family but also the medical staff understand better what contributed to Mrs. Jones' death.

MAKE SURE THE PATIENT HAS AN OPPORTUNITY TO UNDERSTAND WHAT HAS BEEN COMMUNICATED AND TO GET ANSWERS TO QUESTIONS THAT HAVE NOT BEEN ANSWERED.

PHYSICIAN: Do you have any questions you would like to ask me?

MR. JONES: I just can't understand how this could have happened. She seemed to be making progress yesterday. Do you think somebody made some kind of a mistake?

Most people feel that if the outcome is so catastrophic, a mistake must have been made. The physician may suspect that some error in judgment or treatment may have occurred but, not being certain, cannot speculate. In circumstances in which we know that a blatant mistake has occurred in the care of the patient, the patient and, possibly, the family should be told as soon as possible, but we should not attribute blame to anyone. *In such instances, we must guard against any tendency to speculate and elaborate about what happened as a way of comforting the person.* Although the person may find the speculative information comforting, because it provides some plausible explanation for what happened, such discussion may complicate the patient's understanding of the event, especially if it is later found to be inaccurate. It is sufficient to explain the event in a manner that sets the stage for conveying further information when it becomes available.

PHYSICIAN: I really can't say if any mistake has been made. When we have a chance to review your wife's treatment and if we learn something from the autopsy, we will surely contact you and let you know. It's important for us to learn as much as we can about what happened.

[*The son suggests that they go to see Ms. Jones. The father agrees.*]

Concluding the Session

LET THE PERSON KNOW THAT THERE IS A PLAN FOR FOLLOWTHROUGH AND THAT WE ARE AVAILABLE FOR FURTHER QUESTIONS AND CONCERNS.

PHYSICIAN: Ms. Smith will be happy to show you the way. I'll be here in the nurses' station and we can talk a bit more about this when you return. I'll be happy at that time to answer any more questions you may have and if we get your permission for the autopsy, then it will help all of us have a better understanding of what has happened this morning, Again, I'm very sorry for your loss, and if I can be of any further help or if you have any questions, please let me know. Also, I will be in touch with your doctor, Dr. Michaels (the primary orthopedic surgeon), and let him know about what happened. Generally, we give you a call within a day or two to let you know if we have learned any more, but if you want to talk with us before that, I'm happy to talk with you. And once again, I know your loss is sudden and overwhelming and know this is a terrible loss for you and all your family.

DOCUMENT THE DETAILS OF THE DISCLOSURE SESSION IN THE CHART. This note should reflect the time and place of the discussion, the individuals present, the basic information disclosed, and any other relevant information that describes the interaction. In the illustrative case, Dr. Thomas might also describe, in addition to the information disclosed, why he is conducting the session, his discussion with Dr. Allen, his request for an autopsy, and his assurances for contact with Dr. Michaels and further contact with the family in the interim.

4

Adverse Events: What Physicians Can Say About Them

> It is not what a lawyer tells me I *may* do; but what humanity, reason, and justice, tell me I ought to do.
>
> —Edmund Burke (1729–1797)[1]

Physicians should always do the human thing. Something healthy in all of us prompts us to talk about errors, as well as unexpected or catastrophic adverse events. We feel a spontaneous but quite normal urge to express our emotional reactions to the event and to review our innermost thoughts: did we have a role in it, and what were the circumstances that contributed to its occurrence? Are physicians, however, really free to respond in such a human way?

In contrast to so many other serious life situations, the involvement of a physician in a seriously adverse medical outcome triggers the possibility of a lawsuit taking over his or her life and work. Physicians are all familiar with the first advice that lawyers give when briefing them about the legal process: "Don't talk to anyone about it." In pitting that counsel against our own natural reactions, when and how can we ever talk about this major life event?

Before the Lawsuit

A major injury or death to the patient is a tragedy that devastates everybody and often becomes the "buzz" of the hospital, charging the atmosphere with electricity that embarrasses and shames us. Traumatized, we pull back and avoid talking about it, denying ourselves the chance to take any measure of this enormous event.

That it always takes time after such an event to appreciate what has happened to the patient, his or her family, and to us is also human and normal. As this process is engaged, we need some way to express the distress we feel. The healthiest of us needs some understanding from others, especially from those we respect. We need some forum in which we feel safe enough to find and speak aloud the words that capture the nature of the experience. In such a haven we can place the undeveloped negatives of the event in the tray of calm recollection and develop clear prints of what occurred, correcting the distortions of our traumatized memory. By sharing this experience with a trustworthy person in a human manner, we can put both the event and ourselves into realistic perspective.

Dr. Laura West tells of the experience of a young obstetrician in his late 30s after a catastrophic event that became common knowledge in the hospital.

> I don't know if he came to me because I take care of his wife or because he knew I had been through it. He came to talk to me to go over the case; he hadn't even been sued yet. Everybody knew he was going to get sued. So, my efforts, my main goal in the whole conversation was to make him feel good. Do the best you can, you've got a tough job *et cetera*.[2]

Working physicians need such supportive measures. After a bad outcome, they often feel isolated, alone, and in need of acceptance by others and of a vote of confidence in their abilities. Consultation with an older, more experienced clinician can help them gain greater objectivity and understanding and thus begin the healing process from within. Having someone "with them" as they suffer their way out of the shock and distress of the experience is a simple human but incomparable aid in their reclaiming their integrity as persons and professionals. After any serious life event, support from others helps a person open up to regain emotional equilibrium.

Individuals respond to this situation the only way they can—by moving at a pace and in a style that match their feelings of comfort and safety. If, however, an individual is unable to share the experience with another person, he may well become obsessed with the event, unable to shake off his concerns about his role in it or stop replaying the details on his inner screening room. Most physicians help themselves by carefully choosing a confidant who understands them and the nature and meaning of their work.

Without the presence of a lawyer, there is some risk associated with any discussion about events that may lead to litigation. The likelihood of such discussions about a physician's feelings becoming discoverable, however, is quite small. As Dr. West described, physicians do not focus so much on the details of the case—there are other venues to explore those—but rather on the support offered by fellow human beings who can help them reconstitute themselves and restore their self-confidence.

When the Case Is Filed

Lawyers get paid for telling professionals not to talk about their cases to anyone. This is lawyer-talk, their way of ensuring that physicians will not jeopardize their defense by saying something to a third party that may be used against them. Most lawyers will not give physicians permission to do something very human: to talk about the trauma that legal action inflicts on them. They also warn physicians that in depositions, plaintiff attorneys will ask them if they have discussed the case with anyone. Physicians may be charged with perjury if they do not answer that question truthfully. That threat makes many physicians very cautious about speaking to anyone.

This may be sound legal advice but it is questionable psychological advice. Lawyers immunize themselves to the core emotional issues that are touched off by bad outcomes and traumatic legal action. As long as physicians are subject to lawsuits, however, they will experience the sharp tension of being whipsawed by conflicting legal and psychological advice. Lawyers generally believe that feelings should be controlled, as are facts. A physician, traumatized by the adverse event and its aftermath, can reap unlimited help by talking with a trusted confidant. In the words of Dr. Joseph Daley, taking the advice not to talk about it, is "the worst thing that could possibly happen. . . . It is probably one of the most destructive things that we can do."[3]

So Can Physicians Talk?

Only physicians can give themselves permission to talk about the emotional impact of both their adverse medical experience and their lawsuit. Many attorneys and insurers understand that an absolute prohibition of any discussion of an event that becomes a legal case contradicts a person's need to talk about the overwhelming emotional disruption caused by one of the most serious experiences of their lives. Attorneys and insurers may also realize that suppressing these feelings may harm a person's health and ability to function. Physicians may resolve this chronic dilemma by accepting the implied discipline: They can talk about their "feelings" regarding the event but not about the specifics of the event itself. Physicians can respect the concerns of legal counsel and still choose to talk about the problem with a trustworthy and understanding confidant, sharing their overall reactions and mentioning specifics incidentally, if at all. Humans cannot avoid any talk about their reactions to a fatal event without mentioning anything about the nature of what happened. Physicians can, however, accept a literal interpretation of not discussing the specific facts of the case while still expressing their feelings about them.

Experienced colleagues can be helpful by sharing their reactions to their own mistakes or unexpected outcomes. Learning that many of them have had similar events in their lives lessens our feelings of being alone and estranged. Trusted associates can examine the situation more objectively and help free us from the excessive self-criticism that may otherwise immobilize us.

With Whom Can Physicians Talk?

Adverse events and lawsuits share the same genetic character as all serious life events in which individuals benefit from simply being understood by someone else. Although physicians may not easily reveal how they feel, they can prepare themselves, through the relationships they develop with others throughout their lives, to do that when such traumatic moments come. Being human along the way makes it easier for physicians to be human when they really need to be so.

Conversations with one's spouse or attorney merit special protection. Confidentiality concerns aside, spouses and significant others are, of course, first-line sources of support. The closer they are affiliated with medicine, the more helpful they can be. Many physicians find the support and understanding of their physician spouses of enormous value. Their adult children can also offer great help. Sometimes a physician's assigned lawyer can fill the role of trusted confidant. Engaging a personal attorney provides another potential confidant. Family members who are also lawyers or physicians can be helpful. Sometimes a physician's claims professional and risk manager offer this kind of support. Some insurance companies engage professional therapists who provide emotional support to the insureds and become virtual members of the defense team.

Potential sources of support are as varied as are physicians. Dr. Thomas White has had a weekly 6:00 A.M. meeting with two other physicians, of different specialties, for years. They share confidences about their lives and work, including their reactions to their litigation experiences. Some physicians gain support from fellow church members, while others find that they can talk about their litigation with their long-time partner or members of their clinical team. Some physicians find an understanding confidant in their own physician; a lawsuit is an ideal catalyst for physicians to obtain a personal physician if they do not already have one.

Nobody else can do this work for physicians. Physicians need to know those persons with whom they can talk confidently and comfortably about work and personal problems.

During his litigation, Dr. Richard Allen,[4] in observing his depressed mood as well as sleep and appetite disturbances, gave himself a diagnosis of situational depression. He did not seek consultation because:

I felt that there was a finite amount of time that I was going to be involved. I wasn't going to medicate myself. It's funny about doctors. We all think that since we know something about medicine, that we can pretty much work things out and handle it. I did, however, have some long conversations with trusted colleagues, one in particular, which I think helped a lot. We had known each other for years and I felt he was the kind of person that I could trust and he wouldn't talk about it to other colleagues and I knew he had been through a similar situation because he had talked to me about it. He kept saying, "Anytime you want to call me, call me. I'll be glad to talk with you."

Turning to Professional Help

Mental health professionals, including psychiatrists, psychologists, and social workers, can offer some of the most useful support after an adverse event and during the siege of a malpractice case. These individuals, especially if they have some experience of bad outcomes or litigation of their own or that of other patients, can help physicians monitor any symptoms that they may develop, understand their reactions within the context of their own life histories, and support them as they go through the litigation process.

Mike Wallace[5] describes his decision to enter therapy in the midst of his litigation experience.

I give the impression of being fully in command of myself at all times and little by little, I found that I was not. I was worried, I obsessed, I worried and suddenly I found myself thinking about nothing else. Couldn't sleep, couldn't eat, began to lose weight. My wife said, "You know something. I think you're in a depression." And I said, "Come on." And I refused to see a doctor about it. You know, I have a doctor I've been going to for 20 years and we're friends. I finally broached it with him. And he said, "Now, Mike, come on, you're too strong." And it got worse.

Not until some weeks later when he was hospitalized for an infection did a psychiatric consultation reveal a depression for which he finally accepted a referral for treatment.

Many hesitate to seek professional help because of the often-punitive barriers. Whenever physicians renew their medical license or apply for various kinds of credentials, they are asked, in a variety of wordings, whether now, or in the past, they have sought treatment for mental illness, substance abuse, or chronic illnesses requiring on-going care. An affirmative answer risks further inquiries about whether they are competent to practice medicine. They may also be required to release confidential information about their treatment. They may hesitate, therefore, to obtain the necessary consultations for fear that if they do, they will be subjected to a variety of reviews that may jeopardize their career.

This threatening climate is gradually changing, largely due to the efforts of Steven Miles, a Minneapolis internist, and his psychiatrist. In 1996, Miles disclosed his diagnosis and treatment of bipolar disorder on a routine licensing form. The Board of Medical Practice asked for all of his psychiatrist's notes and records. He and his psychiatrist refused because it was "burdensome, discriminatory and an oblique and needlessly intrusive way to evaluate my occupational competence."[6] They maintained that routinely asking physicians to self-disclose diagnoses or submit their records to review does not identify impaired physicians and discourages physicians from getting help.

Partially as a result of their stand and legal efforts, licensure bodies are gradually changing. Most, but not all, state licensing boards have moved from a focus on diagnosis or treatment to questions about occupational impairment.[7] The time frame varies in those states that have revised their licensing forms. Illinois, for example, words the renewal form so that only illnesses that have occurred within the past 5 years and interrupt practice, or that can affect patient care negatively, need to be reported. The current renewal form asks, "Since July 31, 1999, have you had or do you now have any disease or condition that impairs or impaired your ability to perform the essential functions of your profession?"[8]

How one answers such questions is then a question of judgment. Because licensing and other certifying boards are generally very supportive of any efforts physicians make to ensure that their patients receive excellent care, physicians' responses framed in this context underscore their commitment to that competent patient care.

Consultation and treatment for reactions to malpractice suits or bad outcomes that do not impair a physician's ability to practice need not be reported, nor does obtaining treatment for a depression that, although including psychotherapy and medication, does not interrupt one's ability to perform the essential work of the profession. A bipolar illness requiring a period of hospitalization should, of course, be reported. When required, it is usually sufficient to enter a short explanation on the licensing form with relevant information about actions taken to address the problem and reference to the importance of monitoring and caring for one's own health as a component of competent patient care. Physicians should review and, if indicated, seek interpretations to guide their responses to the questions on the renewal forms in their state.

Even if they believe that treatment will not affect their licensure status, physicians tend to put off treatment because of its anticipated demands on their time. They do not quickly or easily address concerns in their personal life even though the long-term benefits of treatment contribute to their health and to the provision of good patient care. Treatment enables physicians to return to equilibrium more rapidly, increases their productivity, and diminishes their vulnerability to physical illness.[9] These are the real dividends of getting help when needed and of taking the risk of disclosing such information when required by a licensing board.

That unanticipated barriers may block one's efforts is shown in the reinforcement by the physician of Mike Wallace of the all-too-common feeling that "I'm too strong to be depressed and can handle it myself" rather than clearing the path to treatment. Ironically, both physicians and their patients are far better served if physicians persist in getting, rather than postponing, the treatment they need at the time they need it.

Recommendations

APPRECIATE THE TRAUMA ASSOCIATED WITH ADVERSE EVENTS AND LITIGATION.

GIVE YOURSELF PERMISSION TO TALK ABOUT THE REPERCUSSIONS OF ADVERSE EVENTS AND LAWSUITS.

ENLIST THOSE PERSONS WHO CAN BE MOST HELPFUL IN PROCESSING THESE EVENTS AND REINVIGORATING OUR WORK AND PERSONAL LIVES.

IF EITHER PHYSICAL OR EMOTIONAL SYMPTOMS DEVELOP AND PERSIST, SEEK APPROPRIATE MEDICAL OR PSYCHOLOGICAL CONSULTATION. Physicians who understand the natural history and impact of adverse events are better prepared than are those who do not to appreciate the short- and long-term symptoms that may emerge in their aftermath and, when necessary, to seek appropriate help.

ON REGAINING EQUILIBRIUM, ACKNOWLEDGE THE EMOTIONS ASSOCIATED WITH THE MEMORY OF THE EXPERIENCE, ORGANIZE THE TRAUMA STORY IN A COHERENT AND ARTICULATE FASHION, AND CORRECT PERSISTENT DISTORTED OR DYSFUNCTIONAL THOUGHTS ABOUT THE EXPERIENCE.[10] When we are isolated and alone, this is an impossible task. By sharing the traumatic experience and the litigation that follows with another trustworthy person, physicians gain healing and a deeper sense of their own humanity.

5

The Interim: Between the Event and the Lawsuit

We experience a bad outcome and immediately begin worrying about its consequences. We regret the incident and are greatly concerned for the patient and the family. We know that they have hit the wall of a life-changing event, and so have we.

Dr. Allen describes his sadness about what happened to the patient and her family. He deeply regretted that he was not there to oversee her care and was convinced that some steps could have been taken that might well have altered the outcome. The long interval of false quiet after the incident exaggerated his anxiety about the aftermath.

> You know the old term "whistling by the graveyard"? You know that someday it's going to show up . . . that thing that's haunting you. When I reviewed the chart, I saw that mistakes were made and, if I'd been in his [the husband's] shoes, I wouldn't have let the matter drop. But I also knew that the paradox of the situation was that even though my name was splashed all over the chart and I was splashed with a situation that I really didn't have that much to do with, I knew I was going to be involved.[1]

Two years later, he was.

Handling Immediate Anxieties After an Adverse Event

Despite widespread impressions to the contrary, both the occurrence of an adverse event and the event's leading to a successful malpractice claim are relatively infrequent.[2-4] Localio and his group[5] estimate that there are 7.6 adverse events caused by negligence to every malpractice claim. Matching medical records and medical malpractice claims, however, revealed that the number of adverse events due to negligence that actually led to claims was 1.53 percent. This difference is explained by the fact that most of the events for which claims were made in this study did not meet the researchers' criteria for negligence. The work of Brennan and the earlier work of Danzon suggests that the severity of injury, rather than any suggestion of negligence, is a central factor in the filing of a malpractice claim.[6,7] This explains why specialty looms large in the claims vulnerability of physicians; surgeons and obstetrician-gynecologists are far more likely to work with patients who sustain serious permanent injuries and death than are pathologists and psychiatrists.[8,9]

Being sued remains a highly contingent event whose occurrence cannot be predicted. Just as a 10 percent chance of rain does not mean that you will not get wet, statistical projections do not necessarily relieve physicians' two-fold anxieties that some event may "mature" into a malpractice claim and that it may be successful. Many factors influence a patient's often long-pondered decision to sue a physician.[10,11]

A surgeon may have a patient who experiences a severe and irreversible complication that requires chronic care. He or she discusses the problem with the patient, takes the necessary reparative actions, and remains in contact. The insurer is informed and an attorney requests the records. The statute of limitation expires but no suit is filed.

Another patient, adequately forewarned, develops a surgical site infection and is successfully treated with only minor residual scarring. This physician follows the same steps as the first one but, within 1 year, this patient files a lawsuit alleging delayed diagnosis and emotional harm.

If no absolute assurance exists about the possibility or probability of our being sued, how can physicians survive the anxiety that floods them during this period? Should they order all thoughts of the situation out of their minds and wait passively until the statute of limitations runs out? Or can they take action to help themselves during this high-pressure interval?

Anxiety and the Role of Control

Most of us manage anxiety by controlling what is controllable. Feeling out of control leaves us feeling exposed to our enemies and vulnerable to stress. First, we must take stock of what we can control in our medical practice and in our personal lives. This is not a small challenge. In case we are sued, we must gather and organize relevant information for our defense. We must monitor fluctuating stress, take care of our personal health, observe ourselves to modulate the tenor of our relationships, implement strategies to decrease our feelings of vulnerability, and attend to everything else in our lives, regardless of whether the lawsuit is ever filed.

In that ideal world just beyond us, we are ready for an adverse event; we have achieved emotional equilibrium by controlling what we can in our life and work and realistically letting go of what we cannot. Doing this puts adverse events and potential litigation into perspective as some of the ever-present possibilities in our professional practice. Confronted with an inability to control a situation, we may increase our efforts to control the uncontrollable by working harder for longer hours to distract us from but not eliminate our anxiety.

Dr. Laura West responded this way to her patient's death. She tried to outwork her worry, attempting to control things over which she may have had little real control. As she was able to shed her needless worries, Dr. West made better judgments about the elements of her practice that she could reasonably control. Even though she was sure that she would eventually be sued, she reassured herself realistically that the documentation was in excellent order and that she could invest herself in preparing herself psychologically to become a defendant. Just before the statute of limitations expired, she was sued along with the hospital for wrongful death. When the complaint finally arrived, she knew exactly what she could reasonably control, felt noticeably less anxious, and possessed a greater sense of mastery, comfort, and self-esteem.

Managing Our Thoughts About the Event

Assessing how much responsibility we have for the outcome is our first and overriding postevent challenge. We manage our concerns about this through our personal resources, being objective and avoiding placing too much blame on others or on ourselves. As the event is investigated, others will reach conclusions about what actually happened that will challenge or possibly reshape our conclusions. A similar sequence of reactions may occur during the litigation process. We prepare best for these by resolving early to be as honest and forthright as we can. Most of us are eventually able to achieve a way of living with the outcome that fits in both with reality and with the final legal judgment. Our work early in the process is achieving some inner resolution and peace about our role in it. Securing this, we enable ourselves to balance our personal and professional satisfactions during a period of heightened stress.

Dr. Richard Allen describes how he endured his long, anxious years of uncertainty: "Even though I knew that the other shoe was going to drop, somehow you talk yourself into thinking you can handle it and (if it does happen) it's not going to be that bad."[12] He worked during the time before litigation at controlling his thoughts about the situation, obtaining relevant information, making changes in his practice situation, and anticipating how he might cope as events unfolded. Although he had an unexpected immediate reaction to being served with a claim, he was nonetheless able to profit by the clear steps he had taken to strengthen his defenses and to create an environment in which he could practice with greater comfort.

Sorting Out Important Facts

The Statute of Limitations

Access to the courts is a time-honored American tradition and a constitutionally protected right. Because this tradition recognizes that persons who sit on their rights too long lose them, legislatures and courts also possess the power to bar access to the courthouse. That is the origin of the statute of limitations. In medical negligence cases, each state provides a time within which a claim must be brought or be barred forever. Legislatures typically set these periods from 2 to 3 years, making exceptions for children, the disabled, and some other situations.

Courts sometimes interpret, at the plaintiff's request, what a legislature meant when it established a time limitation that was considered unacceptable by the plaintiff's bar. Defense lawyers must be familiar with these judicial interpretations, known as case or common law, that frequently extend the statutory time periods.

Physicians' interests are best met by shorter statutes of limitation and by residing in jurisdictions in which the court interprets these time frames strictly. The period of uncertainty during which a claim can be made ends at a definite time, allowing liability insurers to set realistic premiums and to prudently calculate reserves. Statutes of limitations provide physicians with a finite time frame whose close ends the possibility of a case being filed on this matter.

Physicians should resist all tactics that might lead to extensions of time to file a claim. For example, misleading a patient by saying that an unexpected outcome could not be due to an error may extend the statute of limitations. In the eyes of a jury, such efforts damage a physician's credibility and may be a factor in increasing the amount of any award its members recommend.

The good news for most physicians is that the plaintiff's case must be filed by a certain date after the discovery of the incident or it can never be filed. A physician's first question to his or her claims representative is, "How long is the statute of limitations in this particular situation?" Emotionally, however, time is relative and moves slowly if the statute runs for several years.

Insurance Coverage

When Dr. Richard Allen was confronted on his return from his vacation with the unexpected death of his patient, he was certain that a suit would be filed, a feeling he had never had about any previous incident in his career. Admitting, "I had no idea what my limits of liability would be,"[12] his first task was to determine his exact insurance coverage.

Ordinarily, long before an adverse event occurs, physicians should know the terms of their malpractice insurance policy, especially the limits of liability and the scope of coverage. Nothing substitutes for reading it over carefully, and perhaps asking a personal attorney or an independent insurance agent with a strong background in medical liability coverage to do the same. Physicians must understand both their rights and obligations and those of their insurer. Because some insurance companies default or withdraw from the market, physicians must review and monitor on a yearly basis the reputation and financial stability of the company issuing their policy. Too many physicians find themselves scrambling for insurance or completely uninsured because, in opting for the lowest rates available, they failed to anticipate the real costs if their insurer managed its finances poorly or collapsed into insolvency. Insurance, by its very name and nature, should give physicians peace of mind, but physicians must make sure of the sound financial underpinnings of their insurance carrier.

Physicians must learn the technical language of insurance so they can understand whether their policy is *occurrence* or *claims-made*. Until the late 1980s, most physicians had occurrence policies, which covered any incident that occurred during the term of the policy, no matter when the claim for the incident was filed. More frequent now is a claims-made policy, which covers physicians for claims that arise from incidents that both *occur* and are *reported* to the insurer while the policy is in force. A claims-made policy from one company covers the physician for any claim that occurs or is filed during the time span of the continuously renewed policy. If the insurer terminates that policy, and if what is called tail coverage is not purchased or unavailable, any further claims for incidents that occurred during the coverage period are not covered. Physicians who move out of state while a claims-made policy is in effect must clarify whether reporting a claim from a different locality affects their coverage. Most important, the termination of a claims-made policy generally requires physicians to purchase an extended reporting endorsement, which provides the right to report a claim in the future. This tail provides coverage for any incident that occurred while the claims-made policy was in effect but was reported after the policy had expired.

Like Dr. Allen, many physicians are uncertain about the limits of their liability. These are clearly described in any policy as the *limits per claim* and the *aggregate* or *limits per term* of the insurance contract—for example, $1 million for each claim up to an aggregate of $3 million. A risk manager or independent insurance broker can help physicians understand whether the limits of their policy are sufficient.

Other Insurance Considerations

An insurance policy may exclude from coverage certain procedures, practices, and treatments and those involving practice outside the physician's specialty. Physicians must monitor this portion of their policy yearly for any material changes in these terms. The premium is determined by the nature of one's practice and the estimated degree of risk associated with it. An additional premium may be required in some specialties to cover certain practices, such as a psychiatrist who administers electric shock therapy or a dermatologist who performs procedures usually reserved for plastic surgeons.

Insurers expect immediate notification of an adverse event so they can begin to assess the nature of the event, gather the facts, and consider a potential defense. The individual procedures of each insurance company are subject to specific state regulations. In Illinois, the ISMIE Mutual Insurance Company is a physician-owned insurance company that immediately opens a deposition assistance file, which is not considered a claim and is not included in the physician's claims history.[13] When insurers open a file on the case, they appoint a claims representative, one of whose most important duties is to educate physicians about the litigation process. Knowledgeable physicians are always more effective defendants. These individuals familiarize physicians with the statute of limitations and the current tort climate in their jurisdictions. They also inform them about the meaning of and proper response to requests for records or any other actions that are signs of litigation in the making. Depending on the insurance company, claims representatives may also field inquiries from the plaintiff's attorney. A well-trained and well-informed claims representative is also emotionally supportive for physicians who are unfamiliar with or made anxious by the process.

Before a suit is actually filed, these claims personnel may refer physicians to the company's risk manager to help them respond to requests by patients and families for information. They also address appropriate apology situations and respond to regulatory and other inquiries. Because of experiences with hospital risk managers, physicians are sometimes concerned with the divided loyalties of risk managers. Most insurance companies, especially those owned by physicians, retain risk managers whose only interest is helping their insureds to either prevent or successfully defend lawsuits.

After an unexpected complication, a patient may ask a physician to forgive a professional fee, to reimburse their insurance deductible, or to cover a small wage loss. Acceding to these adjustments makes sense if it truly restrains a potential claim. The risk manager will instruct the physician in what is legally necessary to limit the patient's monetary recovery to these specified amounts, that is, to ensure that the patient does not file a malpractice claim after receiving a monetary settlement. Many insurers will supply physicians with appropriate, state-specific waiver forms to use in these situations. Unless these agreements are tied to the patient's promise never to pursue a further claim, the patient may later consult an attorney and bring a lawsuit for further damages. Which of a physician's well-meant concessions could a skilled trial attorney later turn into an admission of liability? Will malpractice carriers cover the claim if a physician made prior financial concessions without notifying and consulting with them? By involving insurers at the beginning, claims professionals and risk managers can guide physicians through the process, even preparing the appropriate settlement and release documents. The earlier physicians make their contact, the better they help themselves and their defense should a claim eventually be made against them.

The policy's conditions for settlement of a lawsuit should be clear. Does the policy allow the company to settle without consultation with the physician? In the event of a case being filed and before settlement, does the policy allow for an appeal? Many physician-owned companies recognize the importance of giving affected physicians a voice in, and sometimes the right to refuse, the settlement decision. If divergent views on settlement exist between the physician and the insurance company, each side may be offered independent appeal processes. Physicians who eventually reach a settlement should know whether the insurer allows them to review, before submission, the brief narrative that accompanies the report of the event to the National Practitioner Data Bank.

Last, old insurance policies should be kept on file in case an "old event" stirs itself and litigation to life. A clear understanding of the elements of the insurance policy, doing homework on the specifics of coverage, and maintaining contact with a claims professional or risk manager will reduce the possibility of surprises and alleviate unwarranted anxiety should an adverse event occur.

The Specter of Nonrenewal

Nonrenewal of medical malpractice insurance is, in effect, a hidden regulatory system that denies physicians due process. Many physicians do not appreciate that their primary malpractice insurance companies spend large sums purchasing insurance from the reinsurance market to cover infrequent, but expensive, larger losses. The malpractice insurance company—the primary insurer—pays only a specified level of monies in damages and, should the award reach a critical level, the re-insurer pays for any excess losses. The relationship between the malpractice insurer and its secondary insurer exerts a powerful influence on whether a physician becomes subject to nonrenewal.

For any one claim, liability insurance companies place at risk only a few hundred thousand dollars of what is termed their *surplus*. Surplus is the amount of money a company has available to pay claims after it has set aside funds to pay all known and incurred but not reported claims. These latter are adverse events that have already occurred but remain unknown to the insurance company and may be reported many months or even years later. Insurers must put aside a certain amount of money to cover such losses that may come from such delayed claims. Because most medical malpractice claims are closed without any payment to plaintiffs, these companies spend a large proportion of their at-risk dollars on defense attorneys and experts. They spend most of their surplus, however, to pay premiums for reinsurance.

In good times, the malpractice insurers are loath to "non-renew" their insured physicians to avoid the bad publicity that could adversely affect their marketing efforts. Hard times are different. Liability insurers become aggressive in non-renewing the policies of physicians because of pressure from the re-insurers who bear the majority of risk. Their contracts with the companies give them the upper hand in such underwriting decisions. When word comes down from re-insurers to "clean up your book of business," the primary insurer may nonrenew the policies of physicians who have a high frequency of claims or a single large payout. If the companies fail to comply, the re-insurer may raise the cost of the noncomplying company's excess coverage or drop it altogether.

State insurance regulators exert indirect pressure on insurers to not renew insureds by demanding that companies increase their surplus before adding new insured physicians to their book of business. The company's board of directors often consists of colleagues who, in physician-owned mutual insurers, for example, then direct the underwriters to drop coverage for selected physicians, often in such high-risk specialties as obstetrics or neurosurgery. This enables the company to accommodate less risky clinicians.

A state's insurance regulations may grant physicians a minimum number of days' notice before being nonrenewed. It is unlikely, however, that they will be given an opportunity to contest or appeal the insurer's decision to nonrenew their policy. Physicians should ask their insurer if any recourse is available to them. With rare exceptions, however, the decision to nonrenew is final and binding.

In Oregon, the state medical association's sponsored liability insurer has since 1985 provided a mechanism for review of its decisions to nonrenew. While retaining its ultimate authority to nonrenew, the company allows most association members facing nonrenewal to participate in the association-operated Risk Assessment and Management Program (RAMP). The association conducts an intensive two-part investigation into the physician's past malpractice claim or claims and examines his or her current practice for common themes or links that forecast a risk for future claims. By changing the risk profile of physicians and monitoring their practice for up to 2 years, the association can justify continuation of the physician's insurance coverage. Only one of the thirty physician participants in RAMP has had a subsequent claim.

Nonrenewal can devastate a practice, forcing physicians to give up practice altogether if they cannot find another insurer. This exit from practice occurs because many states, most hospitals, and most health plans require physicians to have coverage for malpractice claims in minimum amounts, ranging from $100,000 to $3 million per occurrence and in the aggregate. When applying for coverage from another company, physicians are asked if they have ever been nonrenewed and if they have, with rare exceptions, coverage will be denied. The hard truth of the malpractice insurance industry is that one company's refusal to insure a physician means that no other company will accept the risk either.

Practicing for a time without any coverage compounds a physician's problem. Physicians who are sued for incidents when they have no insurance coverage are responsible for both the cost of defense and any resulting monetary judgment. Insurers dread the risk of a physician who had such a gap in coverage more than a previously nonrenewed physician because in some states, the courts force carriers to provide coverage for events that occurred during a gap but became a claim only after the company provided insurance for the physician in question.

The irony of nonrenewal is that it is likely to occur without any due process and often is based on a complex of nonclinical factors such as the frequency and severity of claims, regardless of their validation, and whether a physician was a good witness at trial. Fully competent to practice, such physicians are excluded from their profession by an underwriting decision.

Losing malpractice insurance does not, however, mean that coverage is totally unavailable. A nonstandard market exists for malpractice insurance, whose price tag is determined by market forces. Although insurance carriers in this market cover almost every risk, the coverage is likely to be limited—some write limits of $100,000/$3 million—with premiums two or three times higher than those in the standard market. Nonstandard carriers may also require physicians to carry large deductibles. Physicians who can afford nonstandard coverage and who are free of claims for 1 to 2 years may be able to return to the standard market for coverage.

Getting Our Financial House in Order

Although once adequate insurance served as a firewall against a physician's being consumed financially by litigation, increases in excess judgments now make a malpractice suit potential firestorms that could quickly reduce one's resources to ashes. Physicians cannot wait until the dangerous dry season to make sure that their families or their practices are adequately protected against such disasters.

Defense attorneys tell physicians before any claim is made or suspected that financial planning should begin through consultation with their lawyer and accountant to provide in a realistic manner for their current expenditures and for a secure retirement. Physicians may also consult with lawyers who specialize in asset protection. As absorbed as physicians are in their work and their families, they cannot fail to fireproof and insure their financial houses. This controls their worry about losing when a lawyer files suit against them.

Flirting with Flight

Catastrophic events in practice can traumatize physicians to the extent that they may begin to think about changing their specialty, their career, and even their location. Dr. Michael Gitlin tells of his first psychiatric patient who committed suicide after 6 months of treatment.[14] He describes how he told himself that, "If another patient commits suicide in the next year," he would move to another city and begin his career all over. He fantasized that if he had another suicide in such a short period of time, his colleagues would never accept him as a competent physician. His worst fears were not realized: he was not sued and he did not move. He did, however, suffer the effects of the event for a long time. Another psychiatrist comments about his loss of a patient to suicide, "It reached the point in my fantasy where I was having to leave town, shunned like a leper for the terrible act (the failure to prevent the suicide) that I had committed."[15] Dr. Laura West describes actually changing her practice location during the interim period. Her husband was in a postdoctoral program and would have liked to remain longer but she felt anxious to return to the city in which she had trained and had been highly regarded.

Physicians should not be surprised if similar thoughts flood their consciousness after a negative outcome. They should calmly reflect by themselves and with their families before making such a life-changing decision. This is a time when a conversation with experienced colleagues helps to put such fantasies of flight into perspective.

Flirting with Retirement

During the interim between a bad outcome and a lawsuit, many physicians nourish the thought of retirement: "Why am I continuing to do this difficult work? Why don't I just retire and enjoy life a little?"

Few physicians actually make this choice. If they are serious, however, they must first examine many aspects of their lives, such as insurance issues. If they have a claims-made policy, they should at the time of their retirement purchase a tail to protect their heirs in the event of their death. Many insurance carriers provide, usually after 1 year of coverage, a free tail for retirement, disability, or death. Physicians should review their policy carefully for this provision that gives them the right to earn extended reporting coverage without cost. All retirement planning calls for the assurance that one's financial status can support an adequate and lengthy period of retirement. With a downturn in investment income, some retired physicians have opted to return to practice. In these circumstances, and if they have accepted a free tail from their insurer, they may be forced to purchase that tail to obtain further coverage. Through careful planning, they can avoid any such surprises.

Some physicians who would like to perform volunteer clinical work during their retirement need to check with their insurance carriers to determine whether these charitable activities violate either the letter or the spirit of their free tail arrangement. In some instances, physicians may be required to purchase tail coverage while engaging in such events. They should also be familiar with both federal and state laws that immunize them from liability while volunteering their services in certain clinics for the medically underserved. Even without statutory protections, these clinics may, under their own liability policies, cover physicians in their clinical capacities.

Many physicians may be planning on retirement even before becoming involved in an adverse event and long before they inform their insurer. Because a physician's ordinary limits may cover only the demands of one claim and therefore the demands of two or more claims will exhaust the limits of the policy, many physicians raise their limits gradually before they retire, for example, to $1 million (per claim)/$3 million (in the aggregate) to $3 million (per claim)/$3 or $5 million (in the aggregate). These decisions are made because the amount of coverage available after retirement is determined by a physician's last active policy. Such arrangements afford adequate protection if physicians experience more than one claim in the first few years of their retirement.

This strategy is particularly important for physicians who may be considered low risk. Prior to retirement, high-risk specialists such as neurosurgeons may have a clear estimate of the number of cases that could eventually mature into claims. Low-risk internists, however, are less likely to receive early warning of potential claims. Physicians may not learn about a missed breast lump, for example, until they are 2 or 3 years into retirement. Raising their limits in anticipation of retirement forestalls a great deal of surprise and worry.

A physician's decision to retire or move to a different location may be driven by a sudden rise in unaffordable insurance premiums. The last two neurosurgeons practicing in Southern Illinois, for example, announced in February 2004 plans to leave in the following summer because of medical liability insurance premiums of nearly $300,000 per year.[16] Such precipitant circumstances prevent proper planning and disrupt physicians' personal and professional lives as well as their patients' access to care.

Controlling Medical Practice

While suffering through this period of waiting, physicians may profitably take stock of their practice, reviewing the number and type of patients they see, the number of hours they work, how they share work among the partners, covering call, and how they handle office procedures and staff assignments They may not be able to control all aspects of their practice but, by identifying those that increase the stress of their work environment, they can develop plans to remedy the situation, even if they cannot implement them immediately. During this period,

Dr. Richard Allen reviewed both his financial status and his retirement plans, reflections that led to the dissolution of his partnership and sale of his practice to the hospital.

Living a Balanced Life

While waiting for the other shoe to drop, physicians must go to work each day, often preoccupied with and obsessing about their role in the event that has changed their patient and their lives. They also learn that colleagues and patients, even those who know about their concerns, need them to be the way they have always been: performing optimally and emotionally unfazed as though this demon had never entered their lives.

Medical practice is intrinsically stressful. Physicians find themselves involved in all that is human—birth, acute and chronic illnesses, accidents, and death—that justify medical sociologist Renée Fox's description of medicine as "morally and existentially serious work."[17] She maintains that the pressures that play on physicians arise from their need to "define their work as limitless in time and potential urgency" and the "uncertainties that stem from how much or how little they know." Most physicians, striving to be competent, conscientious, and empathic with their patients, find their already stressful work raised to another power by the constant economic, regulatory, and systemic demands that have become part of contemporary practice. Good training and the lessons of experience increase physicians' feelings of control even as they make them more aware of the unpredictability and uncertainty of their work. When one adds the possibilities of bad outcomes and potential litigation, it is not surprising that physicians can experience spikes in their anxiety.

Physicians are in a double bind of expectation: to be human, just like their patients, and to be superhuman, not like them at all, in never making a mistake and knowing everything. They have little space in which to address, in a healthy way, the emotional character of medical practice and less leisure to reflect on their emotional reactions to the swirling everyday world of their work. Physicians seem to "get the message" during their training that time spent on the human aspects of practice is unacceptable or, at the least, less important than its other aspects. As noted previously, residents complain of too few resources and little institutional support to help them deal with the emotional fallout from their practice errors.[18] The unspoken imperative of medicine is that, regardless of what happens, physicians should be able to "handle it."

When physicians put their training and its supervisors behind them and enter practice, they take on the obligation of monitoring their professional and personal lives and maintaining their equilibrium under their dual pressures of expectation.

New physicians realize that they are now in charge of themselves, that they must take the pulse of their own stress and develop healthy ways to cope with their work's challenges.

Setting Priorities

Clarity about our choices in life, along with our priorities and values and the motivations behind them, helps us manage our professional and personal lives successfully. We make ourselves the obstacle when we do not pay attention to what is going on inside us. Knowledge of these psychological processes is critical to our effective management of stress. Unless we identify the factors involved in maintaining or losing our balance, we feel confused and out of control. No one else can give us the time or the will to think through these personal issues. Naming these factors correctly allows us to regain control over our lives.

Looking at the Capacity to Relate to Others

The simple secret of keeping our balance is found in our ability to relate to someone else in a loving way. Only human relationships sustain, nourish, and give us both refuge and renewal. They are what free us to enjoy everything else we do and to be happy. The things that gratify us in our work take on their glow in our marriage, our permanent commitments, and our family lives. A home provides the safe environment that fosters healthy growth for both adults and children. The inevitable problems of these relationships are healthy, and solving them straightforwardly enables us to manage the stresses of our work.

Monitoring Our Personal Health

Exercise, as we well know, tones us as total persons. We should grant ourselves enough time to re-create ourselves through exercise while we develop a schedule that leaves room for us to focus on things that count. Practical helps abound: taking out a membership in a gym, scheduling regular workouts with a personal trainer, indulging in a long-delayed ambition or hobby such as sculpting or learning to play the piano or tennis, gardening, or taking vacations with family that are unconnected with medical meetings. Late in years, people recall these as among the most important experiences of their lives.

Taking care of ourselves is only practicing what we preach. Surprisingly, many of us do not have a personal physician, so this interval between experiencing an adverse event and the possibility of being sued offers us an ideal time to develop a relationship with one. A personal physician who understands our medical history and how we function as persons also tones us up so we have no need for using excessive denial about our problems. A personal physician is also a rock of refuge when major personal and professional stressors strike us.[19] Unfortunately, because they are close associates or because confidentiality issues and peer concerns plague us, many of us hesitate to confide in our physicians.

An already established relationship with a personal physician frees physicians to reveal their current concerns. If physicians have suffered a bad outcome or major trauma, they may be temporarily in shock feeling that they are going through the motions and not in complete contact or control of their lives. Under such pressures, they may not function as, in retrospect, they wish they had.

Dr. Richard Allen, for example, admits "testing" his cardiologist, as a scientist might, by not volunteering the fact that he had been served with a malpractice complaint the afternoon before he saw him. Had the cardiologist inquired about recent stressors, Dr. Allen would have confided in him immediately. How could this meeting have developed into a more constructive exchange for both Dr. Allen and his cardiologist? The following medical interview and comments might show us the way:

> DR. ALLEN: (after describing the episode that began early that morning): I've never had anything like this happen before in my life. I feel completely different.
>
> CARDIOLOGIST: When did this feeling begin?
>
> DR. ALLEN: I never had even an inkling of this kind of feeling before 4 o'clock this morning.
>
> CARDIOLOGIST: Well, we'll take an EKG and find out what's going on. I would agree with you that it sounds very much like an arrhythmia.

The cardiologist would have been more helpful if he asked, "If you've never had this before, is there anything going on in your life right now that could have played some role in precipitating this?" Dr. Allen, after all, is an internist familiar with the role of stress in the development of physical symptoms. Such an inquiry would have given Dr. Allen an opportunity to talk about what had really happened to him. Even though the cardiologist gives no opening, Dr. Allen is aware that their relationship is a protected, confidential exchange. He also knows that he would not be in the emergency department if he had not been served with the malpractice complaint. He hesitates to confide in the cardiologist, whom he sees on a regular basis around the hospital. It is helpful, however, for him to tell the cardiologist in simple terms why he does not want to reveal what has happened.

> DR. ALLEN: "I'm rather hesitant to tell you about this. I don't know how you'd feel about me if I told you what happened to me yesterday. And I don't know if you've ever had a similar experience. I, however, was served with a complaint for the first time in my life yesterday afternoon and I simply cannot believe it. It's a case that I really had very little to do with and I know I'm just enraged about it. My theory is that this had a great deal to do with how I feel this morning. I've never been so angry."
>
> CARDIOLOGIST: (Let us trust that the cardiologist is empathic as he responds.) "I can understand how you feel since I had a malpractice suit about ten years ago, etc."

or

"Well, I've not had that happen yet in my life but I have treated some of our friends who have had a malpractice case and it was very difficult for them."

The cardiologist's goal is to express concern and understanding while giving Dr. Allen the opportunity to talk more. A nonempathic response would be, "Well, that's really too bad. I'm sorry that's happened to you. Now let's get this blood work and EKG done." This could well lead Dr. Allen to feel even more isolated and injured.

Most physicians would respond with empathy if they knew of Dr. Allen's real concerns, and that must happen if Dr. Allen and his cardiologist are to have a much healthier approach to their respective situations.

After an adverse event, a personal physician can be very helpful by offering support, monitoring symptoms, and prescribing indicated medications and treatments. If Dr. Allen had felt free to reveal his situation to a cardiologist who was empathic and supportive, their relationship would have been a safe haven during the unfolding litigation process. When physicians consult with their personal physician, they are less likely to engage in risky behaviors, such as self-diagnosis and self-medicating, which can be the reactions of physicians under unmanageable stress.[20]

Reevaluating Our Personal Life

A demanding practice, complicated by concerns regarding potential litigation, may blind us to the possibility of reevaluating our lives and work in healthy ways. During this period, we can take the time to evaluate all aspects of our lives and to do something about what we find missing or in need of repair. Do we, for example, live within our means? Are we sufficiently attentive to financial and retirement planning? Do we seek sensible consultation on these matters? Are we sensitive to our family's needs for vacation and leisure time, or do we tend to fit them in on working vacations? Do we give ourselves time to read, think, or practice a variety of stress management techniques such as meditation and exercise? At times of increased stress, our greatest resources are the good habits that we have practiced over the long term and the stability and strength in our personal lives. The interim between a bad outcome and potential litigation offers an ideal opportunity to marshal and draw on these habits and strengths.

Recognizing the Impact of Stress

Stress is not, in itself, an illness. "Complete freedom from stress," Hans Selye tells us, "is death."[21] Stress is the hum of life that, completely tuned out, leaves us bored and careless. Set to fever pitch, it overwhelms and immobilizes us, tipping us off balance physically or emotionally. To thrive humanly, we need sufficient, but not excessive, stress if we are to learn, grow, and live healthy lives. Daily life provides us with sufficient stress to grow professionally by honing our skills and enlarging our scope of knowledge.

We deal with stress in ways that are as different as we are. We take a reading of the impact of stress on us in the *context* of an event that tells us what it is about and in its *appraisal* that tells us what it means to us personally.[22] Does stress invade our family life, our work, or both? Is it desirable, such as becoming a parent, despite the further stress that it generates, or is it totally undesirable? We can accept some stressful events as desirable when we anticipate them despite the additional stress they bring to us.

Are we able to control the event, or does the event control us and make us feel powerless to respond to it? Is this a garden-variety event that falls within the normal and is predictable, or is it completely out of the ordinary and unpredictable? Skiers may not anticipate a broken leg but they cannot classify it as wholly unexpected. A sudden explosion with fire that scorches our home is both out of the ordinary and unexpected. Events that assault us internally cause us stress because they are unanticipated and undesirable and leave us feeling powerless to control them. Events that affect us tangentially cause less stress because we maintain some control through anticipation of them.

Psychological stress is present if the relationship between the demands we place on ourselves internally or those placed on us by our environment externally so tax or exceed our ability to keep them in balance that, unbound, they threaten our feelings of well-being.[23] We make highly personal judgments about each situation that confronts us. We alone can answer the question: "Does the impact of this situation test the limits of my capacity to maintain emotional balance and to respond effectively?" Only we can answer the bottom-line question, "Is this too stressful for me?"

Getting to Know Ourselves

We serve ourselves well by monitoring and identifying not only how much stress we are feeling at any given time but also its origin. In knowing the origin of our problem, we are well on our way to mastering the event. Developing our capacity to cope prepares us to respond effectively when the challenge does come. Ordinary stressors then are less likely to interfere with our ability to work or live a balanced life.

If we are to control and reduce stress, we must observe the impact of external events on our emotional equilibrium. We can be victims of the medical training that told us to deny or suppress our feelings—that is, to literally put them aside so that we can get on with the work at hand. While we must control our personal feelings to fulfill our ethical pledge to put the patient's interests above our own in medical work, we cannot completely dismiss our needs or our emotional lives. Indeed, we must take time after stressful events to review how we feel about the event and whether and how we coped with it. Neglecting to check out our feelings can harden us and drive us into that insensitivity and emotional isolation that undermine our care of patients and our personal relationships.

Learning to Observe Ourselves

Growing up in an attentive and emotionally healthy family attunes us to our own emotional lives. Many of us find it "second nature" to monitor what is going on inside ourselves. Certain aspects of our training and our experiences can, however, dull the fine edge of this gift. We should periodically review the following seemingly elementary and self-evident concepts.

DO WE PAY ATTENTION TO OUR FEELINGS AND HOW THEY VARY OR CHANGE? When we observe some transformation in feeling, do we stop to identify the feeling, and ask, "Why do I suddenly feel this way?" We find strategies in almost all stress reduction exercises to help us, through breathing or counting, to pause, observe, and name the reaction, thereby gaining control over it. Following such simple pathways leads us to deeper self-knowledge. For example, sudden, even faint feelings of anxiety or anger are signals that although things seem normal, something has changed. How intense are these feelings? Are they feelings of mild apprehension or irritation, or are they sharper feelings of intense fear or rage? Do these flow from some change in our work or home life? When did we last feel good? Looking back, we may find that we were sailing along in good emotional balance until we picked up that telephone message that our partner would not be able to exchange weekend coverage. We had counted on going away for a short weekend. We are somewhat irritated and disappointed but we also realize that all physicians have their schedules and obligations. Instead of letting our disappointment steep within us, we should identify its source. Perhaps we should call and thank our partner for considering it and then contact another associate for a possible weekend swap. Doing something positive is good self-therapy for the low-grade fever of negative feelings.

CAN WE NAME THE FEELING? Identifying the nature of the feeling allows us to trace it quickly to the true source of our stress. For example, I suddenly become aware of feeling hurt. If I scan recent happenings, which one might have generated these feelings? Well, I heard earlier today that Dr. Jones has gotten the job I wanted as head of the oncology service. I still feel that I should have been chosen. I am hurt and resentful about being passed over. Even though I cannot change the appointment, this correct "naming" of the feeling is an indispensable first step toward gaining control over my reaction.

HOW CAN WE COPE? How can I adjust to the fact that I have not been chosen? What can I do to feel better about this? Harboring hurt feelings and resenting

Dr. Jones' advancement does not help me. Identifying the source of the feelings does help by letting me begin to adapt so that I feel better about the situation and about myself. I can make the effort to congratulate and offer my help to Dr. Jones. This does not give me the job, but it does lessen my irritation and open me again to the future.

When people judge that a situation, such as a serious illness, holds few possibilities for change, they cope primarily by regulating their emotions. On the other hand, if they appraise a situation, such as occurs in their work, as one that they can change, they take an active problem-solving approach toward it.[24] In most situations, people reduce their anxiety by modulating their emotions and taking action. As physicians, we generally do not remain passive but prefer to *do* something about a problem confronting us. Directly addressing issues acknowledges and diminishes uncomfortable feelings.

Do we pay attention when others, in either our work or our personal life, comment on our behavior, attitudes, or manner of communication? When such things occur, we may excuse ourselves with, "They don't understand how busy I am or how stressful my work is." We should remember that only people who care about us call our attention to something they notice about us. We should stop and reflect, as objectively as we can, on what their observation means. Our behavior is rooted in and expressed through our emotions. Observations from others may sting but they are filled with accurate information about who we are, what we do, and how we feel. Dr. Laura West notes that one of her good friends commented on how anxious she seemed, opening her to a range of behaviors that she could then address.

Do we observe ourselves, as we incorporate subtle changes into our skills or patterns of practice? Accurate self-observation becomes critically important when we are compromised physically or emotionally, or when we enter the rising slope of late middle age and the end of our careers looms ahead. Our primary professional and ethical imperative is always to place the interests of the patient above our own. When we are young, we can see the line between these two clearly and our vigor undergirds our good control of our decisions about these correlated interests. We know, or at least sense, when we make a wrong choice and fail to honor our obligations. Growing older, we may find not only our perception about our own skills dulled but also our sensitivity to fine distinctions in our ordering of ethical obligations flattened. Fatigue, boredom, or disinterest may fray our resolve to stay current, but an unexamined and false conviction that we still command the knowledge and skills to take good care of our patients snaps it completely. We may experience physical problems requiring medications that affect our concentration or our stamina. We may have illnesses or require surgery or treatments that take us away from our practice for significant periods. These scenarios should alert us to the possibility that the balance of our concern is already shifting away from patients and toward ourselves. How we respond to these leading professional indicators almost always has critical repercussions for both our patients and ourselves.

Our failure to observe these changes is called *denial*, a psychological defense mechanism that serves as a shield to protect us from reality, blinding us to what is really happening to us. We embrace denial because it lets us continue to view ourselves as competent and caring professionals. We do not look at the truth that we are slipping and no longer the persons we once were. If, however, we have acquired the lifetime habit of observing ourselves, such unconscious defenses are less likely to constrict our vision of ourselves and we can integrate these changes into our lives.

> Dr. Philip Jackson is a well-respected university-based professor who is highly re-garded for developing innovative surgical procedures as well as for his teaching skills. He noted the onset of parathesias in his hands and observed that he could no longer "sense" the surgical field as well as he had previously. Instead of brushing off the symptoms, he sought consultation that confirmed his worst suspicions of a neuro-logical impairment. He immediately stopped operating and made a significant shift in his professional career that enabled him to continue teaching and participate ac-tively in leadership and administrative activities within his university.

In contrast,

> Dr. Anne Childs, a well known professor and clinical researcher, had a large university-based internal medicine practice. In her later years, she sustained a number of ortho-pedic procedures requiring lengthy absences from her practice. Other physicians in the clinic always covered for her and, as the absences forced her to consider retire-ment, she kept insisting that nothing had really changed; in her telephone contact with some beloved patients, she intimated that she would return in due time to care for them. She neglected to notify her many devoted patients, however, when she accepted formal retirement, apparently presuming that the university clinic would somehow assume responsibility for them. This vague and shapeless withdrawal made it almost impossible to tell how many of her patients lost active medical attention.

Physicians are not the only professionals called on to observe themselves and to make the necessary adjustments to changes in their skills and acuity of judgment.

> A malpractice defense attorney who represented a number of physicians encouraged two of his clients to settle even though their cases were clearly defensible in court. Both physician defendants independently reported their concerns about his advice, as well as their observation of the lawyer's obvious parkinsonian symptoms, to the insurance company. The insurer discussed the physicians' complaints with the law-yer, who admitted that because his illness made him uncomfortable in the courtroom, he was avoiding that arena by urging settlements of these cases.

Failure to monitor the quality of our performance makes us vulnerable to making judgments or engaging in behavior that can result in malpractice claims. To observe and correctly read changes in our skills and judgment is difficult and demanding, but it is ethically essential and pragmatically sensible to do so. Only then can we put patients first and save ourselves from a loss of control and from committing clinical errors that may lead to legal action.

Do we cope effectively? We may respond to stress, in some instances, by suppressing our emotions, withdrawing emotionally from loved ones, isolating ourselves from the nonmedical world, or using such defenses as denial.[25] We are often unaware of how these responses impede our healthy functioning. Sometimes we catch sight of our behavior only as we do of ourselves in a store window, a sudden revelation of what we are like, often at a critical moment. We may unconsciously withdraw, for example, from loved ones, who react in turn by isolating or withdrawing from us. Such a reciprocal dynamic can lead to estrangement or even divorce. Our initial response to a threatening situation may be a clear signal of our ineffective coping style. Sometimes we learn that we are not coping effectively only from observing ourselves directly or through the comments of others. Observing and gaining insight into how we behave under pressure allow us to develop more adaptive coping responses.

Although self-observation may be familiar or even second nature for many of us, others may not be acquainted with it and instead may deny anxiety and anger through distraction, such as excessive work. These latter responses do not work well for our patients or ourselves. Behaviors that we do not observe or discover propel us into a vicious cycle of denial, ineffective coping, and complicated and unhappy lives.

Assessing Other Personal Vulnerabilities

Broadened self-knowledge also identifies our unique and not easily controlled vulnerabilities. Understanding how we can control these parts of ourselves alerts us to their early warning signals so that we can handle them in a healthy manner. This is particularly important when potential litigation introduces its searing stress into our lives.

- *Vulnerability to mood or other psychiatric disorders.* Although the genetic transmission of psychiatric disorders is not well established, strong evidence from family studies suggests that such disorders as bipolar illness may have some genetic basis. It is well established that episodes of bipolar illness and major depressive disorder can follow events that precipitate real or potential losses. It is only prudent to seek psychiatric consultation for early monitoring or intervention if we have previously experienced either a serious depressive episode or any other psychiatric illness or have a family history of such disorders *and* have experienced an adverse event with litigation potential.

- *Early childhood loss*. The many real and imagined threats of litigation include loss of financial stability, self-esteem, and reputation. We may lose our case in court. We always lose valuable practice time when preparing and participating in a lawsuit. Litigation may interrupt our relationships with once close professional or personal friends. The mounting threat of these losses can reawaken and exacerbate conflicts set off early in our lives by the losses sustained through death, divorce, and other unaddressed or unresolved events. Our feelings of increased anxiety about the specter of loss associated with litigation may be a signal to ourselves that we should seek psychological or psychiatric consultation.
- *Personality traits*. Recognizing our prominent personality traits is a large part of getting to know ourselves. Healthy personalities respond to change or stress with a range of flexible and healthy reactions. If we have a restricted repertoire of responses, such as chronically blaming others for our problems or denying they exist although everybody else can see them, we will also turn to these limited and ineffective reactions when we are threatened by the investigation of or litigation from an adverse event. These are not helpful responses, especially when we are called on to disclose error to patients and their families or when we become defendants and must enter fully into an intrinsically adversarial process. When we are aware of how we function psychologically, we can anticipate our responses, guard against our least healthy tendencies, and better prepare ourselves to be effective defendants if litigation is filed.
- *Recent stressful life events*. If we are already stressed by events such as the chronic or acute illness of a spouse, children who are acting out, partners with whom we are in conflict, or problems in our work environment, we can and must anticipate that this waiting period will compound the oppressive stress in our lives. We need to review and identify these separate and unique entities, clarify the feelings associated with each, and respond to them sensibly and separately.
- *Drinking too much*. Too many physicians do not observe how they begin to dampen their anxieties with alcohol or to medicate themselves in other ways during this period. Practiced self-observation enables us to monitor such behaviors when we are stressed and to replace them with more effective ways of coping with these losses. These alternatives include seeking necessary consultations when they are indicated.
- *Social support*. Being well socialized goes along with our being more observant of ourselves, better able to communicate with others, and more open to seeking support from others. Any difficulties in making relationships with others should alert us to our compromised ability to handle the special stresses of the period that may lead to litigation. Our ability to work closely with the

defense team, handle our emotions when confronted by the plaintiff's bar, and, finally, relate well with members of any potential jury are all significant challenges of the litigation experience. Good in themselves, our efforts to develop comfortable relationships with others are a great help in anticipating and dealing with these realities.

Recommendations for Putting Together the Pieces

INQUIRE ABOUT THE STATUTE OF LIMITATIONS RELATED TO THE INCIDENT. The risk manager or claims representative can readily supply this information.

REVIEW OUR INSURANCE COVERAGE. This knowledge helps us in two ways— by allaying anxiety and by identifying issues that need to be addressed immediately. Claims personnel can assist us greatly during this period of waiting.

REEXAMINE OUR FINANCIAL HEALTH. If physicians have planned well, they find, after an adverse event, that they need only review the protections they have raised against any threat to their financial security and their personal assets.

RECOGNIZE THAT BEING INVOLVED IN AN ADVERSE EVENT COMPLICATES THE STRESS WE ORDINARILY FEEL IN OUR WORK. Our ability to observe ourselves is critical in recognizing and managing our reactions more comfortably.

IDENTIFY CONTROLLABLE STRESSORS. The goal is to balance sufficient control with healthy flexibility and our ability to respond to the unexpected events inherent in medical practice. As in the self-help paradigm, the beginning of wisdom lies in knowing what can and cannot be controlled.

WORK TO LIVE A BALANCED LIFE. This interim period offers us a unique opportunity to take a good look at ourselves and to initiate constructive changes in our behavior and goals.

REFOCUS ON OR DEVELOP THE HABIT OF SELF-OBSERVATION. Even a moderately well developed ability to observe ourselves in action and to monitor changes in our feelings facilitates our regaining control and achieving emotional balance.

HONESTY IS THE BEST POLICY. Physicians experience many challenges to their sense of self during this period. The simple proverbial honesty in approaching the investigations and identifying their own reactions proves its value in the sharpened effectiveness of their responses.

PAY ATTENTION TO ANY SIGNIFICANT CHANGES IN OUR PHYSICAL OR EMOTIONAL HEALTH. If we do not have a personal physician, this interval is an ideal time in which to choose one and to cooperate fully with this physician's recommendations. Attending promptly to any changes we observe in ourselves diminishes our risk for medicating ourselves or engaging in other destructive behaviors. The more resolutely we take control of our own health, the more gracefully and artfully we reclaim our physical well-being and mastery over our work environment.

ATTEND TO THOSE PERSONAL VULNERABILITIES THAT MAY BE EXACERBATED BY INCREASED STRESS. Once we recognize and admit these vulnerabilities, we can take the steps necessary to lessen their impact on us.

IF REQUESTS FOR INFORMATION ARE RECEIVED ABOUT THE ADVERSE EVENT, BE ATTENTIVE AND WARY AND, IF IN DOUBT, SEEK CONSULTATION. Because the period between an adverse event and the termination of the statute of limitations can be lengthy, if we are up for recredentialing or for the renewal of our license or insurance, we will receive inquiries about our current professional status. We should read and answer the questions carefully. Although honesty has no peer, it never demands that we say anything beyond the minimum required. If we have no knowledge of a pending claim (a demand for money or services), we should not provide unnecessary information. If, on the other hand, we have had a serious or catastrophic event that may lead to legal action, we should bring this to the attention of the appropriate forum. Managed care entities (such as health insurers and independent practice associations) may also inquire about adverse events. Unless our agreement requires it, we are under no obligation to reveal to them incidents that have not matured into legal cases.

6

The Complaint: A Prelude to Litigation

> Suddenly you're under the kind of scrutiny you've never had. The kind you've given other people but that you've never really had yourself . . . And publicly . . . the words liar, cheat, fraud etc. begin to be bandied about. It was at that time that I realized for the first time how a doctor must feel. A doctor who has spent his time . . . up until the time of that particular suit . . . and now what they are saying is, that you're a killer. It's got to be devastating. A reporter (such as myself), what do we have? We have our credibility, we have our integrity and, all of a sudden you're being called thief, cheat, liar, fraud. It goes to your gut. If you're a doctor, it's the center of your soul; it's the center of your life. If you're a doctor, you're a healer and somebody is accusing you, not of healing but of hurting.
>
> —Mike Wallace[1]

So Mike Wallace describes being sued, along with CBS News and other CBS personnel, by General William Westmoreland, former commander-in-chief of the American forces in Vietnam. The charge was that in a 1982 CBS documentary, Wallace and other personnel had accused the general of "conspiracy at the highest levels" to suppress military intelligence during the Vietnam War.[2] Westmoreland felt that this direct attack on his integrity merited an apology, which the network refused to make. While denying the charge, Wallace experienced it as an assault on *his* integrity, identifying with what countless physicians feel when they are served with a complaint alleging malpractice.

Before the Complaint

Physicians may or may not be aware that their patients and their families remain dissatisfied with the outcome of the treatment or felt that they had not been given the whole story. If physicians fully inform patients at the time of the incident and have documented in detail their final session with them, they have fulfilled their obligation.

Rumblings After the Adverse Event

Sometimes dissatisfied patients and their families simply break off contact with the physician. Some of these patients may have refused to follow up on recommended treatments or medication. When this happens, physicians should carefully document the patient's response in an informed refusal note detailing their conversation about the possible repercussions of refusing the prescribed intervention. Other patients may fail to return for a scheduled follow-up visit. Physicians should document this failure to return, making a clear record of any efforts to notify them of the missed appointment in their letter to the patient. Physicians should be clear about the consequences of failing to follow up, including, when appropriate, a statement that failure to comply could put the patient at risk of serious illness or even death.

When patients continue in treatment after an adverse event, a physician can attend carefully to the patient's concerns and note any changes in their feelings that indicate litigation is brewing. It is not unheard of for plaintiffs to continue as patients even after they have filed suit against their physicians. An inexperienced plaintiff attorney may not recognize that to continue a relationship with the physician defendant may be disadvantageous to their client. During trial, defense attorneys will, with the judge's permission, state that no patients who truly believe they have been injured would continue under the care of a physician they have charged with negligence. In such circumstances, juries may favor the defendant. If physicians have any questions about continuing to see a plaintiff/patient, they should discuss such issues with their insurer's risk manager.

Delay or failure to pay bills is a further sign of patient dissatisfaction. As noted earlier, forgiveness of payment for services may, pending consultation with one's insurance company, be appropriate.

Physicians should also be aware that if any of these patients attempt to call directly to discuss payment, some states require consent from only one party to record a telephone conversation. Physicians should therefore always presume that such conversations with the patient or the family members are being recorded.

After some weeks or months, someone in the medical records department may report that the family has requested the record. Nothing makes physicians more anxious than overhearing colleagues connected with the case exchanging rumors about a potential lawsuit, spiced with the news that one of them is going to be deposed about the case. Although not yet involved, physicians should notify their insurers about these bits and pieces of information.

Americans mistakenly think they have to accept or return calls from reporters and lawyers. There is no imperative to volunteer to speak on the telephone or personally with such callers and physicians should resist any feeling that they should. Even if the patient's attorney reassures the physician that he or she is not the focus of the inquiry, he or she should consult counsel or the risk manager before doing so. Such calls may seem innocuous, but an attorney may use any admissions about the patient's care to strengthen a weak case or even to pursue a claim against the physician without expert confirmation. The physician has become their expert by volunteering an opinion about what a conscientious physician should have done and then enumerating for them those he did not do.

The plaintiff attorney may, in some jurisdictions, forward an attorney's lien to the insurance company, a heads-up that a suit will be filed unless the insurer makes a direct settlement to the plaintiff, a percentage of which goes to the attorney. The service of a lien letter at the Illinois-based ISMIE Mutual Insurance Company leads to a settlement in approximately 2 percent of their claims, obviating the alternative of a lengthy litigation process.[3] If a settlement is not reached, the attorney files a case.

Why Patients Sue Physicians

There are as many reasons for suing as there are patients. Plaintiff attorney Dominic Pellegrino explains a major reason for lawsuits:

> Potential plaintiffs often come in complaining, not about the bad outcome, but about the shoddy way they were treated. Nurses too busy to attend to their needs, physicians too curt to explain what happened, and billing departments too callous to wait an appropriate time after an unexpected death before sending a statement.[4]

Studies suggest four reasons why patients sue:

1. They want to know how and when the injury happened.
2. They need compensation for the actual expenses incurred by the injury.
3. They believe that the organizations and staffs should account for their actions.
4. They want to ensure that others will not be forced through the same gauntlet that they have experienced.[5,6]

Other salient motives include wanting someone to pay for the injury, a sense of suffering an injustice that needs restitution, and a longing to restore a sense of balance.

Maureen Anderson lost her mother to brain cancer in 1978 and, 10 years later, her father while he was hospitalized for elective prostate surgery. In both instances, Maureen felt that the physicians had not sufficiently informed her of the details of her parents' illness and death. Her father allegedly died in his sleep the evening after his surgery. When she received the autopsy report some months later, she learned that he had complained of chest pain, sweating, and vomiting the evening before his death and that the cause of death was a heart attack.

> It felt like somebody tried to put something over on you. I really felt compelled to do it. I wasn't out to hurt the doctor but I just thought it was such poor judgment; it

needed to be brought attention to. My father really put his trust in him, he put his life in his hands and he just didn't do his job. It never really had anything to do with money, it really didn't. I just thought it was time to let him know that and maybe even think about my father again at some point and maybe next time, when a patient says he has chest pain or any symptoms of a heart attack, he'd do an EKG. Maybe that's my little way of helping somebody else down the road.[7]

Although she eventually lost the case at trial, Maureen felt she had gotten her message across to the physician and was satisfied that she had somehow honored her father's memory in the process.

Psychologist Cynthia Davis experienced periodic episodes of nausea, headache, pain, and disturbed vision for over 1 year. After each episode, which was diagnosed and treated as acute conjunctivitis, she noted a slight loss of vision. Eventually, she was diagnosed and treated for acute glaucoma.

I felt not whole and I felt something's wrong with me. And how is this going to affect my life? That was my distress. I was in the doctor's office on follow-up and I was reading a pamphlet for glaucoma and it was commenting on the difference between the usual more gradual onset and acute glaucoma. I didn't know there was such a thing. So I read about the acute glaucoma and I was really taken aback because the symptoms I had were classic. And I know enough about diagnosis that when you have classical symptoms, there should be no reason to miss the diagnosis. And that upset me a lot because I really regretted not having my sight.[8]

She felt that some of the physicians had not only been slow in discovering her diagnosis but also had actually misdiagnosed her and that others had not been wholly truthful with her. The resulting legal blindness compromised her ability to continue her employment. She felt that she was due some compensation, which she obtained in a 3-day trial 5 years after she filed suit.

The Role of Colleagues Behind the Scenes

Sometimes a request by another physician for a former patient's medical records is the first notice a physician receives about a claim. Although such requests may not necessarily signal a lawsuit, the implication can send tremors through the doctor. The request suggests that the patient, without their physician's knowledge, has begun to consult with another physician. When physicians believe that they had a good relationship with patients and had provided them with competent care, they might, if they know and respect them, make contact with the new physician. In the best-case scenario, these latter physicians may be supportive of the care given and play a significant role in diffusing any interest that patients may have in initiating a lawsuit. On the other hand, these physicians may assess the previous care as inadequate and communicate that assessment back to patients in ways that reinforce the patient's dissatisfaction and their intention to sue the original physician. In the worst-case scenario or nightmare, these new-to-the-scene physicians encourage patients to seek legal redress and offer to serve as their expert witnesses.

After reading a pamphlet describing her symptoms, Dr. Cynthia Davis confronted her physician.

> So I said to my doctor, "My symptoms were classic. My previous doctor should not have missed this diagnosis, should he?" And he looked at me for a long time. And finally, he said, "No. He should not have missed this." And then he said, "If you want to sue him, I would refer you to an attorney that I've talked to and worked with before." [My doctor] would not have suggested that if I had not brought it up and he would not have told me that these were classical symptoms. I had to figure that out myself, and that annoys me a bit, too. I felt like he was protecting the other doctor. I didn't want to be mean. While I wanted compensation for my injury, I didn't necessarily want to deliver suffering to the doctor I felt had failed me. So I asked my lawyer, "What would this mean for the doctor? I don't want to ruin him financially." He said the worst thing that would happen is that his insurance rate would go up and that the insurance would pay any judgment, so then I was mollified.[9]

The physician consulted after the first treatment is caught in a dilemma: how can he be truthful and supportive to his patient and be respectful of the previous physician's approach to her condition? When asked by patients to judge another colleague's care, physicians should ask themselves this key question: "Do I have all the clinical information necessary to form an opinion about whether the standard of care was met?" Aside from a detailed review of that clinician's complete medical record of this patient as well as those of previous and concurrently treating clinicians, a physician should speak directly with the colleague, if he or she is willing, whose care is at issue. They should use that conversation to evaluate what may not be entered into the record before reaching any conclusion about whether the standard of care has been violated.

The Request for Medical Records
Without indicating why they want them, patients sometimes request their records directly. Resisting or ignoring such requests may make physicians feel better but in reality this response makes things much worse. The current Health Insurance Portability and Accounting Act of 1996 (HIPPA) privacy regulations provide specific guidelines regarding how physicians are to respond to requests for clinical information about patients:[10]

1. No authorization is required if another clinician requests information about a patient. However, nothing in the HIPAA privacy regulations prohibits physicians from requiring a written authorization from them.
2. Physicians have up to sixty days to respond to a patient's request for information, although some state laws that supersede HIPAA regulations in this area establish a shorter period. Except in emergencies, verbal requests for

information are always insufficient. Physicians should ask patients or their authorized representatives to complete written release authorization forms that indicate that the one requesting the information has the legal authority to do so. Despite some exemptions, it is unlikely that physicians can prevent patients from inspecting and copying their records. Although they should not automatically release any information detrimental to the patient, physicians should be familiar with their state law regarding such exemptions as well as the process through which patients may appeal denial of access.

3. A written patient authorization on an HIPAA compliant form must accompany an attorney's request for records.

4. State laws vary regarding the access to the records of deceased patients. Some states, for example, may require the court to appoint a personal representative or allow access to records to the executor of the estate.

Physicians should review the record very carefully, make a copy, and send it promptly to the patient. The procedure is the same when an attorney makes a request for records on behalf of the patient.

Changing the Record

It is possible that, with the knowledge of their insurer, physicians may have made a legitimate correction to the record shortly after the incident occurred and before the claim was made. Sometimes, as in settings in which residents and medical students write chart notes, the record needs to be amended to correct inaccurate entries or supply obvious omissions. In general, drawing a line through an incorrect entry, noting the error, adding the omitted material, dating the correction, and signing or initialing them are sufficient. Dr. Laura West reports:

> They were saying I altered the record. I used the hospital protocol to correct the resident's things. Put a line through it, put my initials and the date. The lawyer managed to keep eating away, trying to say I altered the medical record. But we worked hard. I gave it my best effort. Later this charge was dropped at trial.[11]

Corrections made after the physician is on notice of the claim automatically raise very serious credibility issues. In the sudden glare of a potential lawsuit, physicians may see something in the chart that "doesn't look quite right," or they may recall a relevant entry that they did not make even though it was in their mind when they made their first contemporaneous notes. Before they do anything, howsoever innocent and correct, they should pause and consider what ramifications may flow from a revised entry. *Altering records before sending them is the single most damaging thing physicians can do. Alteration destroys their credibility and virtually ensures that the claim will be settled for an amount significantly greater than the case is worth.* Settling a claim for this reason escalates risk for the physician involved as his or her liability insurer may view the physician as an unacceptable future insurance risk and drop coverage. Any less-than-innocent alteration can also trigger an investigation that may lead to sanctions by the licensing board.

Attorneys use sophisticated technology to discover even the most ingenious alterations. Searching the documents for alterations, including electronic records on hard drives, is routine in cases of catastrophic injury. The physician involved in a cover-up gives the trial lawyer the gift of a powerful argument that can multiply the cost of the case dramatically.

Such insertions, corrections, and other "improvements" to the record are readily identifiable as later additions to the original record. Putting scientific scrutiny aside, it is highly probable that a third party received and retains a copy of the records in their original preedited form, allowing an easy comparison and discovery of any later alteration.

Thou Shalt Not Alter should be physicians' eleventh commandment. No physician documents perfectly and every physician can recall imperfect, not to say embarrassing, chart entries. Defense lawyers prepare physicians well for deposition and trial testimony about such shortcomings by helping them explain the human history of the records, thereby blurring the impression of ineptitude with which the patient's attorney will try to brand him or her before the jury. Truth, like beauty, speaks best when it is least altered.

When complying with a records request, physicians should also have what is called a "color copy" made to capture the ink and paper color of the original chart, filing it separately from the patient's record. This usually must be done by a copy service. Physicians should supply color copies to their claims professional and defense attorney so that everyone can see and work with basically the same version of the chart.

The Elements of a Malpractice Action

To recover damages in a medical malpractice action, patients must first prove that they are owed a duty of care and that, by a preponderance of the evidence, bolstered by expert witnesses, a physician violated the standard of care in their own or a similar community. Indeed, patients must also prove that this violation contributed substantially to the causation of the injury. Defense lawyers respond through expert testimony that no violation of the standard of care occurred or that the injury was not caused by negligence but was a function either of the natural progression of the disease or of the inherent risk of the procedure about which the patient was informed and to which he or she agreed beforehand. Damages will not be awarded unless the plaintiff meets all standards.

- *The duty of care.* Physicians owe their patients a duty by undertaking their treatment. When they take call for other physicians, they owe a duty of care to those patients even though they may only talk with them by telephone.

Do they, however, owe any duty of care to persons to whom they give some informal or "curbstone" consultation that was noted or the treating physician noted in the chart as if it were a formal consult? "No" is, in fact, the answer in some jurisdictions.

- *The standard of care.* Breaching their duty of care means that physicians have violated the prevalent and recognized *standard of care* or *community standard.* Allowing for differing wording in different jurisdictions, the standard of care is usually understood as *that degree of care, skill, or diligence used by an ordinarily careful physician in the same or similar circumstances in the same or similar community.*

    Many lawyers currently claim that a national standard of care exists, particularly in specialties where national organizations have specified the character of patient care. The American College of Obstetricians and Gynecologists (ACOG) and the American Society of Anesthesiologists (ASA) have, for example, published widely recognized and commonly used guidelines for acceptable care. Plaintiff attorneys and defense counsel frequently refer to these to establish the standard of care as nationally applicable in malpractice cases involving obstetrician-gynecologists and anesthesiologists. This is not to say that a local community standard no longer exists. Defense lawyers are often able to argue successfully to rural juries, whose members receive the same health care as the plaintiff, that the standard of care differs from that in the big city down the road as well as from similar communities in other states.

Do family physicians delivering babies, dermatologists performing liposuction, or interventional radiologists performing invasive cardiovascular procedures have their own standards of care, or are they held to the same standards of care as obstetricians, plastic surgeons, and interventional cardiologists, respectively? Testifying against such defendants, specialists from these latter areas may well assert that if these physicians perform procedures most often associated with the expert's specialty, they should be held to the higher standard of that specialty. Such possible testimony has grave implications for the defendant, as it may be easier to argue that they breached the expert's standard of care, an argument whose impact on a sympathetic jury may lead them to return a substantial award.

Expert testimony must generally be used to prove that a physician has violated the standard of care. Drawn by trial lawyers from a national experts' network, such witnesses often come from different cities or states than the defendant. Most judges allow testimony by out-of-state experts if such experts can demonstrate, to the court's satisfaction, their familiarity with local community standards. Often drawn from the faculties of medical schools, expert professors may be ready to travel to offer testimony that is persuasive to lay juries and is supported by their familiarity with local standards.

Indeed, some medical professionals earn their livelihoods through their frequent courtroom testimony. Their opinions are sometimes used as the foundation for frivolous lawsuits. Until the process of discovery reveals their identity and makes them subject to deposition or interrogatories that cast enough doubt on their opinions to lead to a dismissal, such experts invest plaintiff lawyers with a credibility that allows them to continue with even highly questionable cases without becoming vulnerable to court sanctions.

Physicians can inadvertently admit to a violation of the community standard or cause an injury so obviously due to their negligence that no expert is required. *Res ipsa loquitur*—"the thing speaks for itself "—is the legal term for such situations. Retained surgical sponges or instruments, for example, speak clearly for themselves of negligence in the operating room.

- *Causation.* This is the name given to link the physician's treatment to the injury. Unless an attorney can establish that the physician's alleged negligence was a substantial contributing cause of the injuries to his client, the client is not entitled to recover damages. The causation link must generally be proved by expert testimony. It may also be established by a physician who, in a deposition or at trial, mistakenly responds, "Yes," to the question: "Isn't it correct, doctor, that this injury occurs only when the clinician has been negligent?" By so answering, the physician is serving as an expert against himself.
- *Damages.* Damages fall into three broad categories: *economic, noneconomic,* and *punitive.* Economic damages include lost wages, the cost of present and future medical care, along with impaired earning capacity, and other related expenses of the patient. Noneconomic damages compensate the patient for the pain and suffering that they have experienced. Caps on pain and suffering have been used in such states as Indiana and California to rein in runaway damage awards. Punitive damages are awarded as a deterrent to future similar egregious conduct and to send a message to other clinicians that such behavior will not only not be tolerated but also severely punished. Because trial lawyers so often inflame juries to award these punitive damages in the multimillion dollar range, in recent decades, legislatures have limited the circumstances in which plaintiffs can recover punitive damages in medical malpractice cases.

The Summons: The Lawsuit, a Reality

The summons is a legal document ordering the recipient to appear in court at or within a certain time to answer charges filed in the complaint.

Usually the summons and complaint are delivered by a sheriff, by a private process server, or via registered mail. Because in most cases we do not know with certainty that a lawsuit against us is imminent, we are often shocked and appalled by the impersonal manner in which we are served a document accusing us of negligence. We are further embarrassed by the impact of the threatening impact of the process server's arrival at the office on our colleagues and staff and on our families, if the server delivers the document to our home. Few experiences humiliate or disturb us more, especially if we have small children, than the sight of a uniformed officer handing us a stack of obviously unsettling documents.

Despite the shock of such deliveries, we cannot allow ourselves to become so paralyzed that we deny what has happened or fail to respond, through our lawyer, to the summons by the statutory deadline, usually within thirty days. If the charges are brought in federal court, the time limit is twenty days. By failing to respond in a timely and appropriate manner, we may forfeit our right to a defense. Every year, default judgments are entered against the small number of physicians who fail to respond to a summons in a timely manner. Unless set aside by court process, such defaults mean that the trial lawyer's only task is to prove the damages. Worse still, our failure to cooperate in our defense may lead to denial of insurance coverage for the lawsuit.

The Complaint

The complaint is a list of accusations rendered in the legalese of court papers whose character is unfamiliar to physicians.

The heading at the top of the first page indicates the court in which the papers are filed, such as "In the Circuit Court of the State of Oregon for the County of Multnomah" or, in a federal case, "In the United States District Court for the Southern District of New York."

Beneath the headings is the caption. On the right side, it lists the parties to the lawsuit, beginning with the plaintiff, usually the patient or, in the case of a death, the personal representative of the patient's estate. Listed below are the defendants. Here we find our name, alone or among many, including our colleagues, our hospital, and others. To the right in the caption are words such as: "Action for Damages, Medical Malpractice."

Below the caption are the numbered paragraphs of the complaint. To prosecute a successful lawsuit, the plaintiff is required to plead and to prove the court's jurisdiction, the required elements of the claim, and the patient's entitlement to relief.

In the complaint, plaintiff lawyers cast a wide net of charges, fine meshed to catch even the smallest of possibilities, and then empty it onto the court's dockets. While they can amend a complaint later, most prefer to dump the whole catch, whatever their size or condition, to demonstrate that they do not let anything, big or small, get away. They do this as much to intimidate us as to impress the court.

Our defense lawyers routinely tell us not to take these allegations seriously or literally. But their familiarity with the faux battle pose of lawyers does not reassure us and we often feel more isolated by their seeming lack of understanding for us. To lawyers, allegations are simply a means (the pleadings) to an end (recovery). To us, however, the accusation is personal and enraging in its charge that we "recklessly and with wanton disregard of the circumstances" injured our patient or that we "carelessly, negligently, and unlawfully breached our duty of care."

Because news is predominantly negative, the local newspapers in some jurisdictions publish the complaint, word-for-word on the front page. Our children may come home from school in tears because some other children refer to their father or mother as a murderer. Because defense lawyers are not personally involved in the same way as we are and, by training, are not necessarily sensitized to the emotional turmoil caused by such allegations of fault, they may neither understand nor be able to relate to our outrage at the targeting of our professional performance.

Is the extent of damages always included in the documents? In recent tort reform battles, the trial bar has tried to blunt criticism of its tactics by agreeing to changes in the rules regarding the pleading of damages. In many states, plaintiffs are not required and, in some instances, are not allowed to specify the exact amount of the damages they are seeking to recover. In such states as Illinois, the complaint specifies a minimum demand, asking for "a judgment against the defendant in a sum in excess of $50,000." The media are less interested in running stories about lawsuits filed against a physician that have no speculated dollar value. The public is, therefore, not educated about the volume or cumulative demands of lawsuits filed. In late 2003 in Oregon, plaintiff lawyer demands in the 460 pending physician malpractice claims totaled more than $1.5 billion.[12] To dispose of these claims at the stated award level, each Oregon physician would be forced to pay $300,000.

A common first impulse, after reading the complaint, is to call the patient's attorney in an effort to straighten out "this whole misunderstanding." This is yet another temptation to be resisted wholeheartedly. We should never contact patients' attorneys in an attempt to convince them to dismiss the lawsuit. We may rightly reason that the attorneys have heard only the patient's version of what happened and, that because they lack medical training, they cannot possibly understand the complexities involved in caring for this patient. If they hear our side of the story, we feel, they will surely reconsider. This fantasy, for it is no less than that, highlights the primary difference between physicians and the lawyers who sue them: we are looking for answers and exploring solutions while plaintiff lawyers are advocates whose focus is not a broad and subtle exploration of the true causes of an incident but rather a broad and bold attempt to get as much money out of us as possible.

By talking directly to the plaintiff's attorney, we give them an opportunity to put questions to us without our lawyers being present. We can be sure that any admissions we may make against our self-interest will be used against us. This may seem a good-hearted and commonsense move to us, but it is naïve and dangerous when dealing with lawyers.

Notifying the Insurer

Physicians *must* call their liability insurer immediately after they are served with papers. Failing to do so may jeopardize the insurer's ability to make a proper response or, possibly, cause them to deny coverage to physicians because of their failure to act appropriately. One obstetrician opened the complaint, filed it in the patient's chart, and did not come across it again for almost a year. Another physician, repeatedly observing her attorney's return address on incoming mail, placed it all unopened, in a separate file. Because the physician did not open and respond to this correspondence and the attorney could not make direct contact with the physician, the latter scheduled an appointment with the physician in the guise of a patient. Once inside the office, she identified herself and the physician responded by retrieving the file of unopened mail. Physicians may fantasize that if they deny its filing and do not talk about it, the lawsuit will go away. Such magical thinking complicates their lives in ways as hard to enumerate as they are to imagine.

The company will quickly assign physicians a claims professional, unless they already did that when they reported the case as an incident. Most companies employ experienced professionals who understand the adverse impact of claims on physicians. They are usually courteous, well informed, and eager to be of assistance. Physicians should not hesitate to raise any questions and concerns they have, because they can be assured that these conversations will be held in confidence and are not subject to discovery.

Claims professionals ask physicians to forward as quickly as possible the summons, the complaint, and a copy of the chart. They will also set up an internal file and will assign a defense counsel.

In some cases, as discussed in Chapter 7, the physician's carrier also insures co-defendants who are not part of the physician's practice. Because each person is entitled to an independent defense, it is likely that different claims personnel will handle each separate defense. If this does not occur, physicians should raise their concerns and request different personnel. Because they will want to be able to challenge any assignment of the award to their account, should there be settlement, realistically physicians need their own claims professional to represent their interests.

Preparing a Narrative

Unless, as suggested in Chapter 1, the physician has anticipated their request, claims professionals will ask physicians to write a narrative describing the care of the patient and the events that lead to the claim or suit. This is the physician's opportunity to "tell what happened." As previously noted, this narrative is likely to be submitted to the attorney with the law firm retained by the insurance company to represent the physician and, as such, is considered a confidential communication between physician and attorney. Nothing a physician writes to his attorney or claims professional should be placed in the patient's chart, because this would cause a privileged communication to lose its protection and so become available to the patient's lawyer.

If the insurers structure a narrative process, physicians will answer detailed questions or tell their story in a preset format. Should the claims professional simply ask the physician to tell them what happened, physicians can follow the journalist's five-question approach to an event of who, what, where, when, and why.

The following format lists the most frequently requested narrative information. In preparing the narrative, physicians should ask themselves what they would want to know if they were asked to review and provide an expert opinion in the case.

- Provide information on one's medical school, residency, additional training, length of time in practice, areas of expertise, and familiarity with the specific procedure or treatment that is the subject of this claim.
- Outline the patient's treatment chronologically, beginning with the date of the initial visit, presenting complaints, history, physical findings, and treatment.
- Provide the interpretation and significance of tests and treatment in lay terms, including the name and a description of what was done. Detail any procedure and surgery in lay terms as completely as possible, including the reasons why it was done. Include information on all supplies and equipment used in the course of treatment, including the brand name, model, and type of equipment. Provide similar information as appropriate for each visit thereafter.
- Identify other involved clinicians describing their role and responsibilities in the patient's care. Identify clearly the primary physician. Describe the role of any relevant team members who were involved in making a particular diagnosis and prescribing treatment. Note any disagreement among team members about the diagnosis and means or methods of treatment. List the names and responsibilities of all other personnel including nurses, medical assistants, technicians, and others involved in the patient's care.
- Include if known, relevant personal information about the patient and the patient's family such as the number of children, the spouse, and other relatives. List the family members with whom you have been in contact, including what was said to them. It is of great importance to include all details of the interactions, which may be helpful to the defense of the claim.
- Identify the strengths and weaknesses of the provided care and treatment. What weaknesses can we criticize? Indicate whether the care provided met the community standard and provide supportive data about why it did or did not do so. Recommend specific areas for defense counsel to research.

Assignment of the Defense Attorney

The claims professional will assign a lawyer to defend us against the claim, if one has not already been assigned. Most liability insurers choose a lawyer from a panel, found in every state, of defense firms experienced in malpractice cases or from the one law firm that handles most of the company's trial work. The importance of our relationship with this attorney cannot be overemphasized and is discussed in Chapter 7.

Becoming a Defendant: What Can I Expect to Feel?

> My first feelings after being charged with medical malpractice were of being utterly alone. Suddenly I felt isolated from my colleagues and patients. Since then I have learned, in the course of my own suit and trial and in the research I have conducted, that this feeling of aloneness is not at all unusual, that almost every physician accused of being negligent has a similar reaction. I also understand that what I experienced during the 5-year span of my own case—that it swallowed up my life completely, demanded constant attention and study, multiplied tension and strain, generated a pattern of broken sleep and anxiety because I felt my integrity as a person and as a physician had been damaged and might be permanently lost—are the common reactions of most physicians accused of negligence.[13]

Our reaction to being sued reflects our own personalities, the specifics of our case, and the sum of other variables that make each charge of negligence a unique experience.

Dr. Richard Allen describes his reaction: "It was terrible. It was terrifying. It was depressing. I had acute anxiety."[14] He attributes his episode of atrial fibrillation immediately afterward to the surge of adrenaline that accompanied his intense anger. In addition, he felt that his partner and some of the other physicians began to point fingers at him, whereas some of the physicians who had been intimately involved in the case were not even named in the complaint. Looking back, he felt that he began to carry a burden for years of unexpressed anger that had no direct outlet.

Dr. Laura West describes her reactions somewhat differently. The hospital risk management office alerted her that the complaint was coming. It was delivered to her personally while she was busy seeing patients. She found the lawsuit distracting and upsetting but because she remained distressed by the trauma associated with the case, "it just prolonged my misery."[15]

Physicians who feel isolated are often in invisible communion with colleagues having the same experience: An infectious disease specialist, named in six lawsuits and yet to give his first deposition, has "no particular reaction. I'm often called into a case when the patient is extremely ill. I don't know how I'm going to feel in the deposition." This contrasts with the recently widowed and about-to-be-retired family practitioner who, charged with negligence in the case of an 18-year-old cerebral palsy patient whom she had delivered and treated all his life, sat on her living room sofa all night long "in shock and just stared."

We may feel surprised and stunned or, having anticipated it uneasily for years, we may feel some relief. If there are a number of claims against us, we will react differently to each. If convinced that the charges are inappropriate and unjust, we may feel misunderstood and angry. If we judge ourselves that there may be some basis to the complaint, we may feel devastated and fearful. We may react in any or all of these ways. Our reputation is impugned; our livelihood at risk, our honor is at stake. CBS commentator Andy Rooney spoke for all of us after he was publicly accused of making discriminatory remarks: "It is not clear yet to me whether I have been destroyed or not, but I know that a denial from anyone does not carry anywhere near the same weight as an accusation."[16]

Immediate Responses to the Lawsuit

The varied ways in which we are officially informed of the case can set the stage for our feelings about the entire experience. Dr. Thomas White describes a man dressed in a tee shirt and shorts, apparently representing the appropriate legal entity, demanding loudly to the office staff in front of patients to see the physician immediately so that he could personally serve him with a malpractice complaint. Dr. Joseph Daley's children were present when his subpoena was served at home. He was shocked at his oldest boy's response: "Mommy, does that mean that Daddy has to go to jail?" Other physicians tell of sitting quietly at their desks in the late afternoon after a long day of seeing patients and opening a certified mail package whose contents transformed them suddenly into defendants. Our lawsuit may begin uniquely, but our initial responses will have much in common.

Recommendations

WE SHOULD CAREFULLY AND FULLY HONOR ANY REQUEST FOR RECORDS. We should guide our response by the recent federal HIPAA legislation and relevant state laws.

WE SHOULD RESIST ANY TEMPTATION, LARGE OR SMALL, TO ALTER THE RECORD. Consult the claims representative or risk manager for answers to any questions about altering the record. They often suggest that we include, in our written narrative, any information that is not in the contemporaneous version of the chart.

AFTER ADJUSTING TO THE INITIAL SHOCK, WE SHOULD MAKE IMMEDIATE CONTACT WITH OUR INSURER. Even though we may feel apprehensive and distracted, we cannot ignore the complaint or fail to notify the insurer right away and for whom we review and to whom we forward a copy of the chart.

AS SOON AS POSSIBLE, WE SHOULD GAUGE OUR IMMEDIATE REACTIONS TO THE NOTIFICATION AND ITS URGENT RAMIFICATIONS. Dr. Richard Allen was served his complaint on a Friday afternoon; he reacted intensely and developed an arrhythmia early Saturday morning. Fortunately, he was able to obtain the necessary medical consultation and treatment over the weekend. Others may not have that luxury. It is wise to notify our partners of the complaint so that, should the need arise, they can cover for us. We may not be at our best providing care if we are scheduled to cover the emergency department on that same evening and are preoccupied, not to say obsessed, with the allegations made against us in the complaint. Understanding how overwhelming this turn of events can be, especially if the accusations concern a serious outcome, we need someone to cover for us. On such occasions, sensitive partners may even offer to switch coverage with us before we even ask them.

UNLESS THE INSURER HAS REQUESTED IT PREVIOUSLY, WRITE A NARRATIVE OF THE CASE AS SOON AS POSSIBLE. Due to the lengthy interval between the events and the resolution of a claim, you may need this narrative to help you recall key recollections such as conversations with colleagues, the patient, or the patient's family. These may not be part of the chart but crucial to the defense by organizing the information into a coherent sequence and giving defense counsel a first-person overview of all the facts and circumstances surrounding the claim.

WE SHOULD UNDERSTAND THAT ALLEGATIONS IN THE COMPLAINT MIGHT HAVE LITTLE RELEVANCE TO THE FACTS OF THE CASE. These knife-like statements are finely honed to disrupt and unnerve us by their outrageous and assaulting character.

AFTER RECEIVING A COMPLAINT, WE SHOULD REJECT ANY IMPULSE TO CONTACT THE PATIENT OR THEIR ATTORNEY DIRECTLY TO GET THINGS STRAIGHT. Once the lawsuit is filed, the process of litigation takes over and our only consultation should be with our claims representative and our attorney about such impulses.

NEVER RESPOND DIRECTLY TO INTERVIEW REQUESTS OR COMMENTS FROM MEDIA INTERESTED IN OUR CASE. Instead, we should contact the insurance company that is experienced in guiding physicians through the media minefield.

REALIZE FROM THE START THAT THE PROCESS INTO WHICH WE HAVE BEEN DRAWN MAY BE QUITE LENGTHY. After we have been stung by a seeming nuisance suit, we may not face trial by jury for 3 or more years, whereas a serious wrongful death claim against us may be dismissed within 1 year for a variety of reasons. It is helpful to prepare ourselves at the onset that we may be forced to see the case through to the very end or be surprised by an early dismissal of the case.

ANTICIPATE THAT ACTIVE INVOLVEMENT WITH THE LAW IS ALWAYS TIME CON-SUMING AND FRUSTRATING. The process takes over all our time immediately. Our emotional distress does not dissipate overnight, and we need time to absorb the reality of the situation and to get ourselves and our lives in order. We may have to cancel surgery or other appointments to review the case's chart, meet with attorneys and claims representatives, or research the case. Some of us find it helpful to immerse ourselves in our work. We cannot, however, be so lost in our work that we do not make time to respond to the demands of the complaint and make the appropriate contacts with lawyers and insurers. Refusing to take command of our case and ourselves may offer relief that is temporary at best.

ASK OUR CLAIMS REPRESENTATIVE OR ATTORNEY HOW MUCH TIME IT USUALLY TAKES TO PROCESS A MALPRACTICE CASE IN THE JURISDICTION IN WHICH THE COM-PLAINT WAS FILED. In the same geographical location, the waiting period for a case in a circuit court case ordinarily differs from that in a federal court. Claims representatives usually disabuse us of the fantasy that our case, even if lacking merit, will disappear over the horizon in the morning. We must accept that we are now involved with a process that moves at its own pace where and when it will.

7

Meeting the Lawyers

Another thing that helped. I had a wonderful attorney. She herself had been a neonatal intensive care nurse who had gone back to law school and so she knew ob-gyn. So it was a good team and that helped, too, because I knew that she was on top of things, she took care of things, she was just exceptional.

—Dr. Laura West[1]

The attorney who defends the physician's case is a critical player in determining the outcome of the litigation. His or her professional competence may well decide its success. An attorney who is an expert in litigation in general and the defense of physicians in particular and, most important, who has tried cases factually similar to the assigned case all the way to verdict is best prepared to defend a physician.

Who Will Defend Us?

We may already have a good working relationship with an attorney or be familiar with the reputation of other local attorneys. Lacking previous legal experience and unacquainted with local attorneys, we may agree readily to the insurance company's choice of legal counsel. Colleagues who have survived legal battles can share invaluable information about lawyers experienced and skilled in defending physicians in such sensitive cases as the neurologically impaired infant or failure to diagnose breast cancer. The lawyers who represent state or county medical associations and our national specialty societies can also identify the experienced defense attorneys and firms in our locale. We can share this information fully with claims professionals who are cooperative in securing helpful attorneys for us. For example, although neurosurgeon John Schmidt was attracted by the lower premiums of another company, he remains with his malpractice insurer principally because they continue to provide him with the person he considers to be the premier defense attorney in his region.

Attorneys, like physicians, are specialists. Experts in litigation specialize in trial work and spend most of their time in trial preparation and trial. Even if assigned attorneys specialize in insurance defense, it is important to know that they, rather than just the firm, are also experienced in defending physicians. Professional liability defense is a highly specialized calling that demands an artful mastery of the subject matter, the law, and the courtroom. Lawyers, for example, with hybrid courtroom experience in automobile and general litigation are out of their depth in defending physicians in complex and highly technical professional negligence cases.

We should immediately clarify whether our assigned professional liability defense attorney has tried cases to verdict for colleagues in our specialty charged with similar accusations of negligence. Simply put, we do not want to be the first physician ever defended by this attorney in a "bagged ureter during a lap choly" case. The key to successful medical malpractice defense work is simple: solid experience in this field.

Hesitant to enter unknown territory, we may delay meeting with our assigned attorney. It is far better, however, for our cause and for ourselves to schedule this meeting early, within the first two weeks, if possible, and so to commit ourselves wholeheartedly to one of the most important professional relationships we will ever make. Ideally, attorneys contact us directly, introduce themselves, and invite us to meet with them at the earliest mutually convenient time.

Meeting Our Lawyers: Beginning a New Relationship

Rarely do our lawyers measure up to Gregory Peck's portrayal of Atticus Finch in *To Kill a Mockingbird*. Instead, as in the real world outside the movies, we must settle for someone a lot like us—focused, hardworking, and intensely busy. We want a defense attorney who speaks directly, is at ease in a stressful setting, and, no small asset, has a sense of humor. These characteristics are useful in working with clients and are absolutely indispensable in working successfully with juries.

We may carry some of our feeling at sea about the charges made against us in the complaint as well as our lack of legal knowledge into our first session with the lawyers. During this initial meeting, we begin to get a grasp on our lives again by obtaining information about our situation and the steps involved in the litigation process. We gain a new perspective: this case is no longer happening only to us. As we would in any medical referral, we begin to monitor the professionalism of our defense lawyer and the way our relationship is developing.

We enter this first encounter with the law unsure of the answers to a number of partially formulated questions. What do the lawyers think of our case? Can we win it or do we face ruination? How long will this case take? What are the steps and procedures involved in the legal process? What is our role in them? Are we expected to assist in the process and, if so, how? Do materials exist that we need to review immediately and forward to the attorney? How much time will we need to invest in the case? How much of our income will be eaten away by this case? Are we adequately covered by our liability insurance policy? Will we participate in the selection of experts? What are the consequences of settling or, worse yet, the consequences of losing the case? The fairness of the legal process may also concern us. How can nonphysicians understand complex medical testimony and, as ordinary citizens, constitute a jury of our peers? What if we draw a judge who is pro-plaintiff? We must be confident that our defense team will help us frame these questions fully and that they will respond to them just as fully. Even as we first shake hands, questions arise unbidden, within us.

Are We Comfortable with These Lawyers?

On a journey, especially a tortuous and lengthy one, compatible companions can make all the difference. Do we like them? Do we feel comfortable and in tune with them? Would we ordinarily associate, professionally and ethically, with these persons? Do they project a concern for us or care about us? Do they project empathy for our situation and a desire to help us? Most of us heed our gut feelings for answers to such critical questions. These tell us whether we can work with a partner, a patient, or a lawyer. We can follow the advice of St. Thomas Aquinas to trust the authority of your own instincts in deciding whether we can, with confidence, place our reputation and life in the hands of these people sitting across the conference table from us.

Even in the initial session, we can sense clearly how easily and truly we relate to our attorney. A lawyer's lack of understanding of, or interest in, the case registers immediately, giving a signal of incompatibility that we cannot ignore. A physician who is a foreign medical graduate or who speaks English as a second language must have a lawyer who will take the time necessary to help him or her understand the process and answer questions. We should immediately identify and address any seeming miscommunications. Our feelings about this relationship provide a reliable barometer of its weather and if, despite our efforts to calm it, it remains roiled and unsettled, we should warn our claims representative of the brewing storm.

Are They Competent?

Competence may not be easily defined, but, like good art and bad pornography, we can tell it when we see or sense it. Competence includes a solid knowledge base in a particular area of expertise along with the ability to apply it in a skillful manner. A lawyer's incompetence may not be immediately evident, but a truly competent lawyer cannot be hidden. He or she will, from the first moment, impress us with an unmistakable level of knowledge, organization, curiosity, enthusiasm, and self-confidence. These are the finest of gifts and their pledge encourages us and calms our anxieties.

Are They Experienced?

We must be defended by attorneys who are experienced in medical malpractice law and, as mentioned often, experienced in trying to verdict cases whose care issues match our own. Our defense lawyers should be experienced in trying cases in our jurisdiction. They should also be well acquainted, if it is a federal case, with relevant procedural and evidentiary rules as well as with the judges who preside and the character of the juries in this court system.

As we feel that patients can appropriately query physicians about their experience with a specific surgical procedure, so we have both a right and an obligation to query lawyers about the relevance of their experience to our case. What percentage of their cases have they tried to verdict, and what percentage have they settled? Have they prevailed more frequently than their plaintiff lawyer colleagues? What has been the largest verdict awarded against them? Lawyers known for skill in reaching settlements may not be ideal advocates should settlement negotiations fail and the case proceeds to trial. Physicians often complain about being assigned inexperienced lawyers who seem to be learning their craft. We would never assign a resident to perform, for the first time, a difficult procedure with limited supervision, and we should never allow an inexperienced attorney to plead our case. The modest cost of such representation at the start may escalate tragically by the end of the case. Our insurer is responsible for providing us with the best possible defense. It is our obligation, however, to inform the insurer of our reservations about the experience or skills of the assigned lawyers. Nobody else can or will make this critical decision for us.

How Can We Check Their Credentials?

The experience of attorneys is measured objectively by their credentials and by their reputation in the legal community. We should request their *curriculum vitae* or search the World Wide Web for their law firm's display of detailed biographical information about their members, including their professional certification, designations, and honors and whether they merit an AV ranking with Martindale-Hubbell, a nationwide peer-rating service for lawyers.[2] Lawyers are ranked in the area in which they practice on an A (the highest)–B–C scale for their standard of legal ability, practice qualifications, and expertise. *V* is the highest rating for general ethical standards regarding adherence to standards of conduct and ethics, reliability, diligence, and other criteria of professional responsibility.

The American College of Trial Lawyers, founded in 1950, is an invitation-only society for the best of the trial bar from the United States and Canada. Fellowship in the college is "extended only after careful investigation, to those experienced lawyers who have demonstrated exceptional skill as advocates and whose professional careers have been marked by the highest standards of ethical conduct, professionalism, and civility."[3] Further information can be obtained from the college website.

The International Association of Defense Counsel (IADC) also provides information about the very best defense lawyers.[4] Formed in 1920, it is the oldest and most prestigious organization of attorneys representing corporations and insurers. It provides networking, education, and professional opportunities to its approximately 2,400 invitation-only peer-reviewed members and their clients. The IADC also takes a leadership role in many areas of legal reform and professional development.

Do Their Reputations and Behavior Suggest Their Capacity for a Positive Working Relationship?

Our medical colleagues can supply information and assurances that roll back the unknown about our assigned lawyers. From their own experience, they convey to us in language we understand how these lawyers perform in depositions and in the courtroom and whether they are open to learning new information or, certain that they know it all, are self-complacent and arrogant. Colleagues can also tell us from first-hand knowledge how well these lawyers prepare themselves and their clients and, in view of these factors, whether they are truly supportive and encouraging or merely superficially reassuring. Most lawyers are happy, after getting their authorization, to provide the names of our fellow professionals whom they have defended.

Our personal attorney can also provide us with such key information about local medical malpractice lawyers regarding whether they are prompt and professional in responding to calls and keep their clients informed about case developments, their style in relating to the assigned trial judge or local juries, and whether they respond readily to state and federal reporting requirements. Are they active or passive? Do they prepare well, and do they make, or do they let, things happen?

Will One Attorney, or a Team, Defend the Case?

Some firms rely on younger, less-experienced lawyers to file various motions and to take depositions during the lengthy process of case preparation. As the curtain rises on the trial, the lead lawyer, our most experienced or sophisticated advocate, takes center stage to conduct the courtroom defense. Other firms may depend on the initially assigned lawyer to manage the entire case. It is therefore important for us to know, from the onset, how the case will be managed. From their perspective, lawyers may see nothing amiss if a less experienced attorney accompanies us to our actual deposition as long as the senior trial attorney fully prepares us for the deposition. If we are confident that senior counsel has overseen and had sufficient input in the preparatory process, we may agree to having a less-experienced attorney take the depositions of plaintiffs and their family members. However, as professionals, we may feel downgraded to low priority by such handoffs and delegations. We should not hesitate to raise such concerns with our attorneys, and should our feelings of unease persist despite their reassurances, we should notify our claims representative of our reactions and expectations.

It is surprising and disruptive to arrive for our deposition to find that we are in the company of an advocate unknown to us. Should this happen, we should not continue with the deposition but should ask immediately to speak in a confidential setting with the senior attorney and our claims representative. Too much is at stake to accept a seemingly casual management of an event so critical to our defense.

We need to be familiar with the roles played by other members of the defense team, including paralegals, and seek opportunities to meet the persons into whose hands we are placing our professional lives.

Whom Do Lawyers Represent?

This question will occur to us if there is a close relationship between the insurance carrier and law firm. The carrier may pay our lawyer's fees but ethically and, more important, legally, *we* are that lawyer's only client. They may share in-formation with the insurer that serves the case and does not compromise our coverage. We should receive copies of the lawyer's correspondence with our insurer, including their ongoing evaluations of the case and their opinions of its defensibility and of our potential performance as a witness; we should keep these documents in a clearly designated litigation file that is separate from the patient's chart. However, conversation with our lawyers in which we develop information that could threaten our insurance coverage must remain strictly confidential and our lawyers may not reveal it to the insurer.

Unfortunately, we may at times feel that the lawyers' primary loyalty is not to us but to the insurer. For example, a patient who previously had successful spinal surgery reinjured his back while shoveling snow, a proscribed activity, and had unsuccessful surgery by another surgeon. Alleging that the first procedure was defective, this patient sued the first surgeon, Dr. Joseph Daley.

At the time of this incident, Dr. Daley was balancing multiple financial obligations, including college and professional school tuitions and markedly increased insurance premiums, leading him to have coverage of the "bare minimum of $100,000/300,000." Insurance company lawyers told him that although it would be an easy case to defend, "there's hardly enough money for us to defend you." They "gave me a hard time about how irresponsible it was of me to carry that amount of insurance." Dr. Daley felt that "they were representing the insurance company and their own interests. Instead of putting a lot of time and effort and keeping the meter running, with only $100,000 instead of $1 million, they'll put

ten times less work into it." Feeling intimidated and sensing a lack of support from
his assigned attorneys, Dr. Daley took the initiative and hired his own personal
attorney to make sure that, after such an offer was made, the case was settled within
the policy limits.[5]

The appearance that our assigned lawyers are more committed to the insurance carriers than to us is both disheartening and disadvantageous to our cause. A
legal defense firm maintains close ties with its insurers and knows that the carrier
can influence them to try a case that should be settled or that it may recommend
early settlements out of fear that multiple large awards will endanger its industry
rating. These are a function of the insurer's anxiety that, if their ratings fall, regulators may enter the scene and their market share may slide. Whenever we sense
such a pragmatic dynamic has been invoked, we should raise this issue with our
defense attorney and possibly our claims representative; if it cannot be resolved
amicably, we should consult with an independent legal counsel who is experienced
in medical malpractice cases and insurance coverage matters.

Sometimes the insurance company assigns a single lawyer to represent more
than one defendant in the case. This is legally and ethically acceptable as long as
the interests of each defendant do not clash with or threaten to harm those of the
other defendants represented by the same attorney. If, however, actual or even
apparent diverse interests surface, it is reasonable and sensible to ask whether the
lawyers will protect our individual interests as they resolve the dispute. In these
circumstances, our claims representative should appoint separate counsel and
claims representation for each defendant. We may consult a personal lawyer to
decide whether we should retain another attorney to represent us solely in this
action.

Are They Willing to Answer Our Questions?

Lawyers often begin our session by asking us to tell them in our own words and
in our own way about the case and what we think happened. The ease and interest
in which they interrupt constructively to ask us to make clarifications signify a
healthy beginning. They should also welcome questions from us even if they are
interruptions. Lawyers who wave off our queries or who downplay our need for
participation in our defense thereby telegraph a message about the impossibility
of relating well with them. We have a right to know as much as we can and we
cannot accept a passive role imposed by attorneys who do not seem to value our
contributions or our legitimate questions.

Most of us want to know when and how we will be asked to participate, when
our depositions will occur, and, given what is currently known, when and how
the case will end. Supportive attorneys try to answer questions, encourage participation, voice optimism, and express confidence. They are also realistically
cautious about estimating the final outcome or how many seasons will pass be-

fore it is achieved. They often also share the concerns and experiences of other physicians whom they have defended, using these to teach us about the legal world we are entering and how we can safely make our way through it.

Our only way to inform ourselves fully during resolution of the claim is by reading everything authored or received by our attorneys. They should therefore offer to copy us on *all* correspondence relevant to our case. Such transparency has two distinct advantages for us: first, we are never surprised by developments in the case, and, second, by following the correspondence between our attorney and our insurer, we can verify that our counsel is truly representing our interests rather than just those of the company. It is our urgent obligation to inquire into any communications about which we have not been fully informed. Defendant physicians should, as suggested previously, maintain a litigation file, preferably at home; this information should never be entered into the patient's chart because such a move would destroy its protection as confidential.

What If They Dismiss Our Concerns with, "Don't Worry, Just Leave It All to Us"

Some of us may hear these as words of salvation and, because of our ambivalence about the case and our aversion to any contact with it, we may be tempted to be saved in a "Just call me when it's over" fashion. Lawyers who make such offers deservedly make us anxious about their style in defending us.

Dropping out, in effect, and leaving everything to the advocate raises the already considerable stakes of this experience. At what risk do we place ourselves if, following this strategy, we do not win our case outright? A settlement, even for what seems the best of reasons, must, in most instances, be reported to the National Practitioner Data Bank and usually to our state licensing authority. Such reporting, as is discussed in Chapter 10, may have a strong negative impact on our careers. If there is even the slightest chance of our achieving a positive outcome, we will never regret participating actively in our defense. Nothing less than our professional reputations and our sense of integrity are at risk in litigation. This is highly personal and, as in the case of war and generals, it is far too important to leave entirely to the lawyers.

We feel better when we are working actively as members of a team devoted totally to our defense. Ideally, lawyers recognize the importance of our participation, respect our expertise, and look upon us as their primary experts. They understand that we are in the best position to describe what actually happened and why. Sensible lawyers welcome our questions, using them to expand their knowledge and to solidify our participation in the defense team. Committed and experienced defense lawyers understand that they benefit, as do we, in partnerships built on mutual respect and ordered to a single purpose, crafting and implementing a winning defense strategy.

Do They Have Time for This Case?

Just as we sometimes find ourselves too busy in our own practices, many well-known and well-respected attorneys are too occupied with other cases to attend and to respond adequately to our own. If any of the following occur—our telephone calls are not answered, our letters go unanswered, we are not copied on incoming and outgoing correspondence, underlings submit motions due in the court in a hurried way, and we feel like intruders rather than like clients—we should discuss it with our lawyer; if the problem remains unresolved, we should inform our claims representative of our dissatisfaction and ask for a change.

Points That Defense Lawyers May Make

Defense attorneys introduce physicians into the world of law, giving clues, not always consciously, about how lawyers approach the defense of medical malpractice cases. Attorneys reveal their signature styles during our first conferences, but each will make some, if not all, of the following points:

It Is the Physician's Case

The physician was present at the time of the incident, has a view of what happened, and consequently is the best expert available to the defense team. Lawyers need physicians to be honest, forthright, and competent enough to serve as good educators and team members throughout the entire process.

The Necessity of a Clear and Understandable Rendition of the Facts

Physicians should arrive at their first session with their lawyer prepared, through a detailed review of their office and hospital charts, to provide a crisp and clear account of what they believe happened. Physicians should master the chart from front to back and be prepared to inform the lawyers of which documents would best help them to understand the case, beginning with an immediate identification of any problems about the creation or contents of the chart. They should also share any hesitations, conflicts, alternative treatment choices, or other problems they either anticipated or encountered in the care of the patient. Physicians should also describe all significant conversations they had with the patient or with family members. The better they describe the building blocks of their defense, the more able will the lawyers be to put them in place as the sturdy legal foundation for their case.

At the first meeting, many defense lawyers begin to formulate the case defense. By calculating the key dates of treatment with the case filing date, for example, they may discover a viable statute of limitations defense—that is, that the plaintiff has filed the case beyond the time permitted by state law. The lawyers may appear to be asking questions that have nothing to do with what the physician thinks is important, but the answers may turn out to be crucial to a successful defense.

Informed consent, as discussed in Chapter 1, is also a significant element of defense. As with the statute of limitations, the defense of informed consent, if proved, is a bar to recovery if the physician is shown to be nonnegligent. A chart should contain a detailed informed consent note or even a form, signed by the patient, in which the very complication at issue is discussed in detail and is acknowledged and accepted by the patient consciously as a risk. Physicians should examine their charts and be prepared to discuss this issue in their early meetings with the lawyers.

Litigation Is a Time-Tested Process Aimed at Achieving Justice

The claim by lawyers that justice is really the goal of the process is extremely frustrating. *Truth* is something that may or may not emerge, perhaps only as a byproduct of the process. Physicians are accustomed to viewing truth as the foundation for justice. *Justice* defined as the "conformity to truth, fact, or reason" reinforces this view and contrasts with its other definitions, emphasized by lawyers who argue for fairness and impartiality.[6] The impulse of physicians is to try to convince everyone of the truth of the case. They are frustrated because they feel misunderstood and because others conveniently ignore the intricacies and difficulties associated with how physicians must make decisions, especially in emergency situations. In reality, many colleagues experience unjust outcomes in court that are not related to the medical facts and truth of their cases; many patients' injuries do not even meet the threshold for admission to the courts.

How the Process Unfolds

The lawyer may give the physician an overall sketch as well as the individual steps (Table 7–1) of this process. Physicians are naturally interested in the chances of the case's being dropped or settled early in the process. Lawyers generally have an accurate view of how similar cases play out in the courts, although they emphasize the uniqueness of every case and that no guarantee of early disappearance is stamped even on what appears to be insignificant nuisance cases. It is important to note that almost 70 percent of closed claims are found to be groundless and end without any payment to the plaintiff, that is, that they are dropped, dismissed before trial, or result in a trial verdict favorable to the defendant (Fig. 7–1).

How the Legal System Works

Lawyers describe the specific court in which the case has been filed and the usual period of time it takes to process cases similar to it in this venue. They may give

Table 7–1. The Litigation Process

- *The summons*—A formal legal document, issued by the clerk of the court and usually served by the sheriff. A notification that a suit has been filed.
- *The complaint*—Accompanies the summons and tells in legal terms the nature of the complaint. It may be preceded or followed by a notice in the local newspaper.
- *The pleading stage*—Shortly after the complaint is filed, the attorney begins to communicate with the court by filing motions, a request addressed to the court to do something.
- *The discovery stage*—A process designed to discover information relevant to the case. This includes depositions (oral questions and verbal responses taken under oath) and in some state courts, interrogatories (written questions). The discovery may also request inspection of documents and/or physical and mental examinations.
- *Expert witnesses*—A case alleging medical malpractice proceeds only if each side presents expert opinions that care was or was not a deviation from the accepted standard of care except for *res ipsa loquitor* or informed consent cases.
- *Summary judgment*—An application for judgment on a plaintiff's cause of action before trial where no material questions exist as to the pertinent facts in the case (which a jury would otherwise have to decide at trial). The motion for summary judgment asks the court to decide the validity of the case. If granted, the case is resolved without the need for a trial by jury.
- *Settlement*—An agreement made between two parties to a lawsuit or a claim that resolves their legal dispute.
- *The trial*—This may be preceded by pretrial maneuvers attempting to resolve the case by settlement or some other method. If these fail, the case goes to trial before a judge or a judge and jury.
- *The verdict*—Decision reached by the deciding body.
- *Directed verdict*—A directed verdict may be sought by a party at the close of his opponent's case at trial or at the end of all the evidence. If a directed verdict is granted, the court has decided as a matter of law that a party has failed to prove the essential requirements of his case and directs that a verdict be issued against that party without requiring the deliberation of a jury.
- *Judgment notwithstanding the verdict*—Also known as JNOV (*judgment non obstante veredicto*), a court notwithstanding the verdict reached by a jury may issue a judgment. This may be issued upon generally after the case has been submitted to a jury for deliberation. A party requesting JNOV must establish that as a matter of law, his or her opponent's case must fail, by having moved for a directed verdict.
- *Posttrial activities*—In a civil matter, if a participant fails to receive a favorable verdict, the law permits a number of procedures to appeal the outcome. A posttrial motion must be submitted within a prescribed period of time and is a request to the court to void the verdict usually on technical grounds. A formal appeal may also be initiated to overturn the verdict on legal grounds.

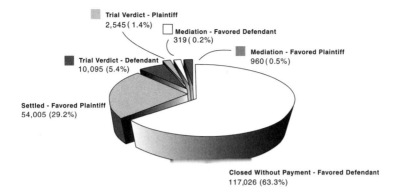

Outcome of 184,950 Closed Claims

Figure 7–1. Outcome of closed medical malpractice claims. National Data (1985–2003), Physician Insurers Association of America (PIAA), Rockville, MD, with permission.

physicians their quick-sketch impressions of the judge, the plaintiff attorney, and the typical jury pools. It is also possible that the case will be filed in a jurisdiction in which discovery is time limited, cases are assigned for trial in eight or fewer months, and the parties are expected to engage in meaningful settlement efforts shortly before the trial date. In these circumstances, the lawyer's approach and the physician's role in preparing the case may be vastly different from what they would be in jurisdictions in which trials are routinely scheduled for dates 2 to 4 years later. The latter docket, characterized by delays and rollercoaster stress, engages and affects physicians in a different way than the fast track protocol.

The Plaintiff Attorney's Best Theory About the Case
The attorneys offer their best estimate of the plaintiff attorneys' case along with its central hypothesis. Before filing the case, the plaintiffs' attorneys make a judgment about the most evident reasons for their winning the case. Because the available case details do not support a charge of negligence, the bad medical outcome is sometimes the only evidence they have. Barry Werth describes how this works in his gripping account of a birth injury case in which, four years after the filing of the case, the plaintiff attorneys finally "cobbled together a workable theory" and were able to retain experts whose testimony "almost, but not quite, corroborated it."[7] The defense attorney's challenge is to anticipate, monitor, and develop strategies to defeat these working theories. Physicians can often help in this critical work by playing devil's advocate, acquainting the lawyers with alternatives to the approach they themselves took in the case and demonstrating how these alternatives may or may not have led to a similar outcome.

The Immediate Plan

The lawyers ask the physician to provide any relevant documents. They may also ask the physician to identify potential experts for the specific situation and professional literature that supports the plaintiff's case and the physician's defense.

Do Not Kill the Messenger

As the case proceeds, the lawyers inform physicians of motions that they win or lose, experts who castigate or support the physician's approach to the care of the patient, and many other temporarily negative case-related events, each of which can at least briefly unnerve and perhaps enrage physicians. The lawyers must keep physicians informed about these constantly shifting events, even when doing so incurs their wrath. Being angry at the bearer of bad news is never helpful. In their first session with physicians, lawyers should discuss the inherent seeming lack of logic and unpredictability of the legal process. Physicians become wiser, more patient, and better defenders of themselves when they understand the vagaries of courtroom culture—that different judges act and react in different ways; that the rules sometimes seem to hinder rather than support the case; and that the constitution of the jury can make all the difference in the outcome of the case. Physicians cannot change the random nature of these events when they occur, but they can manage themselves and their emotions better and save their energy for their defense.

Medicine and the Law Live in Totally Different Environments

Because lawyers have different obligations, they work according to their own construction of the world and a set of rules that fit the goals of the law. Physicians do the same within the universe of medicine. To physicians, the law seems to move forward without much regard for its impact on participants and bystanders. Medicine seems far more focused, demanding that physicians be aware of and respond to events quickly and responsibly for the sake of the suffering patient. This stark seeming diversity of approach may be the most frustrating and alienating aspect of litigation. Howsoever reluctantly, physicians must play in the legal ballpark, accepting and adapting to the rules, processes, and umpires who oversee the process and guide their legal counsel.

Communication Is a Two-Way Street

To succeed in their case, even though they may resent being forced into the process, physicians must agree with their lawyers to maintain open minds and open lines of communication with each other. They must commit themselves to this mutuality at the outset and, as in any relationship, they must work hard to honor and nourish it throughout the course of the case.

Talking About the Case

Although lawyers may approach this issue in various ways, a primary concern is that physicians may disclose information in unmonitored conversations about the case or seem to admit facts in ways that can jeopardize their defense. Lawyers do not want plaintiff attorneys to use apparent admissions in unguarded conversations to back physicians into a corner or as justification to subpoena a colleague to testify against the defendant. Although this possibility is not common, it is a powerful threat.

On the other hand, physicians want to talk about how upset they feel, how unjust the charges are, and their conviction that the law has no business trying medical decisions in court. As mentioned in Chapter 4, *clarifying our feelings is essential to becoming good defendants*. Physicians should understand that lawyers are professionally obligated, in the best interest of physicians, to caution them clearly about the need for prudence in talking about the case. Physicians must also understand their own traumatized state and understand and monitor their own quite normal and healthy urges to express their feelings.

What Should Physicians Do?

DECIDE TO BE A GOOD DEFENDANT. It takes work to learn how to become good defendants. We cannot change the event that has occurred in which contemporaneous, and presumably accurate, documentation exists. Although lawsuits may not change the basic facts of, or our feelings about, the precipitating event, they do intensify and extend our focus on them and, theoretically, provide the setting in which the whole truth will finally come out. The way others perceive and react to the event broadens and deepens our understanding of exactly what happened.

RESOLVE TO BE ACTIVE. We may feel initially impotent, overwhelmed, and uncertain about how, or even whether, we want to actively cooperate. Some physicians are stricken with a fated hopelessness: No matter what we do or how well we do it, we are going to be sued anyway. Monetary awards continue to rise and insurance premiums follow in their wake. Nothing about who we are or what we do seems to make any difference. This *swept away by cruel destiny* scenario depresses us, leaving us feeling vulnerable and defeated before the battle begins. Our cure for the numbing passivity that can set in is through becoming active and going on full alert to defend ourselves aggressively.

Any decision to forget it or leave it to the lawyers joins us to the many defendants who later regret being passive and vow to be more fully involved the next time. Like it or not, our case is personal. Indeed, nothing is more personal than having our integrity, our reputation, and our honor as persons and professionals put on trial. Working cooperatively and energetically with our attorneys engages us in ways that both strengthen our case and control our anxieties. More important, our participation spurs our lawyers and claims representatives to work more diligently, to stretch themselves to look beyond the obvious, and to go the extra mile on our behalf. Our being in the lineup—watching everything, asking questions, helping out, and holding them accountable—motivates them to transcend their best past work.

We probably transfer our habits of control over our professional lives to the defense of our case. Most of us, however, are not skilled advocates and there is no loss of honor or independence in sensibly following the advice of our attorneys. We need to be active team members, in concert with our lawyers, blending our particular medical skills with their legal expertise to the advantage of our common cause. Throughout the process, successful defense attorneys draw on our expertise as medical experts and consultants to the defense team while maintaining control and management of the legal defense. But they must lead the team and they will decide how to use our input in helpful ways.

TELL THE TRUTH. We begin by being honest with our defense counsel. Protected by the lawyer–client privilege, we can speak openly and without fear. The mutual uncertainty of regard in our first meeting may lead us to withhold, for the moment, or to gloss over some of the less-than-flattering information about the case. We should reject temptations to spin the facts, because they will come out anyway, leaving us feeling embarrassed and more vulnerable. Honesty is not only the best policy, it is the only policy when so much is at stake.

The first meeting, according to defense attorneys, is the most important one with their clients. At this first meeting, we not only provide the lawyers with their foundational understanding of the case but we also help them conceptualize the probable plaintiff's theory of the case. We simply must take the time before we meet with our attorneys to learn, memorizing, if necessary, the facts, by reviewing our own notes and the entire hospital chart of the case. We must know and inform our lawyers of the contents of the nurses' notes because these often play a significant role in supporting or undercutting the physician's case. We should also inform the lawyer about any questions that occurred to us at the time of the incident about our medical approach as well as any intuitions we had that the patient was a problem even before the adverse event occurred.

We may also be tempted during the session to blame the outcome on the faults of others. And, indeed, others may be partially or fully culpable and, as we learn later, may not be entirely honest about their role in the event. Our primary responsibility, however, is not to speculate about these perceptions or testimony of others but rather to tell our side of the story honestly and fully. We can only hope that if others are responsible, the testimony will reveal their role in the incident.

Dr. Richard Allen was disheartened when his partner falsely accused him of being responsible for the follow-up of a CAT scan.

> Suddenly the team fractures. It's almost like what soldiers feel when they go into combat. The first duty you have is to your buddies to get through this thing the best way you can. That's the way I feel about medicine. It's kind of a war and you have to help each other out to try to get through it. We're all working toward the same purpose, which is to achieve a good outcome. (A lawsuit) is one of the battles in the war and people should stick together and help each other out and if mistakes are made, we need to be honest about it and help each other with that and don't go around pointing fingers and trying to rat on each other and make the best deal you can for yourself. That's the way I always thought about it and I was very surprised that that's not the way it works.[8]

DO NOT HESITATE TO CLARIFY MISUNDERSTANDINGS. Stress sometimes distorts what we say, so that our judgment that we are conveying our thoughts successfully may be that is vastly off the mark. The attorney may get a picture of what happened that is vastly different than the one we intended to convey. It is prudent to ask our attorneys to summarize for us their understanding of what we said. We should then immediately correct any misperceptions or misinterpretations. Uncorrected distortions have a long half-life and linger on, breeding further distortions.

SET ASIDE ALL THE TIME NEEDED. The time spent defending a lawsuit is never convenient or predictable and we can never get it back. Although it causes unrecoverable economic losses, its greatest impact is the time permanently lost to patient care. Conscious of our time constraints, we may be tempted to resist spending any more of it by responding to our attorneys' requests for information or documents. We may be tempted to use delaying tactics, claiming to be too busy to respond or playing hard to get in scheduling depositions and meetings. We may not realize that we are acting out our anger by being late for depositions or other legal meetings.

We are also irritated by the seemingly casual way in which lawyers view time. We respond as quickly as possible to the demands of patients; they seem to respond to their clients when it fits their schedule and timetable. We have some control over the scheduling of our office hours and procedures, and we resent it when depositions and review sessions appear to accommodate somebody else's schedule rather than our own. We conduct the examination, the operation, or the consultation as scheduled and on time and then they are done; delays and set-overs are the norm in the legal process. Motions and rulings are "continued," as if they were incidental rather than vital events in our case, leaving us adrift in an unfamiliar dimension. We cancel our schedule to give a deposition, only to learn that it is canceled because one of the attorneys is delayed in court.

We mark our calendar to go to trial, only to have the court date rescheduled because the judge is away at a seminar. We go to trial with no certain knowledge of whether it will take two days or a week. Rather than endure endless frustration and grumbling, we serve ourselves and our cause best by accepting philosophically the legal world's attitudes toward time, knowing, as Dr. Allen did, "that there was a finite amount of time that I was going to be involved in this."[8]

FOLLOW THE ATTORNEY'S ADVICE. We all appreciate being heard and agree that listening is an art practiced by two. Because our case is played out in the unfamiliar territory of the court, we must sharpen our listening skills and keep our minds open to what our defense attorneys advise about the strategies, approaches, and timing necessary for a successful defense. We have an obligation to ask questions if we do not understand their advice or if it seems inappropriate or in conflict with common sense.

KEEP THE LINES OF COMMUNICATION OPEN. Just as we expect our lawyers to answer our telephone calls and to keep us in the loop regarding progress in our case, so we should answer their calls and correspondence in a timely manner. Ignoring reminders that we are currently defendants may seem to relieve us of stress but it can harm our case. Open lines of communication with our lawyer guarantee that they will accept and be forthright with us as team members.

EXPECT TO PLAY DIFFERENT ROLES AT DIFFERENT STAGES OF THE LAWSUIT. Our initial responsibility may be limited to gathering the information necessary for the lawyers to begin to prepare our defense. We must read over carefully every document we copy and forward to them. Do chart notes exist that we were supposed to, but did not, countersign? Do nurses' or housestaff notes exist that we failed to review? Do laboratory results or radiology reports exist that we overlooked or skimmed over at the time of the incident? Neither we, nor our lawyers, want to be surprised about unexpected future testimony on such issues by other participants in the case. We need to prepare for our depositions in ways specified by our attorneys. We may be asked to help them choose our experts but will be warned to refrain from contacting them ourselves. We may be asked to help lawyers prepare for the depositions of both the defense and plaintiff experts by researching and formulating appropriate questions. We can also obtain useful background material on the reputations, credentials, and publications of potential experts. Our careful objective review of all depositions—our own and those of the experts—is essential. Our extensive training, experience, and familiarity with the vocabulary and the processes of medicine prepare us to identify and note any errors or omissions in these case documents. Our attorney may recommend that we engage in formal instruction or coaching, if we go to trial, to prepare us for the experience. We may also be asked to help in the development of visual aids for the education of the jury. Our attorneys relying on our familiarity with all the relevant documentation may require our reviewing hundreds, sometimes thousands, of pages of testimony and records. By working closely with our attorneys, we can anticipate the amount of work and time that our involvement will require at each of these different phases and to plan our work schedule accordingly.

8

Coping with the Stress Associated with Litigation

> I will do anything to avoid the law again. I would go to the law if the principle were truly powerful. But for me, it's like going to war. I'm not a pacifist. I believe that if you go to war, you go to war but never delude yourself for one moment on the cost of the war. You have to know in advance that the cost of the war is going to be an order of magnitude greater than you ever thought it would in your worst-case scenario. I expect to take serious wounds to my capital, my self-esteem, and my sense of loyalty to people associated with the case because betrayal becomes a big part of lawsuits.
>
> —Norman Mailer[1]

However we react to the accusation, we have been wounded by an assault from the legal system that now takes over our lives. We are now defendants, and although lawyers and insurers line up beside us, we stand alone in the dock to defend our competence and integrity. Some lawyers tell us that we should not take this charge of negligence personally, that in today's world, litigation is "just the cost of doing business." Perhaps litigation is inevitable, we feel, but it is never less than highly personal. A hurricane may be impersonal but it still devastates everything that is personal to those it touches.

This accusation, rather than the eventual outcome of the case, works a transformation within us that affects how we subsequently think and behave professionally. When we are sued, we must name this new stressor correctly and keep from being overwhelmed by balancing it with all the other stressors in our lives.

Why Physicians Are Upset

Two dissimilar factors explain why physicians feel so intensely about being sued: their commonly shared obsessive–compulsive personality characteristics and the nature of tort law. When these two factors collide, as occurs when physicians are sued, they generate intense emotional disturbances within the affected physicians.

116

Personality Characteristics of Physicians

Human beings often use their obsessive-compulsive personality traits to defend themselves against the threats of life.[2] Gabbard[3] writes of the "compulsive triad" of personality traits in ordinary, normal physicians that makes them vulnerable to doubt, guilt feelings, and an exaggerated sense of responsibility. Almost all physicians possess and draw on these obsessive-compulsive traits as they struggle to moderate their feelings of responsibility for events beyond their control or their feelings of not having done enough.

Under the impact of a lawsuit, these characteristics may morph into exaggerated and destructive tendencies: Where we once appropriately considered options, we are now obsessed with immobilizing doubts; where we once felt guilty over falling even slightly short of a standard, we are now morbidly self-critical; where we once exercised an exaggerated but controlled sense of responsibility, we now condemn ourselves for not managing circumstances well beyond our control. By eroding our self-confidence, these distortions make us miserable. Such a state of mind on our part is exactly what the plaintiff attorneys hope for and depend on: they want us to doubt our competence and to feel guilty and personally responsible, even if we are not, for whatever happened.

Tort Law

The nature of tort law is the other reason that we feel so deeply. A tort is a civil wrong, a perceived harm that demands a civil sanction, usually compensation in money. Torts are distinguished from crimes that are processed through the criminal justice system and whose sanctions include incarceration or death. In tort law, the plaintiff seeking compensation must make a charge of negligence or intentional conduct. If damages or compensation are to be awarded, such an action must demonstrate the presence of the four elements of medical malpractice described in Chapter 6.

A charge of negligence is a savage blow to compulsive physicians who pride themselves on their competence and are acutely sensitive to even the slightest suggestion that they have failed to meet the standard of care. It is this accusation of fault, demanded by the law, this charge that we have failed to meet the standard that damages us most. All of the reassurances not to take this personally do not spare us from experiencing it as a direct assault on our self-esteem and on our sense of being professionals.

Additional Sources of Threat That Generate Stress

We also begin to suffer from intangible but very real threats that ravage our spiritual lives. We usually keep our fears to ourselves until we understand what we have won or what we have lost. Later, we are better able to estimate its final toll.

In the meantime, listing our concerns allows us to gain some control over them and to diminish their impact.

Our Sense of Honor

Our reputation and our good name, those reliable personal characteristics by which we know ourselves and others recognize us, are at the core of our identity. To cherish ourselves, we need to feel a realistic regard for ourselves. A legal charge of negligence sorely challenges our sense of honor, a concept no less real for being invoked so seldom in the modern world. Dr. Richard Allen laments:

> I had guilt about being involved in a case like this. An individual prides himself on his clinical acumen and his attention to detail. It's a blow to the image I had of myself, my code of behavior that I tried to live up to. I'm sure I didn't always do it but I tried to live up to that word (honor) in that the patient who came to me could put his trust in me and I would be his advocate and always try to act in his or her best interest. That was the image that I wanted to convey and also the image that I wanted not only my patients to come away with but also my colleagues that I worked with in the community. It was my impression that I was generally thought of as an honorable person upon whom you could rely and who tried to do a good job.[4]

Mike Wallace mirrors those sentiments: "If you're a reporter, you're a truth-teller and they're saying that you're not telling the truth. It goes to your gut."[5]

A charge of negligence is a well-aimed blow to our healthy narcissism. Two psychiatrists describe their own experience of being sued, "Here are the sense of assault and violation, the feelings of outrage and fear. Most painfully, here is the narcissistic injury, the astonishing wound to our understanding of ourselves as admirable, well-meaning people."[6]

We strive to be that ideal self that embodies our deepest values and goals. We see ourselves as good, beneficent, and caring physicians and we are keenly aware that, even if we fall short of it at times, fulfilling this ideal remains our central motivation. By suing us, someone charges on the public record that we are neither good, beneficent, nor caring, a direct hit on our reputation that, as Mike Wallace observes, ". . . is all we have."[7] Such a public charge may be carried in the media and through public documents and along informal networks so that it becomes common conversation among our peers, the guild of the law, and, indeed, the community at large. We may feel ashamed and may well react by pulling back from our social and professional contacts. We may fear abandonment by our colleagues while inwardly punishing ourselves with self-condemnation.

We can take some solace, however, in that our injured narcissism will motivate us to defend our good name and fuel our efforts to recapture good feelings about ourselves, that central healing of self that is essential to restoring our reputation among our patients and our colleagues. To defend our case is to defend our honor.

Self-preservation

We begin to wonder if we can get through this experience without suffering major losses. Dr. Richard Allen puts it simply, "I didn't want myself to be terribly damaged."[8] Our identity, our physician-hood, overlaps and interpenetrates our understanding of ourselves. Will this malpractice case, we wonder, cause us to lose everything we have worked for? Will we be able to continue to function as physicians? We literally fear for our lives.

The specter of nonrenewal of our insurance coverage, as discussed in Chapter 5, becomes more realistic if we have been sued for significant damages. Whether or not we continue to practice depends, we feel, on the outcome of our case. If we cannot practice, will we have the same good feelings about our self, or will we have to make significant changes in our core identity? Dr. Mary Santos says:

> If I had lost this trial, I would have been out of practice. I have no question because I couldn't have gotten insurance and it would have been (publicized) all over the place. I kept asking, "Would I be able to get insurance?" And they never answered and I knew what that meant.[9]

Physicians may tell their patients that they have a 30 percent chance of having a recurrence of cancer. Although it is a sobering and truthful statement, it is one that, as we believe and most patients agree, also conveys hope. Our lawyers may respond to us in similar fashion, giving us their best estimates of the outcome, telling us the level of damages awarded for similar incidents, and explaining the experiences of other physicians in similar circumstances. Given the overall statistics of adjudicated cases, the estimates of these lawyers may be coldly realistic but they can also give hope.

Our Trust in Others

As physicians, we hold a public trust, reinforced by our ethical code, to devote our knowledge and skill to the good of the persons in our community. Our work is inseparable from human relationships.

Dr. Joseph Daley tells of sitting in his office with a patient who was telling him what a helpful and good physician he was: "You're the only physician I can talk to. Everyone else brushes me off."[10] Across the city at the same time, the constable was delivering a summons at his home on behalf of the same patient. Learning later that day about the lawsuit, Dr. Daley was not only shocked and hurt but also totally surprised. Few people understand how deeply we can be offended when patients, in whom we have invested ourselves, sue us. Some physicians compare the experience with what it must feel like to be raped or stabbed in the back. Dr. Jonathan Shay, a psychiatrist who has studied post-traumatic stress disorders, especially among war veterans, identifies the "deepest danger" associated with any traumatic event as "the loss of trust in others."[11]

By being deeply involved with patients, we make ourselves vulnerable to hurt. Convinced that mutual trust is essential to good patient care, we find that such suits compromise our capacity to continue to give ourselves in the same self-forgetful way.

An orthopedic surgeon described how he had worked diligently, "lying awake at night, worrying," about his efforts to correct, through rod insertion, a young man's scoliosis. A few years after successful surgery, the young man was in an automobile accident that snapped the rod. He sued the rod's manufacturer and the orthopedic surgeon who inserted it. The surgeon was astounded and profoundly hurt, feeling that he had been most conscientious regarding this young man and gone out of his way to help him.

As one psychiatrist reflected ruefully after being sued by patients to whom she had devoted her life and best skills, "I lost my innocence." She was mourning that boon of life, that freely given and accepted bond of trust between herself and her patients at the heart of medical practice. According to Dr. Joseph Daley:

> When something like this happens, there is a jaded edge on the relationship and you never know from then on who is going to foul up a relationship with a suit. I don't think you ever look at patients in the same way.[12]

Our Self-confidence

A suit challenges our judgment and our skill, causing us to question ourselves. This begins almost immediately as one of the most distressing and persistent re-actions to litigation and may not dissipate for many years. Dr. West's ongoing fear that her patients will bleed to death after she closes their abdomen symbolizes this conflict. For two years after her first bad outcome that led to a case that was finally dismissed, she still agonized about the integrity of her closed incisions. Like all compulsive persons, physicians question themselves even when things go well: Is there a better way to do this, and what is the latest research on this issue? A bad outcome that spawns a negligence suit plays on and aggravates this basic human tendency, causing distress that ravages our self-confidence.

Our pride and confidence in managing and controlling our lives bid us to put everything on the table and to resolve the issue immediately. By the time the lawsuit is filed, however, it is largely out of our control. We are suddenly involved in a legal world whose procedural tempo differs radically from any we have ever known. We are suddenly minor team members in a game-like experience that is played according to rigid and alienating rules. We feel vulnerable and powerless because when we enter a process for which we are unprepared, we must depend on others to guide our steps and represent our interests.

Our Financial Health

Because malpractice awards seldom exceed the insurance coverage of the average physician, he or she is in little danger of experiencing significant financial repercussions from malpractice litigation. Unless special circumstances exist or the negligence is particularly gross, the few well-publicized verdicts that each year exceed a physician's policy limits are generally reduced or settled within policy limits.[13] Plaintiff lawyers usually try to name enough co-defendants so that the final monetary judgment is drawn from a pool of a number of sources. However, knowing this does not necessarily relieve us of concerns about the eventual damage award in any given claim.

The Characteristics of the Case

Each case tells its own story and, as we eventually learn, its own "plaintiff's theory" of what happened. Neither gives us comfort. We react one way if the plaintiff died or sustained a permanent injury that requires lifetime care and in a very different manner if a plaintiff's complaint involves a reversible medication side effect or, for example, an enlarged abdominal scar. We react very differently when we are convinced that we made a mistake rather than when we know we encountered an unanticipated complication. We feel differently about the plaintiff who is a long-term and trusted patient than we do about the emergency department patient plaintiff with whom we consulted for a few minutes. We experience more shame and diminished self-esteem from a well-publicized malpractice case rooted in a catastrophic event than we do from one that receives no media attention. We also feel differently about a case in which we are a sole defendant than we do about one in which multiple defendants interpret the same event from differing points of view.

We all know that a delay in decision-making can make the difference between an acceptable and a catastrophic medical outcome. When, however, we are charged with negligence after we make a timely decision that results in a bad outcome, we feel misunderstood and unappreciated and that the case itself is unjust or has been filed for nuisance purposes—that is, in a long-shot effort to manipulate the system and obtain money.

The Current Litigation Climate

Sometimes the specific event in our case becomes a footnote in a rash of novel hysteria-based litigation. Such was the now largely discredited breast implant frenzy of the early 1990s. A plastic surgeon, previously never sued, was named, within a thirty-day period, in a dozen "implant" claims. Who would blame him for being enraged at lawyers and at a system whose unfairness was clear in its acceptance of junk science in what it termed its quest for justice?

Like the weather, the litigation climate in any state can vary greatly from year to year. Of the approximately 10,000 physicians insured by the Illinois-based ISMIE Mutual Insurance Company in 1985, a total of 3,865 were sued, most occurring just before August 15, the effective deadline for new tort reform legislation (Fig. 8–1).

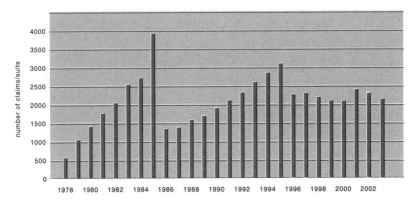

Figure 8–1. The incidence of medical malpractice claims (1978–2003). ISMIE Mutual Insurance Company (Chicago, IL), with permission.

Other Stressors That Already Affect Our Lives

Our generalized distress increases exponentially when that of a case adds to existing stress in our personal and professional lives. The latter includes disruptive or poorly adjusted children who require extra attention, chronically ill spouses, strained marriages, and extended finances.

> For a few years prior to their malpractice suit, Dr. Richard Allen and his partner suffered a significant decrease in income, largely due to the managed care environment in their locality. With his partner close to retirement, they had discussed but not yet implemented plans for alternative practice arrangements. His partner's false allegation that he had informed Dr. Allen about an imaging study was the "the crowning blow" that accelerated their breakup. The disruptions associated with the dissolution of a 26-year partnership only exacerbated the stress they were already feeling from their financial pressures and the malpractice case.[14]

Under the pressure of such multiple sources of stress, we do not want to make decisions we may later regret. We must sort out the respective sources of our stress and then do what we can do, even imperfectly, to manage them. A neurosurgeon who was urged by his insurer to take his case to trial describes his inability to put aside his concerns about his wife's acute and disruptive illness. Knowing himself and his relationship with his family and fully aware of the repercussions, he harbors no regrets for pushing the insurance company to settle the case.

What This Lawsuit Means to Me Personally

Why is being sued more stressful for one person than for another? Why do we feel only mildly disturbed by a lawsuit when our co-defendant seems almost immobilized? Very simply, a lawsuit has a different meaning for each of us. Our reaction is a function of how we personally *appraise* the lawsuit filed against us, a perception that depends on our complex judgment about the lawsuit's place in our life.[15] We instinctively ask ourselves, "What is this all about? Does this affect only my work, or does it also affect my health and my family? How does it make me feel about myself? Do I feel overwhelmed, or can I manage my feelings about it? Do I feel that I can do something about it, or do I feel powerless and hopeless?" How we answer tells us the meaning of the event as well as how we might cope with it. The statements by Andy Rooney that "I do not know whether I will be destroyed or not"[16] and by Dr. Richard Allen that "I didn't want myself to be terribly damaged"[17] reveal how profoundly threatening the charges were to these individuals. We must get the measure of the real meaning to us of the accusation before we can do anything effective about it.

As a group, physicians tend to be active rather than passive in solving problems. Physicians in one study who identify litigation as their most stressful existential experience feel that they have little control over events, experience increased physical and emotional symptoms, and use such psychological defenses as denial, avoidance, and blaming others.[18] Physicians who regard litigation as less stressful than their experience of a spouse's death or divorce feel that they have some control over it, are less symptomatic, and are more active by identifying the sources of stress and changing what they can about the situation.

Reactions to the Stress of Litigation

Plotting the exact point at which stress becomes noticeable during the process of litigation is a function of many contingencies. Some of us identify our most stressful time as when we receive the complaint. Others report feeling its impact later, when giving a deposition or going on trial.

More than 95 percent of sued physicians report that, at some time during the process, they experience at least temporary periods of emotional disequilibria.[19] The most common reactions are inner tension, depressed mood, anger, and frustration. Some develop either physical or emotional symptoms. The most common of these is a cluster of symptoms, very like those of major depressive disorder, that includes changes in mood and sleep patterns, especially insomnia; a loss of interest in usual activities; difficulty in concentration; and, on occasion, thoughts of suicide (Fig. 8–2). Another clutch of symptoms resembles those of what psychiatry terms an adjustment disorder. This includes pervasive feelings of anger, inner tension, irritability, fatigue, headache, and gastrointestinal disturbances. Some physicians may experience the onset of a physical illness or the exacerbation of a previously diagnosed one such as hypertension or coronary artery disease. As noted earlier, Dr. Richard Allen clearly associated the onset of atrial fibrillation with being served with a complaint. Approximately eight percent of physicians report that they use alcohol or drugs to self-medicate their feelings of

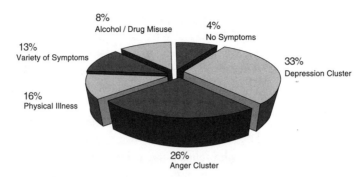

Figure 8–2. Common symptomatic responses to medical malpractice litigation. Summary statistics based on Sara C. Charles, Charlene E. Pyskoty, and Amy Nelson, "Physicians on Trial: Self-reported Reactions to Malpractice Trials," *Western Journal of Medicine* 148(1988): 358–360.

distress. If any of these symptoms persist, physicians should seek appropriate medical and/or psychiatric consultation.

Understanding Our Reactions to Litigation

Feeling that our integrity has been assaulted, we experience rage, sadness, and fear. Our claims representatives and lawyers proffer advice that is easy to give and almost impossible to follow, telling us not to worry and instead to focus on our work. Once again, we begin the process of response to stressful events described in Chapter 2. We are shocked and unable to absorb the full impact of being sued. We are preoccupied and plagued with intrusive reminders of the event, and we draw heavily upon our psychological energy to control them.

Gradually, we regain a feeling of relative calm and can again focus on our work. Then, for example, we enter the emergency department that was the scene of the catastrophic event that led to the lawsuit that forever changed our life. The emotions that desolated us on that last morning of innocence and made us into defendants may overwhelm us again. We must battle these obsessive intrusions if we are to get our work done. Such exacerbations and remissions, always most intense in the immediate postevent period, can strike us at any time, sometimes many times, during the prolonged period of litigation. They seem to retreat as we move away in time from the precipitating incident.

A lawsuit, like war, is not one but rather a series of events. A year into the case, our lawyer suddenly notifies us to prepare for a deposition. Such sudden impositions continue throughout the litigation, filling our days with uncertainty, reigniting our emotions, and then subsiding as mysteriously as they began. We hope that the end of our case will be the end of its traumatic impact on us. The final outcome, however, may be a settlement or an outright loss that assaults us freshly, making us vulnerable to a new cycle of fears and concerns that we must work through. As at the end of a war, we may try to follow everybody's advice to go on with life, but we are, in fact, changed at levels and in ways that we do not fully grasp and cannot easily measure and that others may not understand at all.

Control Over Our Practice: A Challenge from Litigation

The need to control is a prime professional and personal characteristic of physicians. This dynamic, both a strength and a need, must be understood if physicians are to monitor their reactions and responses to the pressure of litigation. In the service of both their personal comfort and their professional competence, they must experience a degree of mastery over and certainty about the decisions they make, which they may alter quickly when the unexpected happens. This professional freedom depends on their observing and managing the ever-present tension of their being both fallible and vulnerable, of being human and so capable of making mistakes and incapable of knowing everything.

The pressure associated with clinical decision making is also a function of patients' expectations and demands that physicians be both infallible and omnipotent. If physicians cannot make a healthy distinction between the reality in which they are immersed and the impossible ideal in which they are draped, they may lose their balance and become anxious and indecisive, almost certainly increasing their risk of making an error.

The long training period of physicians teaches them what they must do, even below the level of consciousness, to maintain sufficiently good control in their daily work. Despite their training and experience, the tension in their professional role, according to medical sociologist Renée Fox, may be a lifelong companion for physicians because the "basic human-associated stresses and dilemmas [of medical work] . . . cannot be eliminated."[20]

Being sued shatters the delicate balance that physicians maintain between their feelings of fallibility and an ideal of mistake-free practice, forcing physicians to work diligently to preserve it. Determining who was in control during an incident and therefore responsible for the bad outcome is the subject of litigation and its draining protocol of depositions, motions, and trial. This issue of who exercised control preys on physicians' feelings of fallibility and vulnerability and the demand, partly internal and partly external, that they be in absolute control over every event. They are suddenly forced to question how much control they actually had over the incident and to wonder about all their past and future choices.

This is the background for the long and wearing process in which the plaintiff repeatedly tries to show that the physician should have foreseen the outcome while the physician, as defendant, pleads the opposite. Each side calls on experts to support or oppose these contentions. The emotional current runs swiftly and shifts without warning; one day, the physician may be elated by the strong and supportive deposition of the expert that confirms the argument that he or she could not have been in control, but on the next day, the physician is outraged to lose a motion for summary judgment, suggesting that he or she still may be responsible for the outcome.

For some, the case ends only when a trial jury finally decides who was in charge and, therefore legally responsible for the injury, thus making compensation for it possible. Physicians, against their will, find themselves strangers in an adversarial environment controlled by others. They feel uneasy, vulnerable, dependent, frustrated with the rules and pace of the process, and plagued by intermittent doubts about their practical and decision making skills. From the start, they must recognize how hard they will have to work to control themselves in an experience that they cannot control.

How Physicians Can Help Themselves: Regaining Control

We respond to litigation's threat to our feelings of control by actively restoring control. We cannot make the lawsuit, now living a life of its own, disappear or change its progression, as shown in Table 8–1, but by helping ourselves to adapt better we can limit its impact on us.

Physicians must start this process immediately because a window of increasing vulnerability appears to open around these events. In a 1995 study, physicians who had a claim-producing event, compared with those who had not, had twice the risk (from 7 to 14 percent) of an additional claim during the twelve-month period following the initial incident.[21] Why would this happen? Physicians may be preoccupied and distracted by unresolved family problems or other problems for an extended period and therefore more vulnerable to mistakes or inattention to their work. Physical and psychological reactions to the initial adverse event and subsequent litigation may compromise physicians' ability to practice optimally, increasing their vulnerability to distractions and making mistakes. The quicker physicians begin to work at diminishing their distress, the more rapidly they will return to their accustomed level of work and self-confidence. They will also lessen their risk of developing the chronic kind of symptoms that can be harbingers of physician impairment.

After being sued, physicians may not always easily regain their former style of addressing problems and need to manage their emotions directly to control their anxiety. Classic examples are physicians who are suddenly unable to take their thrice-weekly run or play their weekly game of tennis. Physicians should not be surprised if, during the long litigation process, they enter phases of feeling overwhelmed and unable to keep up with their usual ways of maintaining their health. While extra effort may help some scale these barriers, others may have to settle for relying temporarily on more passive ways of handling stress.

During the 7-year wait for her trial, Dr. Mary Santos tried to continue her usual leisure-time activities of reading and active sports. At about 5 years into her case,

Table 8–1. Useful Strategies for Coping with Litigation

Obtaining Social Support

- Discuss feelings about the case with a trusted confidant.
- Contact insurance company, medical or specialty society for resources related to support.

Regaining Control

- Inform ourselves about the legal process.
- Introduce good risk management strategies into our practices
- Implement appropriate changes in our practice.
- During periods of increased stress, rearrange our office and surgery schedules.
- Avoid situations that generate anxiety and increase risk.
- Reevaluate our time commitments.
- Participate in relevant continuing medical education.
- Seek consultation on financial and estate planning.
- Participate in such leisure-time activities as active sports and exercise.
- Take regular vacations and time off from practice to engage in other restorative experiences.
- Schedule the necessary time to participate in the defense of the case.
- Actively monitor our emotional and physical reactions and, if indicated, seek appropriate consultation.

Changing the Meaning of the Event

- Nourish the conviction that we are "good doctors" rather than "bad doctors" as portrayed in the complaint.
- Recognize that the tort system is about compensation, not competence.
- Recognize that the tort system is focused on justice, not on establishing truth.
- Be kind to ourselves as we work to understand the "truth" of the case.

she began spending an hour each morning meditating and writing a stream of consciousness journal, chronicling her experiences and thoughts, which she found very helpful.

> I used to listen to a lot of opera but I found that it just didn't sound as good, the food didn't taste good. I lost a lot of weight . . . and even talking to people was very hard. These reactions came in waves, I almost think it was like a battle. I became obsessed with reading about the First World War. I kept thinking about this and all of a sudden, I felt like that was kind of what I was in. I read biographies of Churchill and Roosevelt, people who lived challenging lives. For the first time in my life, I'm not exercising everyday. It's like that part has been taken out of me. It was really abrupt.

Now, some months after her successful trial, she is just beginning to get active again.[22]

A Source of Control: Obtaining Social Support

If we ordinarily feel in charge of our lives, enjoy good self-esteem, and are hopeful and optimistic, we are better armed to deal with traumatic events than if we characteristically avoid reality and blame others for our woes.[23] If we also feel that there are other people who care for us and that their help is available if we need them, we are more likely to fare better in a crisis than if we feel alone or unloved.[24]

DISCUSS FEELINGS ABOUT THE CASE WITH A TRUSTED CONFIDANT. As we discussed in Chapter 4, although at deposition lawyers may try to force us to reveal the names of anyone we have talked to about the case, talking about our feelings to others does not meet the legal threshold for such disclosure. Physicians, in fact, feel increasingly comfortable talking about their reactions to litigation with others. A 1982 study revealed that only 10 percent of physicians acknowledged talking with one of their peers about reactions to their case; 6 years later, almost 70 percent did so.[25]

In any major life event, the single best help for us is the support we feel from understanding and empathic people. It is worth repeating that litigation is the only major traumatic life event in which we are consistently told not to talk about it with others. A lawsuit singles us out as negligent, making us feel isolated and alone. We cannot turn off our profound human need to feel that we are still accepted and appreciated within the physician community. One response is to do the human thing, the healthy thing, and share our feelings with a responsible confidant. In doing this, our goal is not to discuss the clinical details, although we will surely mention some of them, but rather to talk about how distressed and upset we are. Mature colleagues, including some veterans of the litigation process, who understand how we feel about being sued, can help us anticipate the pitfalls ahead and identify the sources of help available to us.

CONTACT THE INSURANCE COMPANY, MEDICAL AND SPECIALTY SOCIETY FOR RESOURCES RELATED TO SUPPORT. Because not everyone has easy or immediate access to understanding and supportive people, medical and specialty societies have developed programs to support physicians in litigation. Recognizing that some physicians are uncomfortable joining support groups or meeting with physicians they do not know, these groups have also developed books, articles, and videotapes, focusing on the emotional and relational impact of litigation, for personal use.

A few insurance companies have well-established support programs available to their members. In addition to providing print resources, the Boston-based ProMutual insurance company, for example, oversees a program that provides informal peer and professional one-to-one counseling and support groups conducted by psychiatrists. The company has a relationship with professionals who offer confidential one-to-one or support group services to their members, and pays for these services without knowing the names of the members who are participating in the program. This program underscores the philosophy that a healthy clinician makes a better defendant who will be less vulnerable to future claims. This approach is supported by common sense and by research showing that a lack of social support often leads trauma victims to suffer a decline in mental health.[26]

Controlling the Controllable in Our Lives and Work

Many of us instinctively know how to bolster our battered self esteem by being active, doing things that reestablish our feelings of control over our work and our lives. We may recognize the measures identified by colleagues as helpful (Fig. 8–3).

INFORM OURSELVES ABOUT THE LEGAL PROCESS. Anticipation is one of the healthiest of the psychological defenses. We can use it by "looking ahead" at the sheer face of Mount Malpractice and adapting ourselves to its conditions so that we can scale it successfully. Developing some idea of the stages of the challenge and of how we fit into our case's defense prepares us to make the tricky ascent as sure-footed members of the defense team.

INTRODUCE GOOD RISK MANAGEMENT STRATEGIES INTO OUR PRACTICES. Risk management means that we actively identify the controllable events that may cause problems in our practice and then design and implement strategies to remedy them.

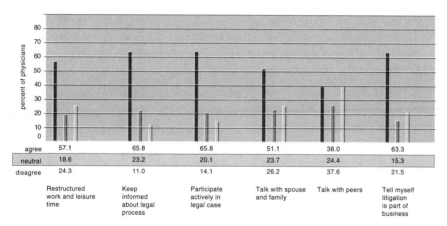

	Restructured work and leisure time	Keep informed about legal process	Participate actively in legal case	Talk with spouse and family	Talk with peers	Tell myself litigation is part of business
agree	57.1	65.8	65.8	51.1	38.0	63.3
neutral	18.6	23.2	20.1	23.7	24.4	15.3
disagree	24.3	11.0	14.1	26.2	37.6	21.5

Selected Coping Strategies

Figure 8–3. Selected coping strategies used by physicians. Adapted from Lisa Kelly-Wilson, Jennifer Parsons, and Sara C. Charles, "Physicians and Medical Malpractice Litigation," *Report to the Council of Medical Specialty Societies* (Chicago: Survey Research Laboratory, University of Illinois, 2003).

Most of us have taken courses in, or heard about, such recommended practices as appropriate documentation, informed consent, the management and flow of information and consultations, the character and conditions of our relationships with our patients and other professionals, scheduling and managing appointments, and the kind of incidents unique to our specialty that give rise to litigation.[27]

We presume that if we follow these recommendations, we will be less vulnerable to malpractice claims. Research, however, tells us these suggestions benefit in reduced claims vulnerability and lower payouts, for those of us who have already been sued—especially in such specialties as anesthesiology and obstetrics and gynecology—more than those who have never been sued.[28] Risk management education gives us concrete things to do that improve us as both clinicians and defendants; many of us, unfortunately, need to be sued before we recognize their pragmatic value and introduce them into our practices.

IMPLEMENT APPROPRIATE CHANGES IN OUR PRACTICE. A lawsuit offers us a fresh opportunity to conduct what may be a long contemplated but also long-delayed review of our office practices, office personnel, and modes of communication. This is the time to fill in the gaps in our procedures and evaluate and reassign problematic staff members.

DURING PERIODS OF INCREASED STRESS, REARRANGE OUR OFFICE AND SURGERY SCHEDULES. We can feel intensely preoccupied, anxious, or emotionally unsettled at certain points in litigation such as being served with our case papers, just before we give our deposition, and when we anticipate or actually enter the trial itself. Observing that our emotions are astir, we can prudently rearrange our schedules, call on our colleagues for help, or cancel activities that may compromise our care of patients.

AVOID SITUATIONS THAT GENERATE ANXIETY AND INCREASE RISK. We serve ourselves better to identify and avoid situations that make us feel anxious or ambivalent. Litigation may increase our anxiety about covering for our partner, taking call in the emergency department, performing certain procedures, or complying with what we feel are unreasonable demands. Situations similar to that which precipitated our lawsuit may understandably trip off anxiety alarms in us. We sometimes feel pressured to compromise our standards by patients or employers who urge us to exceed our expertise or to authorize nonindicated medications or procedures. If we are later sued over any event that occurs during a stressful period in which we are not convinced that we did our best, we compromise our ability to defend ourselves.

Some of us are better able than others to make changes that lessen our anxiety. A plastic surgeon stopped performing hand surgery, the focus of one of his malpractice suits and a nonessential component of his otherwise busy practice. He believes that by avoiding procedures that make him anxious and performing only those procedures with which he feels comfortable, he lessens his vulnerability to undue complications or mistakes.

Dr. Mary Santos was uneasy providing her patients with vaginal birth after caesarean section (VBAC), although it was recommended as a safe procedure by the profession.

> I sort of felt that I was participating in a dangerous activity (although) it was kind of unclear how dangerous it was at the beginning. I was getting very close to saying I wasn't going to do VBACs any more and I had been asking different people all over the country, "What do you think?" I had this sickly feeling that we were doing something that ten years from now we would say "What were we thinking?" My patient repeatedly expressed her absolute commitment to the VBAC procedure during her pregnancy and labor. I had a room next to the OR, I never left her side, anesthesia was present, I had one of my assistants present the whole time. The labor progressed to full dilation, there were variable decelerations, a scalp pH was 7.22, and the essentially dead baby was delivered within 30 minutes. I was never *not* present.

The patient sued, and after seven years, Dr. Santos won a 3½-week trial. Meanwhile, she and her group discontinued offering VBACs to their patients.[29]

REEVALUATE TIME COMMITMENTS. Until the moment we are sued, we may have devoted most of our lives—and time—to our work, perhaps to the detriment of our marriage, family, and social life. Taking a good, hard look at our lives in the total scheme of things—our values, our priorities, our ambitions, our long-term goals—may be difficult but it can lead to our improving the quality of our professional work and our personal lives. Many of us, for example, decide to change our pattern of practice or increase the time we invest in those nonmedical activities that make us feel more comfortable but which we were formerly too busy to even consider.

PARTICIPATE IN RELEVANT CONTINUING MEDICAL EDUCATION. This period offers the perfect opportunity to improve our professional knowledge base and skills, especially in the area at issue in our claim. We can profit from participation in such litigation-specific educational programs as risk management seminars and mock depositions and trials. Such medical and legal–based programs expand our professional competence and introduce us to experts who may serve as important resources for us. Increasing our competence directly increases the capital of our self-esteem and pays a dividend in improving our ability to defend ourselves in the legal arena.

SEEK CONSULTATION ON FINANCIAL AND ESTATE PLANNING. Every malpractice suit seeks compensation for the plaintiff, and we should be prudently concerned about how a settlement or jury verdict may affect us financially. To protect our assets from creditors and maintain our financial security, as discussed in Chapter

5, we must rely heavily on our financial advisors and our lawyers. We must choose only market-proven vehicles to shield our assets.[30] Getting our financial house in order is a great bulwark against anxiety during this period of increased risk for us and our families.

PARTICIPATE IN SUCH LEISURE-TIME ACTIVITIES AS ACTIVE SPORTS AND EXERCISE. We all understand that physical activity is a natural stress reducer. A suit's entrance into our lives may, however, eclipse our daily run or weekly golf game by drawing away our energy or interest in these healthy activities. Such reactions may tell us that we are either depressed or unduly preoccupied. Regardless of the cause, we take better care of ourselves by renewing our efforts to engage in some physical activity. If we do not have the energy to play tennis, we may participate in a workout or a personal training session. Reading and listening to music are good changes of pace when we are unable to exercise. We may interpret any long-term interruptions in our ability to use our leisure time constructively as our way of telling ourselves that we need professional consultation.

TAKE REGULAR VACATIONS AND TIME OFF FROM PRACTICE TO ENGAGE IN OTHER RESTORATIVE EXPERIENCES. Many physicians take time off only in conjunction with medicine-related educational activities. The long haul of litigation offers us the opportunity to reexamine and break away from this habitual response and to set time aside solely for leisure activities and vacation for us and our families. It takes enormous energy to run the legal gauntlet and still maintain emotional equilibrium and focus on our work. There is no better prescription than a good rest and a true vacation to relieve our accumulated fatigue and restore our zest for life and work.

> Dr. Thomas White's faith is "the most important part of my life." Coincidental with his recent lawsuit, he began yearly service at a mission hospital in Africa. He extols the gratifications associated with this work in which he does what physicians are trained to do, "save lives." African patients, who have a much higher rate of stillbirth and understand death as part of life, express gratitude for his life-saving efforts. He contrasts this with American patients who sue when a "stillbirth" occurs even when completely out of his control. Although mission work is inconvenient and economically costly to his practice, he feels this experience provides him with incomparable support to his professional commitment and an unparalleled opportunity to strengthen his spiritual life.[31]

SCHEDULE THE NECESSARY TIME TO PARTICIPATE IN THE DEFENSE OF THE CASE. We spend no time in our lives more wisely than that we give without stint in preparing for depositions, the various motions, and the climactic trial itself. If we are prepared and perform well, we may not prevail or win every one of these challenges, but we feel far better about ourselves than if we approached any of these tests in an ill-prepared or a casual manner. We may resent the time and money we seem to lose on such preparation but if, despite its frustrations and inconveniences, we do everything we can to be a "good defendant," whether we win or lose any of these engagements, we will prevail in the long run.

ACTIVELY MONITOR OUR EMOTIONAL AND PHYSICAL REACTIONS AND, IF INDI-CATED, SEEK APPROPRIATE CONSULTATION. We are better off when we take charge of our lives, observing our functioning and taking the necessary steps to maintain our good health, than if we leave others worried and wondering about whether we can do our work. We may develop symptoms that persist or are not easily managed. Not uncommonly, we invoke strenuous denial about our own symptoms, but we are better off if we can put aside our nonobjective distortions, acknowledge, and name our reactions accurately and, if necessary, seek appropriate professional help.

Controlling Our Thoughts: Changing the Meaning of the Event

NOURISH THE CONVICTION THAT WE ARE GOOD PHYSICIANS RATHER THAN BAD PHYSICIANS AS WE ARE PORTRAYED IN THE COMPLAINT. Eighty-seven percent of physicians in a recent study say that "telling myself I am a good physician" is their most frequent coping strategy for dealing with litigation.[32] This is not just an empty incantation but rather a statement that, based on a review of our overall careers, we can make truthfully. All of us have had bad outcomes, have made judgments we regret, and have made choices we would now reconsider. Nonetheless, most of our patients have done well and benefited from our care. We may have only one malpractice claim in our entire career. For a host of reasons beyond anyone's control, we may eventually settle it out or even lose at trial. Viewing this lawsuit in the context of our entire career keeps it, and us, in healthy perspective.

The psychological energy we spend doing this is a wise investment that we make repeatedly by reminding ourselves of our competence and successes. Knowing that we are competent and good at what we do, enjoy good relationships with our patients, and are esteemed by our staff and colleagues: these convictions provide a sturdy shield against the volleys of accusation loosed at us right up to the last day of the trial.

RECOGNIZE A FUNDAMENTAL TRUTH: THE TORT SYSTEM IS ABOUT COMPENSA-TION, NOT COMPETENCE. Even though almost no case can be tried without testimony from expert witnesses who either support or criticize our approach to the care of the patient, we recognize that such testimony is far from the last word on assessing our competence. Some cases are based on clear incompetence but, of itself, a lawsuit does not necessarily establish that fact. The goal of any lawsuit is to obtain compensation, and, in many cases, the hope of the plaintiff attorneys is that the outcome is so tragic, that the events that led to the outcome are sufficiently murky or complex, or that the jury becomes so sympathetic to the injured patient that, regardless of the facts, the provision of compensation will seem inevitable and irresistible. This understanding of the real world purpose of tort law allows many physicians to interpret their involvement in litigation as just part of doing business.

When Dr. Cynthia Davis was deciding whether to file a lawsuit because of what she perceived to be one of her physician's misdiagnosis, her lawyer assured her that her suit would not cause her former physician any personal suffering. His insurance rates might increase but the insurance company would pay any judgment. "So I felt better about that," she said, "that there was a system to handle these kinds of injuries."[33]

RECOGNIZE THAT LAWYERS AND PHYSICIANS VIEW LITIGATION IN DIFFERENT WAYS. Very good lawyers may caution us that, in our lawsuit, "the truth may or may not eventually come out." Lawsuits do not usually happen because something is clearly right or wrong or because the facts are clearly evident. They are born out of differing views of the same events. For those of us who have read depositions and have been on trial, one of the most disappointing, and sometimes shocking, discoveries comes from the participants who, from our perspective, under oath, distort or completely violate the truth. It is more philosophical than cynical to face the hard reality that as much as we want and need the full truth to surface, we may have to settle for less than that.

BE KIND TO OURSELVES AS WE WORK TO UNDERSTAND THE "TRUTH" OF THE CASE. Our legal and insurance counsels spend many hours reviewing our perception of the case along with the differing views of various experts and others. They try to prepare us for how the opposing side, and eventually a jury, may view or react to the case or certain facts associated with it. It is not always easy to take a retrospective look at alternate ways of approaching the care of the patient, of using a surgical technique that may have fewer potential complications, or of choosing another option in communicating that would have made a difference. It takes time, a measure of humility, and hard work to examine and to absorb these other scenarios. We also need to be patient with ourselves as we work to expand our perceptions and thereby become better defendants at the same time.

Dealing with Our Relationships During Litigation: Unnamed Defendants

Dr. Joseph Daley admonishes his younger colleagues:

> I tell them to be prepared to have this intruding on their daily life and to warn their spouse about what is coming and ask for their understanding because I think that's

the thing that's hard to accept. You're just brooding all the time. You're in the middle of doing something that you enjoy doing and suddenly the suit pops up and the whole process just keeps going. You're not as happy or as interested in doing fun things that normally you would be doing with the kids. Sort of withdrawn into the inner self. Even after the case is resolved, it will persist.[34]

Our Marriage

Lawsuits markedly affect our most intimate relationships, especially our marriage. Our first decision is whether we are going to share that we have been sued with our spouse or our closest intimate, a decision that sets the stage for our emotional life during our long passage through the lawsuit. What we choose to do, of course, is a function of the strength of our relationships as well as of our personality style. Most of us choose what, for various reasons, suits us even though this choice will influence and perhaps alter our life dramatically.

Ideally, we find our richest source of support in our spouses or others close to us. We share our innermost feelings with our closest confidant and feel not only understood but also cherished by their responses. They may not always appreciate our obsessions about the medical details, but they do know how deeply we feel for the affected patient and family and sense and understand the emotional costs of being charged with negligence.

Only our spouse knows the dedication we feel or how hard we work to maintain our competence. They reinforce daily our own efforts to reassure ourselves that we are good physicians. Empathic spouses not only absorb our irritability but also share our worrisome nighttime vigils while maintaining a daytime calm in our family life, shielding us from unreasonable demands, and managing our social life. Supportive spouses understand rather than resent the time preempted from leisure and family activities by the multifaceted obligations of defending ourselves legally. We may be too preoccupied at the time to notice the generosity and graciousness with which they support us and maintain a balanced environment around us.

Spouses reveal their dedication when they actively join themselves to our battle to defend our integrity and honor. A dermatologist's wife describes becoming almost an expert in malignant melanoma, the clinical focus of her husband's lawsuit. She searched the literature, developed summaries for the defense team, attended depositions, and, at the time of trial, filled the courtroom with a supportive group of family and friends. The message to the jury that eventually acquitted her husband was of how highly he was esteemed by his colleagues and his community.

Not everyone is so fortunate. Some physicians characteristically keep work issues to themselves, not wanting to bother their spouses by making them privy to such concerns. When they are sued, they may be too ashamed or traumatized to share their deep feelings about their work with their spouses if they have never done it before. The stories of those physicians who choose to handle the situation on their own and muffle their suffering, as they habitually do, in silence, overwhelm their ability to tell them or to recount their side effects. This falsely shrouded suffering can manifest itself in an array of behaviors and symptoms that, easily misinterpreted by even those close to them, undercut them and complicate their lives. How are spouses to understand when their physician spouses, usually as in control of their world and in command of their feelings as a Gary Cooper cowboy hero, become increasingly preoccupied and irritable, replacing any interest in sexual or romantic life with growling ruminations on sleepless nights, seeming to become different persons supplanting their interest in their families with their absorption with a secret they hesitate to share—that they are being sued for malpractice?

Spouses cannot miss our backing away into emotional distance, our spending ever more time at work, and our coming home, persons cut off seeking solitary rest. Such combustible scenarios flare up easily into misunderstandings, accusations, and even bitter arguments. Such a wartime atmosphere can endure for months and sometimes years. It is not uncommon for spouses to feel so shut out of intimacy with us that they suspect that we are involved with another person. The possibilities of unnecessary pain and even separation are high unless we reject passivity and fully incorporate our poorly informed but long-suffering and frustrated spouses into full partnership with us in suffering the trauma of being accused of negligence.

It is possible that after sharing our distress about the lawsuit, we are disappointed in our spouse's lack of understanding and inability to offer us support. Just as we need our spouses to understand how preoccupied we are and how unhappy we feel, so they need us to understand and appreciate their bewilderment and the world they are trying to hold together. To secure the objective of protecting and strengthening our marriage during the sometimes protracted siege of litigation, we must recognize just how hard and how patiently we must work together to enlarge our mutual understanding.

> Dr. Henry Clark managed his first malpractice suit well, developed no real symptoms, and, within a year, settled for a minimum amount of damages. Seven years later, a fellow physician filed a complaint against Dr. Clark on behalf of his birth-injured child. Dr. Clark was devastated and poured his heart out to his wife of 20 years. She responded by telling him that his work was becoming too preoccupying, not worth the cost to him, and that he should give up his obstetrical practice. He felt that her response totally missed his concerns since, even though it was fraught with difficulties, he loved his work. She made no real effort, in his view, to understand his concerns. She seemed to dismiss his distress and began to complain to him about his lack of sexual interest and his withdrawal from family activities. During this period, feeling increasingly alienated from his wife, he confided in his office nurse who seemed solicitous of his concerns. Within eight months, he separated from his wife and began an affair with the nurse that eventually led to marriage.

Our Family

During litigation, we apply ourselves earnestly to keep our emotional balance at work so that we can offer our patients our full attention and skills. When we go home, our feeling that we can lower our guard can result in our being moody, irritable, and short-fused with those closest to us. We may opt out of long-planned family events, criticize our spouses for minor inconveniences, yell at the children, slam the door, or kick the dog. We may attempt to soothe our discomfort with excessive drinking or television viewing, isolating behaviors that further complicate our relationships

Our best approach requires that we work at becoming aware of our own reactions and better at monitoring our effect on others. Such self-knowledge gradually enables us to reduce abrasive behaviors and to make constructive changes in our responses to others. At the least, we can begin to talk calmly and openly about what we are experiencing so that our spouses and families can understand the reaction that otherwise puzzles and frustrates them.

Being sued affects and changes family dynamics. Our maturity in managing this event and our family relationships may ultimately lead to strengthening our initially tested family ties.

Our Children

Older children, who may be physicians themselves, offer significant support to their sued parents. Shielded as children from our problems, they may be parents themselves and understand adult burdens. If we have recognized and appreciated their growth, we can be fortified by sharing our distress about our malpractice suit with them.

Older children often demonstrate an amazing capacity for understanding and solicitude. Serving as confidants to one or both parents, they are able to mediate and alert one or the other about their sometimes separate concerns. A grown daughter may tell her father of her mother's feeling that he does not appreciate how hard she works to manage their life so that he will not have to bear that burden. So informed by a daughter, the father may respond with positive tactics, such as a weekend get-a-way with his wife or a special dinner with close friends at which the conversation will broaden everyone's perspective on their current life stresses. So, too, the son can talk to his father about the latter's excessive ruminating and drinking alone, suggesting such positive alternatives as a golf game together, helping to snap the bad habits before they bring further sadness and disruption to the family. The active support of older children deepens family relationships, endowing them with a richness that, lacking such a crisis, they might not otherwise achieve.

Younger children must be informed in ways that match and do not excessively tax them based on their age or their capacity to understand. We may offer young children simplified versions of what is going on: Daddy or Mommy is having problems at work that may make them seem upset but they do not mean to be irritable and unhappy with the children and it is certainly not their children's fault. The success of this approach depends on how well we monitor our feelings and behavior so that when we notice, for example, that we are overreacting to the child's untidy room, we can explain our reaction and apologize immediately.

Special problems arise when the lawsuit receives media attention. Children need to have available some explanation that they can understand easily and tell their friends and that they can use if others taunt them with news reports about litigation involving a parent. This can be complicated if the lawyers who initiated the action are the parents of their friends. Part of what children need to learn is that when people are sick, sometimes bad things may happen. These injured people can get money from the insurance company to take care of their problems only if they sue the physician. This does not mean that we are bad physicians, that we deliberately hurt people, or that we are criminals. There is no chance of our going to prison because of this, but these episodes in our family life may last for a while and we may have to go to court before we can get everything settled. Some version of this explanation usually allays their anxiety. Children have an amazing capacity to sense our feelings and the more open and, at the same time, protective we are of their feelings, the healthier it is for all of us.

Our Social and Professional Life

Our prelitigation manner of relating to our extended family, our medical colleagues, and our friends and acquaintances will be mirrored in our postlitigation relationships. The more intimate we are with members of our extended family—parents, siblings, aunts, and uncles—before we are sued, the more easily we can confide in them after the suit is filed. We may share our situation with close friends and trustworthy staff members, or we may continue in our usual style of confiding only in those closest to us. As all of us know, even with the best of intentions, it is difficult to change our behavior.

> Dr. Paul Young describes his family as a "typical" midwestern clan. The men in the family hunt and fish together, talk politics, and enjoy exchanging barbs and jokes. The women talk about children, recipes, and vacations, without mentioning their individual troubles. Learning that his anesthesiologist cousin had been sued, he felt impelled, given his own experience with litigation, to schedule a fishing trip with him so that they could talk. He describes fishing for most of a weekend, talking constantly, but never once broaching the subject of either his own or his cousin's lawsuit. Although neither changed their usual style of relating and they were aware that talking about their concerns might have been helpful, they nonetheless each expressed satisfaction about sharing the weekend "away."

Colleagues may suspect we have been sued after we experience a widely known catastrophic outcome but hesitate to mention the subject. Sometimes it is helpful, especially for senior physicians or department chairmen, to approach colleagues, of whose suit they have knowledge or suspicions, and offer to talk with them about it. They can be especially helpful if they have been through the process themselves. Our partners and other colleagues can be even more helpful, as we have noted, if they know that we are in the midst of a lawsuit, switching coverage, for example, because they understand that we need extra time to attend to it. Uninformed, they will not know that our request for time away is to attend our trial and not just a vacation. It is far better to be accepted with understanding and support than to invite hard feelings into our lives because of our frequent unexplained absences.

Sometimes we sense that one or more of our colleagues, especially those who are well-meaning family friends of the potential plaintiff, are involved in the case. They may have made remarks to the patient that proved instrumental in the plaintiff's filing of the lawsuit, they may be serving as an expert witness, or they may have a social relationship with one of the litigants. There is no easy cure for the disruption this can introduce into previously harmonious relationships.

Dr. Cynthia Davis had a good friend who had repeatedly expressed her concern about Davis's eye problem. Finally, she insisted that Davis consult with another of her friends, an ophthalmologist who Davis later sued.

> So I thought, I cannot tell her that this has happened. She was upset that she didn't act in time, didn't refer me soon enough; how is she going to feel now if the physician she referred me to screwed up? And so while the jury trial was going on, she called me several times and she said, "What's going on, how's everything, how are you doing?" And I told her nothing about this because I had resolved not to tell her anything. I didn't know she knew. I wouldn't have told her. She was withholding and I was withholding. My motivation was to protect her. Her motivation was she was very angry with me because I hadn't told her. Then afterward, she called me and said, "Okay, I know all about it, tell me, I'm very angry. A friend wouldn't do this; I can't trust you; we're done." That was very stressful. So she and I met and we didn't exactly resolve it but at least she resolved to be my friend. And so it was touch and go, a little tentative, tense for the next year but it's behind us now. I wouldn't say we're back as close but we're back as friends.[35]

Such rifts and estrangements in the medical community are among the unintended, but very real, consequences of the litigation explosion. On the other hand, the support of colleagues who, on principle, willingly serve as expert witnesses on our behalf is heartwarming. None of us could successfully defend our case without the testimony of colleagues who are willing to study the case and place themselves and their reputations on the line to stand by us.

Personal physicians constitute unique resources for physicians who have been sued, as mentioned in Chapter 5, offering not only support but also sensible advice on managing our health and minimizing the stress associated with a lawsuit.

We must manage our relationships with the office staff in our own way. When we tell our staff about our situation, their knowledge of the stages of litigation and what it demands of us makes them supportive, solicitous, and protective.

Dr. White still wonders what his staff thought about the noisy summons delivery. Now that his case is successfully dismissed, he thinks about asking them what they thought of him during those hectic years of legal involvement.

Our relationships within our church or faith community can also give us significant support. We can pray and share our predicament with our priest, rabbi, or minister, with our Bible study group, or with other members and leaders of our religious community.

Others of us, especially obstetrician-gynecologists, tell our patients of our lawsuits, especially when they are highly publicized, and offer them the option to choose other physicians. Such informed patients almost overwhelmingly appreciate knowing about the lawsuit, express confidence in us, and respond with their support.

Dr. West reflects about her recent loss at a highly publicized trial.

> If I lose some patients, I'm too busy anyway. I tried to be an example, actually for my younger physicians, and show them life goes on. I'm sued, I'm humiliated, and I'm on the nightly news, the radio and the newspaper. But, guess what, I'm still earning a living, I still have my family, my patients are sending me flowers and writing me sweet notes. Some left. But I don't know who they are. My partner got the same thing. So, it didn't in the long run make any difference other than I think we're both a little embittered, I maybe more than she is, in that we like to practice medicine, even though you say to yourself, "I'm not going to care about these people anymore," but you still do. [36]

Seeking Consultation: When We Can Do It Better with Help

Sometimes we may be overwhelmed by our involvement in litigation, and the stress is intensified if we are preoccupied with other personal or professional problems. We may observe changes in our behavior, our mood, or our ability to focus and concentrate or are gradually drinking more after we arrive home, angrier and more isolated. We are unpleasant company, irritable with our spouses and children, and we cannot miss the way our staff seems to be giving us "plenty of space." Our pleasure in our work and our life in general is greatly compromised because our case is not moving toward resolution. We find that our once reliable means of reducing our irritability and stress, such as jogging, taking naps, reading, listening to music, or working out, now fail us. Can we possibly do anything about this situation? In fact, we are the only ones who *can* do something about it.

We may, however, finally need to face the truth: We must become, at least temporarily, a patient, a person who both suffers and endures. We generally perceive this state as being one of dependency, with its implications that we lack control and that we are, in some measure at least, failures.[37] It is not uncommon for us to minimize our symptoms [38] or, in situations in which we observe ourselves accurately as having either a physical or an emotional problem, to delay getting help, arguing that we need to be sure of the diagnosis. How many of us have talked our colleagues into running a laboratory test or taking a radiograph or magnetic resonance image, or done so ourselves, to verify a suspected condition before checking in with our own physician? Armed with our tentative diagnosis that maintains our sense of some control over the situation, we can then safely seek consultation with our physician, already anticipating what the further workup and treatment will involve so that we experience less anxiety than those unprepared for such examinations.

We often fail to take the advice we give to patients with suspected hypertension, depressive symptoms, or periodic chest pain that they need to be evaluated and treated properly. We know that safe and effective treatments are available that will not interfere with, but rather enhance, our ability to work comfortably. Why, then, do we still resist seeking such a consult? Because we feel threatened when we depend on another's judgment, or, as noted in Chapter 4, we fear unnecessarily the consequences of seeking any treatment that may trigger an examination of our licensure status. Such evasion does not serve us or our patients well.

Unfortunately, our personal physicians sometimes conspire against us for being our worst enemies as we struggle to get help. Let us return to Mike Wallace.

> "My own physician, to whom I still go, missed it completely." He had discounted the journalist's complaints about depression, thinking him "too strong." "And it got worse. Finally, it got so bad, I wanted out of there real bad." Thinking it would get his mind off his obsessions about his trial, he traveled to Ethiopia on assignment. Upon his return, he was hospitalized for severe flu-like symptoms but also for "feeling down, shooting pains in my arms and so forth. . . ." He was told after consultation with the chief psychiatrist, "Mr. Wallace, you're having a clinical depression." He accepted the recommendation of antidepressants and psychotherapy. After his trial, feeling relieved and less depressed, he left therapy against the advice of his psychiatrist. "Within a week, I was playing tennis, fell and broke my wrist and, boom, I was back in a depression. It really was the same thing all over again." He returned to therapy, was successfully treated, and now still requires, what he refers to as, a periodic "lube job."[39]

Obtaining Psychotherapy

Some of us may not experience a major illness during the litigation but do experience disturbing symptoms and preoccupations. The threat posed by litigation may open up old wounds related to earlier life experiences of loss or of misunderstandings that remain unresolved. Formal psychotherapy, either individual or in a group setting, can be enormously helpful in successfully managing such situations.

We may also take advantage of previously noted opportunities offered through our insurer or we may individually choose a therapist who can offer support and understanding as we work through the trauma we sustain through the adverse event and the litigation that follows. Because finding the right therapist may take time, friends or colleagues may help us find the appropriate resource. One physician tells of consulting with three or four therapists before finding the one with whom she felt that she could work. We need first to feel safe, valued, and understood before we can plumb the true feelings in our depths. The risk involved in locating the professional who can really help us, if needed, is worth taking. Mike Wallace says of his psychiatrist, "He saved my life."[40]

The Focus of Psychotherapy

Therapists who treat sued physicians will recognize the themes that Horowitz[41] describes in the therapy of those who have suffered a traumatic event. Even those of us who do not seek therapy can identify with these motifs, the ideas and feelings related to the adverse event that generated our case and that may persist long after the resolution of the case. Many physicians find help useful in dealing with these feelings common to the process of litigation and find that if they do, they become more effective defendants.

Fears of the Same Thing Happening Again

Previously cited data support the idea that our being sued sensitizes and motivates us to make changes in our practices that we believe will prevent the same event from recurring. We should not, however, allow phobic avoidance to motivate us— that is, out of fear, rather than in a reasoned evaluation of our total situation—to make significant changes in our personal or professional lives. We should discuss all of our options with a third party, perhaps a neutral therapist, before we stop doing, out of fear of being sued again, certain kinds of work, performing selected procedures, or drastically altering our clinical time.

Shame over Our Vulnerability or Feelings of Incompetence

We may experience some difficulty putting this one event, in a career of thousands of successful events, into a reassuring and realistic perspective. Indeed, we may require objective help from somebody else to achieve this healthy sense of proportion. This mediation allows us, within a safe environment and with an empathic person, to take a look at ourselves in relationship to the event in its context.

Intense Anger

Being named in a malpractice suit unleashes rage, sometimes at the patient but, more often, at the many agents of the suit—the lawyers, the system, or the media. Although this rage is by no means all negative, we cannot allow its energies to overflow our lives and we must learn how to direct it into pursuits. Saul Bellow shares his feelings:

> You don't know what to do with your feelings of outrage. You say to yourself, "It's hopeless for me to be outraged." So it's just a waste of the emotional energy. But at the same time, you feel old-fashioned Shakespearean outrage. Murderous. These people . . . took pleasure in pouring it on because I was a writer. You have these classic emotions. I'd say Shakespearean or Dickensian, that you're helpless and these guys are giving you a going over so you feel outrage. And then you realize how foolish it is to be outraged because it generates a lot of emotional energy and it isn't doing you any good at all.[42]

Although ranting about the "system" may be understandable, it is far more healthy and useful for us to volunteer our time to work for our colleagues and our cause within the insurance company and medical society or in supporting our distressed colleagues.

Extreme Sensitivity to Guilt

To avoid taking on more responsibility than we may have for what happened, we must assess our role as objectively as possible, making the adaptations necessary to assess, accept, and absorb the reality of the situation. While some of us may be able to do this for ourselves, others may require a helping and supportive hand to achieve enough distance to examine the event thoroughly and realistically.

Rage at Those Exempted

The system, as many of us characterize it, places unfair demands on us, holding us to a higher professional standard than any other group in society. Why are some of us, such as Dr. Allen, caught in the law's net while the patient's primary physician, the orthopedic surgeon, escapes it? Being angry at such situations wears away at us, interfering with doing our work well and offering us a warning to find alternative ways to cope with this consuming rage.

Unresolved Grief

During a lawsuit, we always lose something, sometimes many things, including the patient through death or severe injury, our reputations, our referral base, and our smooth relationships with our patients and colleagues and with our family and friends. We need time and perspective to assess the actual losses we experience because of the outcome and time beyond that to resolve our feelings about them. We place ourselves at the greatest risk if we surrender to pervasive despair about the entire malpractice environment, becoming negative and passive in ways that deepen our depression, making our last state worse than our first.

Discovery: Gaining a Foothold for the Defense

> When my adversary has drafted his writ against me, I shall wear it on my shoulder. And bind it round my head like a royal turban. I will give him an account of every step of my life and go as boldly as a prince to meet him.
> —Job 31:36–40[1]

Within a time schedule set by the court, our lawyer responds with an appearance, that is, a letter to the plaintiff's attorney setting down the ground rules agreed to by both lawyers. These terms of engagement allow the defense to challenge, through filing arguments, the "sufficiency" of the plaintiff's case. This instrument also defers a formal filing of the answer to the charges until this phase, known as the "pleadings," is completed.

Our lawyers eventually file an answer, which includes specific denials of each and every allegation of the complaint coupled with a request that the court dismiss the claim in its entirety. These pleadings can be amended throughout the discovery process up to and including the trial phase. We should not be surprised, during this period, when plaintiffs amend their complaint or we amend our answer.

Forms of Pretrial Discovery

Both in every state and in federal court, parties to a lawsuit engage in some form of discovery. The goal for both sides in discovery is to learn everything possible about each other's case before trial so that they can make intelligent decisions about how to manage the case.

Interrogatories

Pretrial discovery can take the form of written questions, or interrogatories. Each side asks the other to respond, under the seal of an oath, about background facts and information concerning the parties and any witnesses who may be called in the event of a trial. This first purpose of the process is to narrow the case's factual issues and to assist the lawyers in developing questions for depositions. In jurisdictions where "requests for admissions of facts" are allowed, interrogatories also produce valuable evidence to support requests that are used to establish that certain key facts are not in dispute. We usually participate in our lawyer's drafting interrogatories to the plaintiff and responses to the plaintiff's interrogatories to us.

Requests for Admission of Documents

To simplify the trial procedures that govern the introduction of documents as evidence, lawyers may use a "request for admission of genuineness of documents" whose purpose may be, for example, verification of the identity of medical records from another state. Discovery can also include "requests for production" that, as with interrogatories, are designed to flush out the opponent's documentary evidence. In most states, these requests are exchanged under oath, so anything less than full disclosure can result in monetary sanctions and the striking of allegations or answers, actions that can be legally damaging for those sanctioned.

Our lawyer uses this process to obtain all medical records concerning the plaintiff regardless of where or when the treatment occurred. Such a complete medical record history of the plaintiff may reveal the actual, or a contributing, cause of the injury that the plaintiff has attributed solely to our negligence. Lawyers may also use materials from the record to test the credibility of plaintiffs in their deposition.

Disclosure Before Trial

Most states and the federal court system allow broad discovery with disclosure of the findings before trial. Each side discloses the names of their witnesses, including experts. After the lawyers for both sides depose or question these witnesses under oath, they provide summaries of their proposed testimony. By the time the case is ready for trial, each side knows almost everything about the strengths and weaknesses of the other side's case. In view of full dockets and limited courtroom space, judges encourage broad discovery as a way to motivate the parties to settle or request dismissal before the case goes to trial.

We should actively familiarize ourselves with the rules relating to disclosure and the pretrial depositions of experts in our particular state. Oregon is one of the few states that prohibit pretrial disclosure of expert witness identities or their testimony. This limited discovery approach, known with mild cynicism as "trial by ambush," is the exception rather than the rule. In limited discovery, defense lawyers do not have the opportunity to depose the other side's expert and must conduct their cross-examination without benefit of pretrial preparation. Familiarity with experts from previous trials, however, gives defense attorneys some sense of their style and credibility.

Exploring the merits of the opponent's case in discovery may consume a substantial portion of the time it takes to resolve a claim. The trial therefore becomes less a forum for learning the other side's evidence and more a venue for determining which side has the most persuasive facts, opinions, and arguments.

Depositions

Judges give attorneys wide latitude in pursuing avenues of discovery, allowing them to ask questions and elicit answers about many matters that they would not admit into evidence in a trial. Such questions are justified by the evidentiary rules that foresee that the answers to these inquiries may lead to other admissible evidence. Physicians should expect attorneys on both sides to cast wide nets in their pretrial searches.

Our Deposition

It is almost certain that we will be deposed during the discovery process, that is, be questioned, under oath with a court reporter present just as in the courtroom. Attorneys for both sides are present and participate in our examination and cross-examination. Our deposition testimony is evidence that will influence, perhaps decisively, the outcome of the matter at issue. Even though depositions are taken in a setting less formal than the courtroom, in the lawyer's office, for example, and without a judge or jury present, it does not mean that we can lower our guard or approach the experience casually.

We learn how best to collaborate with our attorneys and come to appreciate that, just like us, they possess skills that serve us well in some ways but not in others. Because each case is different, our experience of doing well in one deposition does not justify our lowering our vigilance or lessening our preparation for a future one. As Dr. Laura West tells us, familiarity with the process is not the only criterion for giving a good deposition:

> I was smarter at giving a deposition the first time I ever did than with some of the other ones that I've given. Just try to do what you're supposed to do. Just answer the questions, don't give any other information. My deposition in this last case was poor. I just didn't stay on track. Maybe I had been up. I don't know if I had taken call, I just wasn't at my best that particular day. The best things to do are just know the case backwards and forwards and do exactly what your lawyer says. They know the law.[2]

General Directions for Our Deposition

Nothing less than thorough preparation for our deposition, including practice questions and answers, as well as testing our reactions to techniques used by plaintiff lawyers to upset and unnerve us will suffice. Our lawyer will outline the contents of a good deposition and offer us a list of key points to follow in preparing ourselves to perform well. The following generally helpful suggestions are not legal advice; we should follow the lead of our attorney in specific circumstances.

TELL THE TRUTH. Just before jury deliberations begin, the judge instructs the jurors on the law and on how to judge the credibility of witnesses. In many jurisdictions, the standard instruction is that witnesses shown to be false in one part of their testimony are to be disregarded in all other parts. A single untruthful answer, even if given without intent to mislead or deceive, can destroy our defense. To give a truthful answer we must both hear and fully understand the question. We make a mistake whenever we assume that we know what the questioner means when they ask us: "She said you were not paying attention the second time she brought this up. Is that true?" To answer that question truthfully, we must understand who "she" is, when "the second time" was, and what "she brought up."

MANAGE OUR FEELINGS. Most of us are angry about being sued and about accusations that we failed to take proper care of our patients. Experienced plaintiff attorneys look for ways to agitate our already roiled feelings to make us express our anger and frustration. Venting such emotions not only shatters our calm attitude and demeanor but also, more decisively, robs us of our ability to listen and respond accurately to questions. Successful defendants immunize themselves against the implied criticism, sarcasm, or derision with which opposing counsel may lace their tactically hostile questions. We should respond to the disagreeable questions of the lawyer with an enlarged calm and increased self-control. Hostility may be the other side's sole weapon. If we are not cowed by such hostile approaches into making mistakes or errors in our testimony, these histrionic maneuvers may subvert their own case.

LISTEN TO THE QUESTION ASKED AND ANSWER ONLY THAT QUESTION UNLESS SOME FURTHER EXPLANATION IS REQUIRED. Imagine a target with a bull's eye surrounded by concentric circles. A well-experienced attorney tells us that our answers should be aimed at and limited to the bull's eye and we should shape answers that will be precisely on target.

QUESTION: When did you finish your residency?

INAPPROPRIATE ANSWER: I finished my residency at Stanford University Medical Center in 1987.

APPROPRIATE ANSWER: 1987.

QUESTION: Have you been sued before?

INAPPROPRIATE ANSWER: I've had no other lawsuits but I have reported several incidents to my insurer that never became suits.

APPROPRIATE ANSWER: No.

TAKE TIME TO ANSWER THE QUESTIONS. Some questioners try to get us to say more than we need to by asking, in staccato fashion, questions that can only be answered "yes." They then append a key question, banking on our giving the automatic "yes" answer. Accepting the cadence of the questioner, we may later regret our hasty and erroneous answer. By listening with care to each individual question, we can avoid making the serious admissions that these trap-like inquiries are designed to manipulate out of us. If Rule One is never to feel rushed in a deposition, Rule Two tells us never to worry about how much time we take to think through and understand questions. This is why setting aside sufficient time for our depositions allows us to feel relaxed and unhurried.

AVOID THE NATURAL IMPULSE TO TEACH. We know a great deal about the medicine of our specialty and are usually highly experienced in delivering care in a safe, efficient manner. Some lawyers appeal to this expertise and prompt us to educate them, playing the unsophisticated dumb country lawyer, fumbling the vocabulary, mixing up the anatomy, and appearing unfamiliar with the chart. Beware of lawyers bearing such gifts and educate them only at your own peril. The best deposition witnesses follow their lawyer's advice and answer questions narrowly, volunteering as little information as possible and withholding correction of even inaccurate science and loosely constructed hypotheses.

QUESTION: Since 80% of women who have a CA-125 of less than 15 units have the likelihood of malignant disease, how do you explain your failure to consider that your patient had ovarian cancer?

Inappropriate answer: Well, that is not correct. The data suggest that patients whose CA-125 is greater than 35 units have a greater likelihood of malignant ovarian cancer and. . . .

APPROPRIATE ANSWER: I am unable to answer the question as you have stated it.

RECOGNIZE THAT HINDSIGHT IS NOT ADMISSIBLE. It is almost second nature for physicians to evaluate their care of patients openly and honestly and to value the judgments and criticisms of their peers. In retrospect, much can be said about any and every decision we make in real time with limited information. In a lawsuit, however, the focus is on events as they occurred at the time of the incident. Our lawyer will prepare us to answer this line of questioning, but we must restrain ourselves from peering back through the lens of the plaintiff lawyer's "retrospectoscope."

QUESTION: Doctor, wouldn't you have avoided severing the patient's common bile duct had you opened the patient immediately rather than continuing laproscopically?

INAPPROPRIATE RESPONSE: Well, yes, I guess I could have prevented the bile duct problem if I had opened the patient immediately.

APPROPRIATE RESPONSE: In the circumstances at the time, my decision was both clinically appropriate and in keeping with the community standard.

GAUGE THE ATTORNEY'S EXPERIENCE. Not all plaintiff lawyers are skilled in prosecuting medical malpractice claims. Lawyers without trial experience may and do bring negligence cases to trial. During discovery, inexperienced lawyers often make serious mistakes. They may, for example, ask questions that expose their own theory of the case: "Isn't it true, doctor, that someone in the OR warned you several times that. . . ." This alerts our counsel to investigate which staff member in the OR may have issued a warning. The plaintiff attorney may also unwittingly reveal problems that could confront us later as a witness, giving our defense counsel the opportunity to remedy the situation with us before trial.

The Plaintiff Attorneys' Goals

PLAINTIFF ATTORNEYS NEED TO ESTABLISH WHAT WE KNOW AND, MORE IMPORTANT, WHAT WE DO NOT KNOW. If, during our deposition, the plaintiff lawyer fails to pin us down on key facts or does not establish our lack of knowledge about them, we may be able to present previously unrevealed information that can turn a trial in our favor.

PLAINTIFF ATTORNEYS WILL TRY TO CAPITALIZE ON OUR LEGAL NAIVETÉ AND GET US TO MAKE ADMISSIONS THAT CAN BE USED AT TRIAL.

QUESTION: Doctor, are you familiar with Smith's text on orthopedic surgery?

APPROPRIATE RESPONSE: Yes, I am familiar with it.

QUESTION: Well, then, doctor, you recognize this text as authoritative, do you not?

INAPPROPRIATE RESPONSE: Yes.

APPROPRIATE RESPONSE: It is one of many useful texts.

This may seem like an innocent enough question about a text that, in scientific terms, may be authoritative. Legally, however, an affirmative answer may also be a potential bombshell. The plaintiff attorney can use our "yes" and our endorsement of it as an authoritative text to turn it into an expert witness against us by reading passages that contradict what we have said on the stand or in our deposition.

PLAINTIFF ATTORNEYS MAY ASK TRICK QUESTIONS TO CAUSE US TO MAKE AD-
MISSIONS THAT CAN BE USED AT TRIAL.

> QUESTION: Doctor, are you aware that when my client told his current doctor that
> you performed the surgery that left him crippled, Dr. Brown just rolled his eyes
> and shook his head?
>
> INAPPROPRIATE RESPONSE: Well, Dr. Brown has always been critical of my work
> and is responsible for generating several other lawsuits against me.
>
> APPROPRIATE RESPONSE: First, I was not aware of that. And second, I know of no
> reason why Dr. Brown would act that way. My care was completely appropriate
> and my patient's injury was an unfortunate but known side effect of the proce-
> dure, which I covered fully in the informed consent conference.

The inappropriate response opens up new lines of questioning. The lawyer may
then ask what inspired Dr. Brown's criticism as well as about the other cases we
mentioned. Neither of these lines of inquiry would have opened up had we answered the question appropriately.

PLAINTIFF ATTORNEYS GAUGE OUR STRENGTHS AND WEAKNESSES AS WIT-
NESSES. Are we easily rattled or confused under intense questioning? Do we take
the bait proffered by the plaintiff lawyer's challenges to our competency or in his
insinuations that we are reckless or greedy? These lawyers also recognize when
we are charismatic, unflappable, and articulate professionals. The credibility of
the witnesses can determine the outcome of any case. If we have performed well
in a deposition and the plaintiff's witnesses perform poorly, the plaintiff attorneys may re-think whether they should continue with the case.

PLAINTIFF ATTORNEYS MAY USE OUR DEPOSITION TO IDENTIFY OTHER WITNESSES,
DOCUMENTS, OR EVIDENCE OF POTENTIAL VALUE. We may testify to the complex
jumble of events surrounding our decision to perform an emergency cesarean
section during a particularly difficult delivery. While the plaintiff lawyer will attempt to pin us down on the facts, as we believed them to be, he will also search
our testimony for mention of other witnesses whom they may call as potential
defendants or as witnesses who may contradict our version of what happened. The
plaintiff lawyer may even ask us for the names of persons, other than our lawyer,
to whom we have spoken about the case.

> QUESTION: Doctor, please name any individuals with whom you have discussed
> this case.
>
> APPROPRIATE RESPONSE: Aside from my lawyer, I have mentioned that I have
> been sued to some individuals and may have told them how I felt about it but I
> have not discussed the facts or circumstances of the case with anyone.
>
> APPROPRIATE RESPONSE: No one other than my lawyer.

PLAINTIFF ATTORNEYS MAY TRY TO MAKE US HOSTILE WITNESSES. Making us hostile witnesses means that the lawyer wants to make us a witness against ourselves by using our answers to undermine our own testimony. The plaintiff attorney attempts to achieve this goal by posing dilemma questions. Most of us profit from some instruction from our attorneys on how to recognize and respond appropriately to these questions.

> QUESTION: Doctor, isn't it correct that if the physician uses reasonable care, this result (referring to the patient's injury) does not ordinarily occur?
>
> INAPPROPRIATE RESPONSE: That's correct.
>
> APPROPRIATE RESPONSE: Although the result may not ordinarily occur, when it does occur, it is most often due to the inherent risk of the procedure.

Careful dissection of the question lays open its internal dilemma. Does this injury ordinarily occur? When it does, is it always the failure of the physician to provide reasonable care? By answering affirmatively to this double-pronged question, we qualify ourselves as expert witnesses against ourselves.

PLAINTIFF ATTORNEYS MAY USE THE DEPOSITION TO PRESERVE THE TESTIMONY OF SOMEONE WHO MAY BE UNAVAILABLE FOR APPEARANCE AT TRIAL. The time between deposition and trial may be lengthy and a key witness may not be able to testify in person because of illness or commitments scheduled long before the trial date was set. In such cases, their deposition, especially if available on videotape, is used instead.

The Defense Attorneys' Goals

DEFENSE ATTORNEYS FILTER OUT INAPPROPRIATE QUESTIONS. During our deposition, our interrogators may ask us questions that call for an objection. We must recall that the court reporter takes down each and every word spoken by anyone during the process. Objections made in timely fashion by our lawyers will be on the record, allowing a judge to rule later on their merits. In some instances, our attorneys will instruct us not to answer a specific question.

> QUESTION: Doctor, what was the finding of the hospital peer review committee concerning your care of my client?

Our attorney will interrupt the process and object on the grounds that this calls for us to reveal privileged information and will instruct us not to answer. The plaintiff attorney may then choose to contact a judge for a ruling on the objection "in real time." If the line of questioning is crucial to the plaintiff's case, they will have to argue the point, interrupting the deposition, which will have to be "continued" at a later time. Alternatively, the plaintiff attorney may note and seek a later ruling on the objection. Our attorney makes the call on whether we answer the question that prompted the objection.

In some instances, our attorneys will object to the *form* of the question and still allow us to answer it. If such objections to form are not made at the time the question is asked, they are waived. It is important to understand this because our attorney's objection may preclude the use of this question and answer during the trial to impeach us, that is, demonstrate that we have contradicted ourselves.

DEFENSE ATTORNEYS PREPARE THEIR CLIENTS CAREFULLY. Defense lawyers prepare themselves and their clients carefully for a deposition. Our lawyers may suggest that we participate in witness school, in which instructors spend many hours preparing us, both substantively and stylistically, to answer the questions that are certain to come up during our deposition. According to a risk manager with a large malpractice carrier, however, not every attorney prepares their physician clients so thoroughly before their depositions. Dr. John Schmidt ruefully describes his own experience.

> The attorney for this particular case was a weakling, who, in my experience, was not very adept or experienced, not very verbal and vocal about things, and didn't play hardball with the plaintiff attorney at all. And just sort of sat there. He did not have a lot of objections during the time and, I thought, kind of just let me be strung out. So, I almost felt abandoned by my attorney. I'm not sure what legal malpractice is or not but I know good attorneys versus not so good attorneys. I thought he would be very adequate in my defense and I thought he should do OK, but much to my dismay, it did not turn out that way. So, I've usually had someone in other cases who was trying to prepare me, give me the proper advice in advance, of what to read, what to expect, and how the deposition would be conducted. But at that particular deposition it was just the opposite and that didn't turn out well. I realize that a deposition is different than a trial. I think that during the deposition, latitude is far greater, that they can ask what they want and say what they want and things can be stricken at a later time. But it sure is difficult to sit through.[3]

Tips Defense Attorneys Give Physicians to Prepare for Deposition

- *Pay close attention throughout the deposition.* By answering too quickly we may "step on" our lawyer's objection.
- *Pause slightly at the beginning of every answer to make sure we understand the question and to give our lawyer time to object.*
- *Listen to the objection.* Our lawyer is giving us important information about how to answer the question.

QUESTION 1: Doctor, didn't your nurse call the patient's mother and tell her not to worry about the situation?

COUNSEL: Objection, the witness has no personal knowledge.

MESSAGE: *The message to us is clear.*

INAPPROPRIATE RESPONSE: Well, the nurse is a very caring person so she might have said that.

APPROPRIATE RESPONSE: I do not know.

QUESTION 2: Doctor, you had a great deal of difficulty visualizing the operative site and you did take the opportunity to clear the field before proceeding, isn't that correct?

COUNSEL: Objection, compound question.

MESSAGE: *This is our clue to ask the examiner to rephrase the question or break it down into two parts.*

QUESTION 3: Isn't it true, Doctor, that the radiologist's report of my client's mammogram was crystal clear?

COUNSEL: Objection, the question is vague and ambiguous.

MESSAGE: *This is our clue that we need to ask for clarification.*

APPROPRIATE ANSWER: The report stated:_____. I would not equate that with your characterization that the mammogram was crystal clear.

- *Be prepared to see the plaintiff at deposition.* All parties to a lawsuit have the right to be present when another party is examined under oath. In an attempt to make us uncomfortable, the patient may sit directly across from us. The plaintiff attorney also believes that to testify in the client's presence makes us more cautious or conciliatory. Our attorney will intervene if the patient is overtly disruptive by, for example, grimacing or making sounds that serve as commentary on our answers. We must simply ignore them, whiting them out, and focus our attention on the attorneys and their questions.

Dr. John Schmidt arrived at his deposition to find not only the attorneys present but also his patient's widowed husband and his two teen-age daughters.[4]

> They sat there looking at me, and what a bad guy I am, I killed their mother. So this intimidation with family members around during a deposition was very memorable, obviously with all those eyes looking at me, peering at me, staring at me during that same time. I was aware of that as being a ploy. It had happened before. I learned my lesson early on about intimidation. . . . Teenage daughters, tears running down their eyes about Mom, and what a bad doctor I am again, and you did this, you didn't do that. That was particularly memorable with the young daughters there. The husband always sneering and leering at me. So that particular deposition

was one of the most trying ones I have ever had just because of the daughters being there and their emotional reaction. . . . And the questions typically being offered and asked about me, my background, and hearing all these things about, "Well,
doctor, you've been sued 14 times" and these questions going on about that and
the significance of it or lack of significance. So those kinds of things you take to
heart so much and it's so grinding, just so intolerable. There is no way to squirm
out of it. There is no way to not answer the question. You're there. You've got to
step up to it.

- *Unless advised against it by our attorney, be present during the patient's
  deposition and those of key plaintiff experts.* Exaggerating is always more
  difficult in the presence of the very professional being criticized. It is by no
  means unusual for us not to know what really went on at and around the time
  of the incident. Charts tell only part of the story. Frequently, the patient's
  version of events is totally at odds with that of the hospital. For such reasons, many defense attorneys insist that their clients attend the plaintiff side's
  depositions.
- *Be prepared for other attempts to intimidate us.*
- *Be prepared for the possibility that the plaintiff attorney may videotape our
  deposition.* There are advantages to videotaping. On cross-examination at
  trial, opposing counsel can project the actual deposition testimony side by
  side with a transcript of our answer so that the jury can evaluate both our
  demeanor and the content of our answers. Videotaped sworn testimony may
  be admissible if, for some reason, a witness is not available for the trial. Juries
  have a much greater sense of the witness's credibility when they can view
  the actual question and answer exchanges. If we are in a jurisdiction in which
  depositions are routinely videotaped, we should be prepared well, working
  with our attorney to make the best presentation possible.
- *Understand the difference between close-ended and open-ended questions.*

CLOSE-ENDED QUESTION: You did not tell the patient about the risks of this
surgery, did you, doctor?

Clearly, the questioner is attempting to elicit a concession from the physician.

Signal flags are raised by questions that begin with, "Isn't it true that . . . ?"
or "You don't disagree that . . . ?" or "Aren't you saying that . . . ?" These
are efforts to pin us down or to concede a key point.

Attorneys generally ask open-ended questions when they are simply interested in obtaining information. Our temptation is to provide too much information. We should respond by asking for clarification or in a way that forces
the questioner to ask for more precise information.

OPEN-ENDED QUESTION: Doctor, what did you tell your patient about the risks of
surgery?

APPROPRIATE ANSWER: I told my patient that there were some risks.

QUESTION: Which risks?

INAPPROPRIATE ANSWER: Well, as with any surgery, there are risks, and this was a particularly difficult procedure that I am now much more familiar with. However, I don't see what that has to do with the lawsuit, which in my opinion has no merit whatsoever.

APPROPRIATE ANSWER: Infection, bleeding, damage to another organ, even death.

- *Listen for questions that contain assumed facts.* Sometimes lawyers ask questions embedded with some fact or series of facts. The question appears to be seeking information about who was in the room but, in fact, the attorney is maneuvering to have us confirm that we alone made a decision crucial to the case.

QUESTION: Who was in the operating room when you made the decision to continue laproscopically?

OBJECTION: Object as to the form of the question. The question is compound. You can ask him who was in the room and then ask him whether or not he made a decision at that time.

Compelled to answer the question, we may say the following:

APPROPRIATE ANSWER: I made no decision alone, and the following people were in the room.

If our attorney does not object to the compound nature of the question, we should take the initiative and give the following answer:

APPROPRIATE ANSWER: I cannot answer the question as you have phrased it. Please break it up into two separate questions.

- *Listen carefully to the questioner's cadence.* We need to be sensitive to the questioner's pace and phrasing of questions. Experienced plaintiff lawyers may vary their cadence, asking two or three questions very quickly and then asking one in a slow manner. They may also jump from one subject to another. If we do not listen carefully, the change in pace and abrupt shift in subject matter may throw us off. Expecting a logical progression, we may be lulled into anticipating questions that never materialize. It is not useful to formulate answers while questions are being asked. It is far better to focus on the one question being asked and then to take the time to formulate the best answer. Our lawyer may have past experience with the plaintiff attorney and may help us understand how to deal with his or her typical style. The key is being alert to being lulled into a sense of complacency or so mesmerized by the pace and tempo of the inquiry that we lower our guard and lose our attention and concentration.
- *Pay attention to efforts by the plaintiff attorney to get us "off script."* During the preparation of our deposition with our counsel, we concentrate on

organizing the chronology of events as well as an account of all the actions we took on behalf of our patient. That familiarizes us fully with the case and enables us to answer all questions truthfully and in ways helpful to our case.

The good plaintiff attorney may use any of the previously discussed tactics in an attempt to pull us "off guard" and "off the script." They may ask such questions as, "Can you explain, doctor, why . . . ?" or "Please give me all the reasons that you . . ." or "What was your plan going into the case?" *We do not want to answer these questions quickly.* The examiner's chance of striking gold rises exponentially whenever we respond to issues that we are not prepared to discuss. In this instance, we want to respond truthfully but in a limited way. If we are asked questions for which we are poorly prepared, we may begin to improvise responses and drift into areas dangerous to our defense. Our lawyer should prepare us for such questions, as they may be a part of our deposition.

- *Do not get angry or show irritation if the attorney repeatedly asks the same question.* Sometimes the attorney will pose the same question, with minor variations, over and over. Usually this is an attempt to trick or frustrate us and turn us into an angry, frustrated physician who is no longer able to perform well.

The Defendant's Goals

As every guide or lecture presentation on the subject emphasizes, deposition preparation is vital to a successful defense. Good preparation demands time from both physicians and experienced lawyers. The physician must also be rested and in total command of the chart and accompanying materials.

OUR PRINCIPAL GOAL IS TO FINISH THE DEPOSITION WITHOUT MAKING A MAJOR MISTAKE. A deposition free of material error leaves the factual underpinnings of our presentation to the jury intact and provides our defense expert witnesses with a firm basis for their testimony. We accomplish this when we answer questions truthfully, behave professionally, and demonstrate mastery of the medicine and documentation in the case. Our performance need not, however, be perfect. We must remember that lawyers are professional advocates who practice the art of questioning every day. We can always review our performance critically, finding areas in which we can improve. Should the case go to trial, we will have ample time to address such issues with our defense attorney.

WE WANT THE PLAINTIFF ATTORNEY TO BELIEVE THAT WE ARE FORMIDABLE OPPONENTS. We want the attorney to know that we give the jury an impression of us as competent, caring physicians who practiced within the standard of care and did everything possible to provide appropriate care for our patient. If the case comes down to who is more credible, and with all things being equal, jurors frequently side with the physician over the patient. Smart plaintiff attorneys will factor this into the chances of winning a verdict and, as noted previously, following a strong physician performance in a deposition, will often drop the case. Doing well in our deposition gives us a sense of strength and resolve helpful at trial. We have engaged the enemy and we have performed with distinction. We solidify our defense by completing our deposition without major mistakes.

10

To Settle or Not to Settle

In general, the discovery process gives all participants a realistic view of each side's chances to prevail at trial. Only about 7 percent of cases nationwide are finally tried to verdict. Before or during trial, as noted in Figure 7–1, approximately 29 percent of the malpractice cases nationally are settled with awards of monetary damages to the plaintiff.

Why Settlements Happen

Both sides agree to settlements because, after weighing their respective chances of success, they conclude that a predictable outcome is preferable to getting nothing (a defense verdict) or being hit with a large jury award (a plaintiff's verdict). Although both sides want an outright win, there are many reasons to stop short of trial and enter into negotiated settlements.

The Insurance Company's Interest in Settlement
Controlling risk is a primary factor for the insurer. Because a settlement establishes a known amount of money that must be disbursed, it reduces the insurer's risk of being confronted with a large, unplanned award. On receiving notice of a potential malpractice claim, the insurance company immediately evaluates it,

estimating potential damages in the event of a plaintiff's award. Over the ensuing months and years, it puts money in reserve to cover the loss if it is settled or is resolved through a plaintiff's verdict. This amount is adjusted according to the latest information on the potential value of the claim.

The financial implications for the company are enormous if a verdict's award greatly exceeds the amount of money that has been placed in reserve for the claim. The company's financial stability may be threatened if such an outcome occurs frequently. Insurance regulators may also scrutinize their finances, rating companies may take adverse actions, and potential insureds, hearing about possible insolvency, may decide to take their business elsewhere. Every insurer (whether physician owned, mutual, reciprocal, or a stock company) wants to avoid tipping off this cascade of events.

Some insurers retain the ultimate authority to settle a claim based on both the defensibility of the claim and its potential to yield significant damages through a negative trial outcome. Some insurers will not settle clearly defensible claims solely to avoid the costs of litigation on the principle that a reputation for aggressive defenses discourages unfounded malpractice suits. While some companies reserve the right to settle to themselves, others allow physicians the right to consent or refuse to settle. Physicians should be clear at the time they purchase coverage about their rights contained in the policy's "consent to settle" provisions.

The Court's Interest in Settlement

In every court, judges are responsible for stewarding scarce judicial resources and clearing overburdened dockets. They may therefore pressure the parties to come to an accommodation as quickly as possible, ideally before trial. Various forms of mandatory settlement efforts, including arbitration, mediation, or similar processes, are used to achieve such settlements.

> The judge in Dr. Mary Santos' case tried to get us to settle because she said, "I know somebody who went through this, he lost, he never practiced again and his marriage broke up." For several days she kept saying, "you should settle, you should settle." It was a tremendous amount of pressure on us to settle. Finally, the lawyer told her we weren't going to settle. Later, Dr. Santos discovered that the physician described had been the judge's husband.[1]

The Plaintiff's Stakes in and Motivations for Settlement

When the odds are against having a successful outcome, the plaintiff often accepts a pretrial settlement. Juries tend to like physicians, and in close cases, they may give them the benefit of the doubt. These unfavorable odds make going to trial a "gamble" for plaintiff lawyers, who can invest upward of $250,000 of their own monies to pay the experts' fees and related litigation expenses of the case. Most plaintiff lawyers accept cases on a contingency basis and receive their fee only if an award is made. Losing at trial, they lose their investment because most plaintiffs cannot pay them for their services.

Even plaintiffs who believe they will prevail at trial may make a settlement decision based on whether the state awards prejudgment interest, that is, interest on the judgment beginning on the date the lawsuit is filed. Jurisdictions lacking prejudgment interest increase the likelihood of defense appeals against plaintiff verdicts because there is no penalty for drawing out the case. The defense knows that while waiting for the appeal the plaintiff may also wait a long time with no distribution of monies or no accumulation of interest. Wanting money immediately is a strong motivator for plaintiffs to settle even when both sides expect them to be successful at trial.

The Defendant's Stakes in and Motivations for Settlement

Defendants settle to avoid the negative consequences of losing the trial. A jury may, for example, return an award that is greater than their insurance coverage, confronting them with possible financial ruin and bankruptcy. An adverse judgment may also jeopardize their future insurability, generate adverse personal and professional publicity, generate a report to the National Practitioner Data Bank, and lead to licensure or credentialing investigations. While they can appeal an adverse verdict, in some jurisdictions they may be forced to post a bond in the full amount of the judgment to keep the plaintiff from executing on their assets during the appeal period.

Except in situations where liability is obvious and damages are significant, discussions about settlement normally occur after the completion of discovery or just before or even during trial itself. Each insurance company has its own requirements about seeking settlement, but they generally demand the assembly and review of all pertinent documents; the completed depositions of both fact witnesses, including defendants, patients, family members, other clinicians, and experts for both sides; the completed exchanges of interrogatories and requests for admission; and the resolution of motions for summary judgment. The lawyer and claims representative usually exchange information about these developments and share opinions throughout the entire discovery process. Reaching the point of potential settlement, the interested parties, including the defendants, weigh the strengths and weaknesses of their case, after a review of the pertinent elements, and reach a decision about entering into settlement negotiations.

Questions to Consider Before Settlement

IS THE DOCUMENTATION OF THE CASE ADEQUATE? The clinical record should support the defense's contention that we met the standard of care in our treatment of the patient. Does the clinical record, taken as a whole, reflect the care we gave to the patient and indicate that we demonstrated adroit decision making and good clinical judgment? Using our chart as a basis, can expert witnesses testify that our treatment was within the standard of care? Are key questions that reflect on our credibility, such as documentation of after-hours telephone conversations with the patient or patient's family or notes concerning our informed consent session with the patient, resolved in our favor? That such issues be successfully attended to is reflected in the familiar admonition: "If it is not in the record, a jury will not believe that it happened." If we do not have complete and accurate records, we may be forced to consider the merits of a negotiated settlement.

ARE THERE ANY SERIOUS ERRORS, OMISSIONS, OR ALTERATIONS IN OUR DOCU-MENTATION OF THE CASE? The medical record must be accurate and reflect contemporaneous care of the patient. Have all the dictated notes and reports been dated and signed? Do changes we have made conform to the appropriate hospital medical records documentation standards as described in Chapter 6?

Inappropriate alterations include removal of such sections of the chart as laboratory results and electrocardiogram strips, whose inclusion might weaken our defense. Our claims professional, defense attorney, and the plaintiff attorney review the chart carefully to determine if their condition merits a move toward settlement.

WILL WE MAKE A GOOD WITNESS? If we are to prevail at trial, we must perform well before the jury. Our deposition offers us a good measure of how we will conduct ourselves at trial. We can review our deposition, videotaped, if possible, and assess our performance with our counsel. Even if we did not do as well as we wished, our attorney can coach and rehearse us to correct help our deficiencies.

Dr. Mary Santos and her lawyer had concerns that she might not make a good witness.[1]

> So I said, well, let's do a video and I looked really bad. The other thing they did was sent me this guy who is a psychologist and lawyer. He helped me prepare. He was very useful. He came like two or three Sundays. At trial, when the jury went out, they came back and asked to go over my testimony . . . and actually it was perfectly clear.[2]

Ideally, we want to demonstrate an intimate familiarity with the record to the jury. We want to present a logical, coherent account of the events surrounding our patient's care, teach the jury about medical information in a lucid and easily understood way, and reveal ourselves as conversant with the relevant medical literature. We want our demeanor to communicate compassion, understanding, patience, and professionalism. We want to appear as professionals who are well trained, well experienced, and well respected in the community—in short, as someone they would like as their physician. We damage our case by being arrogant, defensive, easily frustrated, and impatient, or confused or disorganized. We need to evaluate in the company of our counsel and as objectively as possible, whether and what we can modify about our personal characteristics.

Dr. Cynthia Davis speaks of her former ophthalmologist, who was defending himself at trial.[3]

> He probably thought he was dignified. I'm sure the jury was interpreting it as arrogance. He could not help but portray himself in that way because he was dressed so nicely. Yet, what could he do? He was a doctor. He couldn't not be a doctor and come dressed badly. I don't see that he could do anything else.

Our appearance and clothing are not the only things that influence the jury's perceptions of us. Our attitude, emotional balance, and respect for the proceedings themselves communicate who we are and what we are like.

DO THE EXPERTS PROVIDE STRONG SUPPORT? Even with an outstanding chart and a stellar performance on the witness stand, we still need strong supporting testimony from qualified experts if we are going to prevail. We must play a central and active role in evaluating and selecting our defense experts. We can also provide helpful and objective input about the strength of the deposition performances of plaintiff's experts.

Effective defense experts impress jurors as plain spoken, skilled at explaining complex medical matters, well versed in current and accurate knowledge about the subjects of their testimony, and having an open mind. Such experts may concede valid points in cross-examination instead of obstinately "digging in." Good experts generally practice medicine full-time in clinical settings and have first-hand knowledge of the circumstances we confronted in the case. They do not come across to the jury as advocates for one side but as professionals assisting jurors to make a fair and impartial decision. Experts who are known to testify for both plaintiffs and defendants seem more objective to jurors and therefore more credible. Lacking credible defense experts, we may be forced to settle.

DO RISK FACTORS EXIST THAT PORTEND AN EXPLOSIVE VERDICT? Because of the complexities of both the medical treatment and malpractice trials, there is no way that we can control all of the contingencies that may come to light in discovery. Because nonmedical situations can play a significant role in determining whether a settlement is indicated, we should examine any risk factors that may pose problems at trial with our counsel.

The defense misread an additional risk factor in a case in which a mental health professional violated the ethical imperatives by having sexual relations with a number of his patients. He had also prescribed psychotropic medications to each of these patients. The defense mistakenly focused solely on the possibility that a jury would view these sexual encounters as matters between consenting adults, in short, as mitigating factors to excuse the physician. It failed to consider the impact of his excessive prescribing on the verdict. The jurors viewed this pre-scribing practice as predatory by taking advantage of these patients, making them vulnerable and unable to object to the sexual advances, and as therefore directly harmful to them. They awarded significant damages to the plaintiffs.

Sympathy for the patient is another major factor in juror behavior. Plaintiff's counsel may take cases of questionable liability to trial confident that once the jurors see the patient's pain and difficult life circumstances, they will react with sadness, compassion, and pity toward them. The arousal of such emotions com promises the jury's ability to render a fair and impartial verdict by manipulating them to favor the plaintiff for their injuries even if the physician is not respon-sible for them. The sight of a child with cerebral palsy, strapped into a wheelchair and parked not ten feet from the jury box everyday for six weeks, gives pause to any lawyer defending the physician involved in the case. Such a calculated place-ment of the victim, regardless of the science and medical evidence in favor of the defendant, may increase the likelihood of a multimillion dollar award and be a stimulus for reaching a more predictable settlement.

Medical malpractice cases were published in the local paper when Dr. John Schmidt was faced with a decision about whether to settle his case.[4]

> I thought, "Oh, small town, only neurosurgeon, the plaintiff is a prominent person in the community. If this goes to trial, it could be a losing situation. If you know that it is not a matter of right or wrong but it is a matter of what the jury perceives. And I thought I could be castigated and I could be strung out again and I'd better just cut my losses right now because even though I was as innocent as could be, the poten-tial for loss was great." At mediation, two of three saying there should be a goose egg in terms of me, the third said it was worth at least a quarter of a million dollars. This lady wasn't employed, they were people of means, they owned a factory, and there was a sympathy cause there because of the teenage daughters. Again, to cut our losses, I, and the attorney, felt the same way the insurance company did, and my insurance company has always said that the final decider should be the physician. So, we settled.

MIGHT THE AWARD EXCEED OUR POLICY LIMITS? In Chapter 5, we explored such ramifications of an excess verdict as nonrenewal of our insurance coverage, a powerful consideration when we are deciding whether to settle a claim. We be-come aware at some point in the process, of the potential at trial, for an excess award. Because someone else will be required to pay a bill that our policy will not cover, seeking settlement may be not only prudent but also necessary.

At this point, perhaps on the advice of defense counsel, we may retain a pri-vate attorney, if we have not already done so. Ideally an experienced plaintiff or defense lawyer, this attorney evaluates our exposure and advises us about demand-ing the insurers settle within our policy limits. On accepting the demand, the insurer will enter into negotiations with the plaintiff to settle within our policy limits. An insurer who rejects such a demand and lets the case be tried to a verdict that is in excess of our policy limits provides us with the legal basis for a "bad faith" settlement claim against them. When this happens, the plaintiff attorney ordinarily takes an assignment of our claim against our own insurance company and drops us from further involvement, except as a witness, in the matter. In effect, the plaintiff then "steps into our shoes" to pursue the insurer for the amount by which the verdict exceeded our coverage and may be successful.

CAN A LARGE AWARD JEOPARDIZE OUR FUTURE COVERAGE? When adverse market conditions limit our choice of liability insurers, concern that a large verdict may result in nonrenewal of our policy may drive us to settle.

Dr. Santos reflects:

> I had $10 million dollars' coverage. We sort of figured they were looking for something maybe not over $100 million but, as you know, there have been several cases in Pennsylvania and New York that are now $100 million. So we sort of think the number they were looking at was going to be $80 million. My immediate instinct was I'm going to fight this one. I kind of felt like I shouldn't have settled the other ones. I always had this sensation that I should not have settled. I knew the plaintiff attorney wanted to settle. My defense attorney told me, "Whether you want to settle or whether you want to fight it, we will be with you." And then I felt so hazy about settling, but the really hazy thing was, if I did settle, would I be able to get insurance? And so in a way, it's a kind of moot question if you settle. Because then I wouldn't be able to get insurance and I would effectively be out of obstetrics. After choosing trial and reassured by my attorney, "We are really going to have fun doing this," I successfully defended myself. If I had lost at trial, I would have been out of practice. I have no question because I couldn't have gotten insurance and it would have been all over the place.[5]

With standard carriers unavailable or unwilling to insure physicians who have experienced a large jury award, we may be driven into the nonstandard market, where premiums can be twice or three times the amount we currently pay. Settlement can reduce the risk of nonrenewal, especially if continued renewal by the insurer is incorporated into the negotiations.

> "I was devastated," said Dr. Laura West, as you always thought, could I have done anything differently, did we do the right thing, should we have done this? Always second guessing yourself. We had good experts. The insurer thought the case was defensible and we should go to trial. My partner and I said, "Great, we don't think we did anything wrong but this doesn't look good. It will not be a jury of our peers; these are going to be the average Joe. This was Cook County." I said, "We're going to lose." We said, "No, we don't want to go." Well, the board who makes the decision are doctors who have been sued and they said, "No, this is going to court." So we had to go to court. I used an attorney I had used in the past who had great creden-

tials but as it turns out is not a good court room attorney and I think that contributed to our losing. But I think we would have lost anyway—but we really lost it. Anyway, we did a good job, we trained hard, and we spent hours of trying, reading, and looking at illustrations. As it turns out, the insurance company did what they promised. They said you didn't do anything wrong, this was our decision and you won't be penalized. If the insurance goes up, it will be like everybody else. And that's what happened.[6]

WILL THE COSTS OF TRIAL BE PROHIBITIVE? Defending cases through trial is an expensive proposition for a liability insurer. Lawyer and expert witness fees and other defense-associated costs normally run into six, and sometimes, seven figures. Insurance carriers rarely gravitate to settlement simply to avoid these expenses, which they view as part of doing business.

A two- or three-week trial keeps physicians from seeing patients, performing surgeries, or providing evening and weekend coverage for their patients. The tasks of rescheduling other patients, explaining their absences, and feeling guilty about the burden this places on their partners and employees exact a financial and emotional toll on them. Even though some policies provide a token reimbursement for the time physicians lose to a case, trial costs are nonrecoverable and can have serious ramifications for those in solo or small group practice. Physicians may believe that their case is defensible and that their counsel and experts are ready and able, yet they opt to settle to avoid the excessive costs of going to trial. Recognizing the odds and the risk, some physicians respond to other personal and professional pressures and make the difficult decision to defend themselves at trial anyway.

The plaintiff attorneys who sued Dr. Mary Santos were aware of another claim against her partner and were pressing for settlement.

> I definitely think they are sort of timing experts. For example, my partner had another case immediately after mine, which started within two or three days of mine ending. Now they didn't have that case, another firm did, but they aligned the cases so they knew that it would be exceedingly difficult for a practice with two physicians out when, in fact, we were doing sixty deliveries a month among three physicians here. And they took one out for a full month and another one out for almost three weeks. They had about three days in between so they really tried to make us settle by forcing us. . . . Neither I nor my partner would agree to settle. During the trial, I operated all day Monday. I saw patients early in the morning and I saw patients late at night. Financially, it's tough to float this boat without doing this.[7]

ARE THERE OTHER LEGAL FACTORS THAT MAY INFLUENCE OUR POTENTIAL FOR SUCCESS? Medical malpractice lawyers are familiar with "locality trends," that is, the influence of local circumstances on successfully defending a claim. This particular aura of a venue is a function of a wide range of socioeconomic and cultural factors, including the makeup of juries. Lawyers are sensitive to these circumstances and alert us when they feel such trends may influence the outcome of the trial.

On the eve of trial, we may learn that some consider the judge assigned to our case to be "pro-plaintiff." As our lawyers are conducting *voir dire*, or jury selection, they may discover how unsympathetic the panel is. We may learn, just before putting on our case, that a key expert is no longer available to testify. Settlement may be thrust upon us because of forces that are outside of our defense team's control. Our commitment to try the case to verdict is no longer an option, and we must accept settlement as disappointing but a necessity.

Pretrial Settlement Negotiations

Most jurisdictions require us to participate in some sort of pretrial settlement negotiation that may range from being pro-forma, nonmeaningful activities in which we may not be involved to important moments in the resolution of a case in which we will almost certainly participate.

Settlement Conferences

During settlement conferences, lawyers report their findings to date and, in conversation with the judge, discuss whether the parties have attempted to resolve their differences and whether, in the opinion of the parties, the direct involvement by the judge or another person would assist in resolving the case. The judge usually concludes with an admonition to continue discussions and to report back to the court as the trial date nears.

Arbitration

In arbitration, each party selects an arbitrator, who then selects a third person to join them in evaluating the case. In what amounts to a minitrial, the arbitrators hear each side's evidence and legal arguments and then render a decision that may include an award. Most arbitration decisions are not binding, that is, the parties are free to accept or reject their decision. Because in the latter case no resolution is reached, the parties proceed to trial. By accepting the arbitrators' determination, the parties forego their right to a trial by jury.

Arbitration can take place more quickly in jurisdictions where the dockets are crowded. Arbitrators may be able to address complex clinical issues more effectively than a lay jury and, in a jurisdiction that may be known for explosive jury awards, arbitration awards are historically much lower. Arbitrators, often attorneys themselves, are less likely than are lay jurors to be swayed by the sympathy component to the case.

On the other hand, arbitration gives the plaintiff attorney the opportunity to examine the witnesses and is much more likely than a jury trial to award some money. If the arbitration is nonbinding and either party is dissatisfied with the award, he or she may reject the arbitrators' recommendation and proceed to trial. Arbitrations can also be costly in lost practice time and the expenses of attorneys and expert witnesses.

Mediation

Mediation is an entirely different form of dispute resolution. A judge or private mediator usually meets separately with the parties in an attempt to find common ground for a settlement number. Mediators ask the parties to outline the strengths of their case and the weaknesses of their opponent's case, strive to narrow the factual differences that could be significant in resolving the dispute, and, finally, reach a settlement amount that the parties would be willing to accept. Armed with this information, the mediator shuttles back and forth between the parties until the matter is resolved or the mediation breaks off.

In mediation, as distinguished from arbitration, each party comes to the table with a notion of what it will take to settle the case and the skillful mediator nudges the parties toward common ground until a mutually acceptable figure is reached. If such mediation fails, nothing that the parties say or do is admissible in a subsequent trial. This encourages openness and an honest assessment of the case's strengths and weaknesses. Physicians may be able to play a substantial role in the mediation process and have some idea of the amount of money that will settle the case. Last, mediation usually takes less time than arbitration and requires physicians to spend only a limited amount of time, often less than a day.

Pretrial Screening Panels

In the early 1980s, tort reform legislation in many states created pretrial screening panels, composed of lawyers and one or more physicians who generally share the defendant's same specialty. As in arbitration, panels may take testimony, admit documentary evidence, and listen to lawyers' arguments. The full panel makes a nonbinding agreement about whether the care rendered was within the community standard. Some jurisdictions try to discourage patients' option to go to trial by allowing the findings of the panel to be admitted at trial as evidence that the standard of care was met. Critics view this largely out of favor process as giving the plaintiff "two bites of the apple" and as expensive because of the need for expert testimony.

Dr. John Schmidt sat on such a mediation panel a number of times.

> There used to be mediation panel composed of docs chosen by both sides with lawyers also chosen by both sides. They reviewed all the data and decided whether the case had merit or not. The panel also placed a monetary value to the case. And I sat on mediation a number of times and the tenor was always, "Oh see, this suit has got some merit" as the plaintiff attorney would say. "We've got to pay for that somehow, they should be granted some dollars, we should get at least $10,000 to $20,000 out of this."

And I'd say, "Bullshit, a goose egg is a goose egg. If they are not deserving of it, there is no reason to continue with the suit or grant someone money, even if it's a piddily amount." And the good old boy system prevailed with the plaintiff attorney saying, "We've got to get something out of it. We've got to cover some of our costs." Wrong, wrong. But that was the tenor, that was the feeling of how it should have been, and that's where the mediation panels turned out to be a mockery of justice and the physicians sitting on them. That was all stopped, probably 8–10 years ago.[8]

The Mechanics of Settlement

Most insurers require our written authorization to settle the case. Our defense counsel, often in company with our claims professional, approaches us about settlement authorization.

Physicians need be aware of the sometimes surprising twist of the process. Although they may or may not be consulted about the final dollar number, physicians will ordinarily consent to settle for an amount up to the limits of their policy. They may later discover that the insurer negotiated a settlement that is within the policy limits but many thousands of dollars more than the physician thought it was worth. Although physicians should ordinarily be consulted before the final amount is determined, they must be prepared emotionally when this does not happen.

Sometimes parties who are far apart on a settlement amount can use a structure to come to a satisfactory compromise. Structured settlements constitute a form of annuity. The patient is guaranteed a monthly or yearly amount of lifetime compensation and, in some cases, at a reduced amount, for the life of the surviving spouse or relative. Some injuries, such as birth-injured infants or severely injured adolescents, require full-time care, expensive medications, numerous physician and hospital treatments, and equipment for transportation. An annuity costing $2 million to $3 million can buy an income stream some ten to twenty times greater than its original cost. The cost savings for the defense are obvious, and numerous insurers can financially support the 40- to 60-year payout provisions. The annual or monthly payment also serves as a restraint for the plaintiff from wasting a lump sum award. The insurance company can also structure the plaintiff lawyer's fee in the form of an annuity that serves as a retirement plan.

Other Ramifications of Settlement

Settlements are generally negotiated for amounts well within our policy limits. Although settlements terminate the case against us, they do not provide the clean break we would desire. With the passage of the Health Care Quality Improvement Act in 1986 (Title IV, Public Law 99-550), any medical malpractice payment, of any size, made to a plaintiff on our behalf must be reported to the National Practitioner Data Bank and be forwarded to the state licensing board for further investigation, if necessary.[9] Although we are not found legally guilty of malpractice, the implication that we have erred in some way lives on in these postsettlement realities.

The National Practitioner Data Bank

The alleged purpose of the National Practitioner Data Bank is to encourage greater efforts in professional peer review and to restrict the ability of incompetent practitioners to move from state to state without discovery of previous substandard performance or unprofessional conduct. Any evidence of such behavior by physicians, dentists, and other health professionals, based on medical malpractice payments, adverse licensure actions, adverse actions on clinical privileges, or their professional society membership, is reportable to the data bank and to the appropriate state licensing board. Such data are then available for review by authorized eligible hospitals and other health-care entities.

Most of the reports to the data bank are medical malpractice payments. From the onset of the data bank on September 1, 1990, through October 9, 2004, the names of 193,538 MD physicians, 11,948 osteopathic (DO) physicians, 1,545 MD residents/interns, and 236 DO residents/interns had been forwarded to the data bank in association with medical malpractice payments.[10]

In response to intense lobbying by the medical establishment at the outset of its implementation, the law states that "a payment in settlement of a medical malpractice action or claim shall *not* be construed as creating a presumption that medical malpractice has occurred."[11] Nonetheless, the fact that our name is permanently placed on a federal data bank when settling a malpractice case suggests otherwise. Even though there is no implication of substandard practice, for the balance of our career, we will be subjected to inquiries about our malpractice history every time we change jobs, request privileges, or present ourselves for other professional advancements. Most physicians believe there is an inherent flaw in this law and resent that such negative implications should be attached to any settlement.

When our name is forwarded to the data bank, a report verification form is immediately sent to the reporting entity and a practitioner notification document is sent to us to verify the report's factual information. It is in our best interest to review the information and, if we find it incorrect, to initiate a dispute of factual information to the data bank. A process for further appeal exists if the dispute is not resolved in our favor. Any report that puts our name on the list of the data bank indefinitely should, at the very least, accurately reflect the incident that initiated such action.

The law requires hospitals to query the data bank every two years about their staff or others to whom they grant clinical privileges. They must also query the data bank when they are considering an applicant for a medical staff appointment or for clinical privileges. State licensing boards, health-care facilities, individual practitioners, and, in special circumstances, attorneys who have filed a claim against a hospital may also query the data bank, although they are not required to do so.

After the case, the defense attorney can write a detailed summary letter for the physician's file that can be used to respond to and clarify any future inquiries about the settlement.

Physicians and the Data Bank

Initially, physicians felt insulted, angry, and very concerned about the establishment of the data bank. The feeling remains that a data bank entry is a blot on their record that could conceivably cause them problems. Many physicians' names are now on the data bank list, mainly as a result of settlements, and although physicians still feel anger and resentment, they have also become resigned to this as just another cultural burden imposed on the profession. Most physicians also expect that it is only a question of time before they personally are reported to the data bank. Many conclude that the data bank's failure to make the distinction between settlement payments that do not presume the occurrence of malpractice and the other disciplinary reports that it acquires is weakening the effectiveness of the data bank and undercutting its goals.

Deciding to Settle Our Case

We should attend to the emotional factors that can influence our decision to settle. Because of the diverse motivations for settlement, we serve ourselves well in considering the following questions.

DO WE HONESTLY FEEL THAT OUR CARE OF THE PATIENT WAS WITHIN THE STANDARD OF CARE? Contemplating whether to settle is, for many of us, a moral conflict. If we think that what we did was right, how can we agree to participate in a process that awards money to a patient who, in our opinion, received good or even superior medical treatment? A settlement in which there is no technical admission of guilt nonetheless gives the impression that we played some role in the outcome. Feeling vulnerable but innocent of malfeasance, we believe that such payments are made only in cases of blackmail or extortion and cannot be associated with a court of justice. Feeling outraged by pressure to settle, we sometimes respond with greater resolve to "take this to the mat." We must pay heed to this moral outrage even though it is only one facet of the settlement decision. These feelings arise from and accompany our passion to defend our honor. They are also relevant to our insurance company's stance on our right to consent to settlement. If we act against these intensely personal feelings without examining what we are telling ourselves through them, we may end up with feelings of disappointment and regret. Such feelings led Dr. Mary Santos to lament her previous settlements and energized her resolve to go to trial.

The finality of a settlement means that we can never revisit it. Can we live comfortably with the decision to settle when we know we did nothing wrong? We must weigh all of the personal and professional factors and take into account all of our feelings to remain true to ourselves if we are to achieve a sense of peace about a settlement.

DOES SETTLING JEOPARDIZE OUR RELATIONSHIP WITH OUR COLLEAGUES, PART-NERS, OR PRACTICE ARRANGEMENT? The tenor of our relationships with our col-leagues is a major factor in our comfort at work. When bad things happen, we can easily begin to point fingers toward those who were with us in the room or pro-vided us with information that was used in our decision making. The glare of a lawsuit puts all of these relationships into sharp relief, often leading colleagues to put self-preservation first by finding somebody else to blame.

We may come away from settlement with unresolved resentment about taking the blame for everyone involved. While it may be difficult, we may seek an ob-jective review of the case, including the role of all participants, before deciding on a settlement. A settlement reached without such a review can breed deep feel-ings of resentment, bitterness, and permanently broken relationships.

WHAT ARE A SETTLEMENT'S FINANCIAL IMPLICATIONS? We often settle to avoid the risk of excessive financial loss that may occur if we do not. Our degree of risk, as noted before, may depend on whether we are the sole defendant or whether our corporation or partners are also named, on the potential costs of a trial in lost time and income, and on the potential of a significant award to foreclose our abil-ity to obtain reasonable, if any, insurance coverage. We must also factor in the possibility that a judgment exceeding our coverage may make us personally li-able for the excess portion of the award and place our family and personal finances at risk. We must discuss these issues thoroughly with our financial and estate advisors before we agree to settlement. Sometimes our financial risk is so great that we have no choice but to authorize a payout.

DO WE HAVE PERSONAL REASONS FOR SETTLING? Many of us have circumstances that supercede all other considerations for settlement. We may be preoccupied with a family illness that precludes us from devoting the time necessary to go to trial. Our spouse may feel overwhelmed by the potential risks associated with our going to trial and, for the sake of our family relationships, we may choose their concerns over our own. We may have issues of personal health, as Dr. Richard Allen did, that outweigh other risks that may evolve from settling. We must con-sider all of these uniquely personal factors before we make the final decision.

They were asking for a total of a million dollars, $225,000 from me, $300,000 from my associate, and the rest from the radiologist. At that point, from a financial point of view, I knew what my downside was. I had to make a decision once we got through the deposition phase about whether or not I wanted to pursue a court trial to totally exonerate myself or accept a small settlement that they would pay on my behalf. It was much less than the two hundred thousand or so they were suing me for, I think it was in the realm of $50,000 that my attorney explained to me. He said, "Look, if you've been splashed with a case like this and all they walk away with is $50,000 that's almost exoneration. You can go to court and you can attempt to settle for nothing. However, you also have to look at the downside of that. You don't know what a jury trial's going to do. They may look at the facts again and decide that you were really more involved than you were and all of a sudden a much higher award is obtained and you really haven't accomplished that much. And also, if you're going to drag yourself through the emotional mess of that court case again." And I began to think about that and I said, "You know, one episode of atrial fibrillation and a trip to the emergency room is enough in one's life if you don't have to do it." I was just afraid that those court appearances and the anxiety that it could provoke might tip me over again. So, I decided discretion was the better part of valor. My health was the number one factor. Had I been a healthy 30-year-old person, I probably would have pursued it. I truly felt I got blind-sided by this and upheld my end of the bargain pretty much throughout the entire process and was a victim of circumstances. I just was very angry about that and probably would have pursued it.[12]

WHAT DO OUR SPOUSE AND FAMILY THINK ABOUT A DECISION TO SETTLE OR TO PROCEED TO TRIAL? In the final analysis, our highly personal decision to settle necessarily affects our financial health, our emotional life, and our relationships with others. As we consider this decision and its long-term implications, we should discuss all of its elements with our spouse or significant other. What we decide and how we react have a large impact on how we feel and behave and on how we relate to those closest to us.

We may feel great relief, have no problem putting it behind us, and go on with our lives. We may be able to look on the settlement as a cost of doing business to be paid and reports to the data bank and the state licensing agency as necessary burdens to be borne. We may nonetheless experience the lingering feelings that Dr. Joseph Daley describes, "Even after the case is resolved, it persists. I still feel it is a very unjust case."[13] We may feel a certain fatalism about settlement paired with a resentment that influences our attitude and care of patients and sours us on our profession. If we are well schooled in self-observation, we can identify, isolate, and modulate these reactions.

Whatever our choice, sharing our decision making and concerns with our spouse and family provides us with the input and support we need to make a well-thought-out decision with which we can live comfortably.

11

The Trial

> It was only after I was sitting there in that courtroom and I realized that that prosecuting attorney, and that judge, and these people on the jury—they had an immense amount of real power. And the band of brothers . . . I hated their guts up there anyway . . . the judge, and the defense attorney . . . and the prosecution's attorney. They're up there doing what they are paid to do and what they love to do. They're laughing. Westy is sitting slumped. I am in a depression.
>
> —Mike Wallace[1]

From October 11, 1984, until February 18, 1985, CBS News reporter Mike Wallace and U.S. Army General William Westmoreland stare at one another in a New York courtroom, the honor of each at stake in legal combat over differences in the reporting of certain incidents in the Vietnam war. The emotionally burdened protagonists, almost overwhelmed by the adversarial nature of the trial, come to resent their advocates' obvious ease and bantering old boy exchanges in the embattled atmosphere of the courtroom. Crowded to the side of the stage as the curtain rises on the trial, they feel stripped of their presumption that they are the principal figures in its drama. The lawyers move easily into the limelight, sure of themselves, accustomed to playing the leading roles in a small ensemble cast whose influence is enormous.

The Decision: Trial

Our decision to go to trial is tested right up to the bailiff's calling the court to order on its first day. We may be moving inexorably toward trial because, given the circumstances of the case, the opponent's settlement demands are at least unreasonable and perhaps outlandish. Claims professionals tell us that an unlikely jury award will exceed the proposed amount. Although not without risk, going forward to trial in these circumstances favors our side. We may also be moving to trial because we are completely supported by the testimony of our experts who, as locals, may even be known to the jurors selected to hear our case. In addition, our responses at deposition and during pretrial run-throughs raise our confidence in being good and credible witnesses.

We also recognize that plaintiff's experts will testify that our care fell below the community standard and that the patient's injuries are serious. We know that if we are found negligent, the award could be significant. Nonetheless, our defense counsel and our claims professionals assure us that the odds favor a defense verdict. We are then prepared to go forward, convinced that we did nothing wrong and eager for the public vindication we feel we deserve.

Setting the Trial Date

We may know the trial date as long as ten weeks and as soon as a month ahead. It is not unusual for such dates to be postponed because of the court's schedule or the availability of the judge and other officers of the court.

Courts in some jurisdictions assign a trial date 1 year to eighteen months from the date the complaint is filed. This forces the parties to complete discovery and engage in whatever pretrial settlement activity is warranted before then. Such a compressed time frame may cause difficulty for an opponent inexperienced in prosecuting medical malpractice cases. Gathering effective trial experts is a serious and time-consuming task. Those without much experience often turn to the "1-800 hire-an-expert" services advertised in the trade journals of trial lawyers. Often unscreened and uncontrolled by either professional societies or state licensing boards, these experts have been known, for sufficient compensation, to testify to nearly any theory of any case.

At times, cases are dismissed on the trial date itself because the plaintiff's attorney is unable to secure an expert or the expert resigns at the last minute. In these circumstances, our counsel may offer a negotiated dismissal whereby the defense waives the right to collect its costs, the filing, deposition, and witness fees, which usually are less than $500, in return for the plaintiff's full and final dismissal of the claim.

An Introduction to the Court

It serves us well to dispel some of the mystery of the court, familiar only from the movies and television, by acquainting ourselves with it before we actually take our place there.

The Courtroom

Most courthouses were built before the middle of the twentieth century. Some courtrooms are like a cathedral, with ornately carved appointments and sturdy furniture, emphasizing formality and the law-and-order atmosphere that breathes mystery and authority into the life of the community. In older courtrooms, the players are arrayed as if at a square table, with the judge and the witness chair at its head, the jurors to one side, and the contesting parties and their counsel seated opposite either the judge or the jury. Modern courtrooms are more functional and egalitarian and, with the increasing use of computer terminals and projection systems, mating battle zone with surgical suite, in which intense emotions are counterpointed by the high gloss and high-tech background.

We can ease more comfortably into the role of defendant if, after our trial is scheduled and before it begins, we visit the courtroom with our attorney to help us anticipate and learn something about its environment.

The Players

Today's guardians of the law, in the manner of high priests celebrating the mysteries in ancient temples, perform courtroom rituals that only the initiated understand. Mixing Latin phrases with technical and complex words alien to all but the brethren of the judiciary, these tribunes conduct the court's business from formidable daises segregated from the public by the bar of the court. Those admitted to the bar may pass through it into the sanctuary-like realm of the trial, where, together with jurors and witnesses, they celebrate the ancient ritual that divines whether we are at fault and, if so, how much we are to pay as compensation for the patient's injuries.

THE JUDGE. Attired in somber black robes and gazing down from imposing benches, judges occupy the supreme position of power and authority in the courtroom. Their role is to rule on motions, objections, and arguments of the parties and to instruct the jury on the *law* applicable to the case. State court judges are either elected by the people or appointed by the governor. They remain in office by prevailing in pro-forma elections in which they usually have no opponents. The president of the United States appoints federal judges for life and, once confirmed by the U.S. Senate, they are removed from office only by retirement, death, resignation, or the impeachment process. Federal judges enjoy a lifetime tenure that theoretically frees them to render difficult and often unpopular decisions without regard to political consequences.

Judges may have prior experience on the bench when, as lawyers, they sit *pro tempore* to hear motions or even to conduct trials. Most, but not all, are members of the trial bar before becoming judges. Many factors influence judicial appointments as, for example, when liberal governors offer judgeships to plaintiff lawyers, famous for their activist political organizations. Appointments are also given to district or state attorneys and criminal defense lawyers.

Some judges are easygoing, intervening only when absolutely necessary, but generally allowing the lawyers to try their cases with a minimum of interference. Others, professing to move along the proceedings, involve themselves in every phase of the proceedings, interrupting questioners and lecturing the lawyers on the finer points of trying cases. Temperaments aside, we benefit greatly if our judge knows the law of medical malpractice and has a record of being upheld on appeal.

THE ATTORNEYS. Some plaintiff lawyers dramatize themselves as mavericks. Fringed in buckskin, Wyoming lawyer Gerry Spence strides into courtrooms as if onto the set of the movie *Shane*. Many identify with the underdog just as they also identify themselves with the mythic lone hero of that old film. They often take big risks, rolling the dice at trial on moves that, if successful, will yield them not only courtroom victories but also large contingency fees.

Other plaintiff attorneys, impeccably dressed, low key, and professional, rarely offer objections, request sidebars, or cause delays in the process. They solidify their credibility by their focus on the seriousness of the proceedings, their time management, and their respect for the jurors.

Defense attorneys typically choose to be quiet and restrained. Dressed conservatively and unremarkably, they strive to project strength, stability, and professionalism.

Both plaintiff or defense attorneys share a dedication to preparation and attention to detail. Before a major trial, they often sequester themselves for two or three weeks, with all the relevant materials, to be fully prepared to plead the case.

In some jurisdictions, the lawyers are allowed during the trial to approach the area in which the jurors are seated, the jury box, as well as the chair from which witnesses testify, the witness chair. Perry Mason–style, such lawyers can draw intimately close to witnesses or jurors, the point blank range from which they can better intimidate or more easily engage the powerful dynamic of sympathy that is vital to winning a large award. In other jurisdictions, judges restrict the lawyers' questioning and arguing to a circumscribed area around a neutral podium in the well of the court.

THE PLAINTIFF. Plaintiffs, like jurors, are Everyman. The defense prefers robust plaintiffs whose apparent health raises questions about their need for compensation. In many cases, however, the plaintiff's injuries advertise themselves boldly and unmistakably. They may be disfigured, have obvious incapacities, or even be bound pitifully to a wheelchair. Opposing counsel will attempt to dramatize their condition for maximum impact on the jurors. Physicians must maintain their professional composure even in the presence of patients whose real suffering is both disturbing and unnerving even when they know that they did not cause it.

THE DEFENDANT. We are also principal players in the courtroom drama. Escaping the emotional and financial challenges of the trial may be an alluring fantasy, but we cannot exempt ourselves from participation in the trial. An empty chair next to defense counsel would symbolize our absence and send the wrong message, perhaps contributing to a significant award for the plaintiff. We need, in a sense, to follow Spencer Tracy's advice to young actors: "Know your lines, be on time, and don't bump into the furniture." We need to project our professionalism by being fully present, well focused, emotionally controlled, and clearly prepared to participate appropriately.

Many days or even weeks may pass in the trial before we take the stand to testify. Meanwhile jurors form their impressions of us on the basis of our actions and demeanor. At the very worst, jurors should have formed no fixed opinions of us before we take the stand. That is better than a negative impression, which we may not easily or completely overcome in our comparatively brief time on the witness stand.

CLERK OF THE COURT. Clerks for judges sit either directly below or to the side of the central bench. Clerks function as keepers of a judge's chambers, as persons who, for example, can facilitate or block a lawyer's access to the judge's inner sanctum. They perform their work at the pleasure of their judges and are often seen passing notes to the latter about relevant matters. Most lawyers understand that good relationships with court clerks are essential, and we will observe them enjoying what appear to be friendly exchanges with them during trial.

THE BAILIFF. The bailiff calls the courtroom to order, serves as a link between the jurors and the court, and provides first-responder security should any disruption arise in the court. Often retired law enforcement officers, bailiffs seem self-contained and rarely speak to any of the participants. They are privy, however, to much, aside from deliberations, that takes place in the jury room.

THE COURT REPORTER. The court reporter sits within hearing distance of the witness chair to record the courtroom proceedings. Some face, and others sit facing away from, the witness. On occasion, the judge or one of the attorneys will ask the reporter to read back a portion of the testimony. One appreciates their quiet contained art as they flip back through a stack of folded brown paper barely 3 inches wide and, translating hieroglyphic-like symbols, accurately repeat words spoken hours, or even days or weeks, earlier in the trial.

THE COURT WATCHERS. We may also observe a cluster of strangers in the spectator seats who become regulars, raptly absorbed in the full course of our trial. These court buffs not only add background color to the otherwise tense and purposely drab atmosphere but also may play an important role in the proceedings. Good trial lawyers cultivate these court veterans, sometimes retired lawyers themselves, who often give sage advice to the lawyers on such subjects as the makeup of the jury, the impact of our counsel's opening or closing arguments, or observations on the habits and whims of opposing counsel.

We may well notice other trial lawyers present to observe the tactics and performance of the defense and plaintiff attorney. They may fill the courtroom, especially during closing arguments, to scout attorneys they may face at later trials or to learn from the styles and strategies of more experienced trial lawyers.

Last, family, friends, staff, or associates may be present for some part of the trial to lend support. They come and go as their schedules permit during long trials, but they convey both encouragement to us and a belief in our personal and professional integrity.

Immediate Preparations for Trial

Reviewing Relevant Documents

Armed with a definite date and the belief that we will prevail, we begin by repeatedly reviewing the medical records and ancillary documents as closely as before our deposition. The goal is to achieve the same degree of proficiency we did in our anatomy class, that is, a thorough mastery of content melded with an ability to recite most, if not all, passages from memory. We must read and re-read our own deposition. Consistency between our deposition and trial testimony is crucial to a successful outcome.

We must also review the deposition testimony of both the plaintiff and the experts. This allows us to understand how each side views the strengths and weaknesses of our case and prepares us for the plaintiff attorneys' certain witness stand challenge of such fault lines as they may identify in our deposition. We are prepared to defend where we know their perceptions will lead them to attack. We must also carefully review the depositions of the other key fact witnesses. Often, the credibility battle is won or lost on seemingly inconsequential matters such as when a telephone call was made or what was said during a late-night conversation. Nothing else sounds like the simple truth, and our ability to confidently address the issues to which we know others have testified allows us to speak it in a way that members of the jury are most likely to hear it.

Preparing to Testify

We should practice both our direct and our cross-examination. Lead counsel may conduct the former, whereas partners or associates in the firm can play the role of the plaintiff attorney during cross-examination. If the exercise is to be meaningful, the attorney acting as the plaintiff lawyer may use a style and tactics much like those of our prospective examiner. If we have already encountered this person during depositions, we should speak up if we believe that the training substitute does not match the original. In these sessions, we want to familiarize ourselves with what we are likely to encounter while on the stand during the trial. Plaintiff attorneys do not necessarily display or use all of their weapons or ammunition in depositions and may well reserve some for the trial itself. To surprise or unnerve us before the jury, they may use an entirely different style, structure, or content and vary the pacing of their cross examination. Our lawyers should know the opposing attorneys well enough to prepare us for when we are examined. We should so thoroughly integrate that knowledge within us that we can communicate in a calm, collected, and confident manner to the jurors.

Depending on the case and the potential size of an adverse verdict, our counsel may, in association with professional coaches, videotape and critique us. We may even participate in a full-scale mock trial. Our counsel will choose persons drawn from communities whose demographics match those of our likely jury pool. Both the process and the outcome will closely approximate reality. Our attorneys will then adjust our defense strategy to the results of this quasi-trial.

Anticipating Delays

The postponement of scheduled trials is commonplace. The assigned judge's current trial may be taking longer than expected or the opposition may be experiencing difficulty in scheduling its crucial expert. In any event, the prospect of such delays means that we reschedule patients and surgery, rearrange coverage, and adapt to all the psychological disruptions involved in what seem the almost casual changes commonplace in this world that is so unlike our own. We have heard of trials being delayed but, hoping against hope, we count on this date as a time when in a public forum we can finally present our side of the story. Then a new trial date is set and we must promptly readjust ourselves emotionally.

The Trial

The trial, as outlined in Table 11–1, finally begins. It dawns on us that, as eagerly as we anticipated going to trial, now we are worrying about what the jury will think about us and our care of the patient. Will they judge us to be good doctors?

Our Appearance and Demeanor

Jury members base their initial impressions of us on our looks and bearing. Colleagues wearing trial campaign ribbons typically advise us to dress as approachable professionals. We can settle any doubts by dressing as we would in our offices.

We should feel confident enough to be ourselves, just as we are, in the courtroom. We sometimes learn, through what we or others observe about us, that we have some rough edges that may either put others off or be easily misunderstood by them. We should work on these, consulting with others, if necessary, to correct or minimize them before the trial begins. Willingly or not, we reveal ourselves through our behavior—the way we sit, listen, or look casually about—in every moment of the trial.

Table 11–1. The Trial Process

- Pretrial Conferences—Opponent lawyers meet with the judge to discuss procedures and ground rules for the trial. Either side may present motions relating to the conduct of the trial.
- Jury Selection—The judge and each side, if permitted by the judge, question each prospective juror to establish if they can render a fair and impartial verdict.
- Opening Statements—Each side, with the plaintiff's attorney usually presenting the first statement, outlines what they believe to be the facts of the case and what their evidence will show.
- Plaintiff's Case—Plaintiff's counsel conducts the direct examination of witnesses and medical experts testifying in support of the plaintiff's case. Defense counsel cross-examines each witness. The plaintiff's attorney has the option to conduct a re-direct examination and the defense attorney may conduct a re–cross-examination, if necessary.
- Motions—The defense may ask for a dismissal or directed verdict, or both sides may argue motions to govern further proceedings.
- The Defense's Case—Defense counsel conducts the direct examination of the defendant, other fact witnesses, and medical experts who will present evidence in support of the defense's theory of the case. The appropriate attorney will then conduct appropriate cross-examinations, re-directs, and re–cross-examinations.
- Closing Arguments—Each lawyer summarizes his or her view of the evidence and suggests the conclusions that jurors should draw for a verdict in their favor. Because the plaintiff has the burden of proof, they usually argue first and last.
- Directed Verdict—The defense may argue that the plaintiff has failed to prove the essential requirements of the case and therefore the judge should direct a verdict in favor of the defendant.
- The Verdict—The jury renders their verdict. It may be for the defendant or plaintiff. If a decision cannot be reached in a reasonable period of time, one or other side may ask for a mistrial or, unable to come to a decision, the jury may be hung. If this happens, at a later date, the case is set for a retrial or the parties come to a settlement.
- Appeals—The losing party may, in a specified period of time, file posttrial motions that may request a new trial, change the amount of the damage award, or a judgment contrary to the jury's decision. Depending on the judge's decision, an appeal may be entered generally to review the legal rulings made during the trial to determine if errors had been made.

Plaintiff Dr. Cynthia Davis was also prepared for trial.

Well, I met with my attorney twice. And he prepared me. Here's what they're going to ask. Here's what I want you to do. Here's how I want you to dress. Here's how I want you to behave. Now behaving and dressing were most stressful. That bothered me . . . I had to behave in ways that weren't so for me. At the time, I was wearing corporate uniforms and, really, I looked quite stylish. I had to dress down. Flat shoes. And I just felt that I had to portray myself as kind of pitiful. And that was stressful because it seemed dishonest and yet I know it's part of the game . . . it was a value conflict for me—the dishonesty, and yet, you know, it was a game and so I played. . . .

And the attorney said, "They cannot see you reading. They cannot see how well you can or can't use your eyes.[2]

Our testimony is a significant part, but only one part, of the overall defense, and jurors watch us closely as we react to other witnesses as well as to court rulings and to the arguments of opposing counsel. Much as we must maintain a professional but caring manner in dealing with patients or emergencies in our everyday work, we need to control our feelings of disappointment or elation at the turn of any of these events. If we appreciate how jurors emotionally transfer their experience with their own physicians to physician defendants, we can understand why they expect to relate to them with respect and professionalism. Their personal physician rarely expresses overt anger, hostility, or satisfaction at someone else's expense. Manifesting such behaviors eats away at the benefit of the doubt that jurors may be ready to grant us. They make judgments about whether we are genuinely interested in the proceedings, noting how attentively we listen to the testimony of others, whether we take notes when appropriate, and whether we relate to them in a pleasant, noncommittal way. There is no way to fake any of this because our daily unself-conscious behavior delivers a consistent message about us. In the face of the trial's stress, we must invoke our professional calmness, comporting ourselves as neither above nor beyond the proceedings, committing ourselves, as fully as they do to fulfilling one of our greatest civic responsibilities.

Pretrial Conferences
Like operas, trials generally begin with overtures filled with familiar judicial music: the added preliminaries of new motions to be heard, past rulings occasionally revisited, issues related to jury selection, and, at times, attorneys disappearing for extended periods into the judge's chambers to resolve points at issue.

It is helpful to remember that in the courtroom, lawyers are playing on their home field and that they appear relaxed and comfortable with each other as they begin what, for them, is the game they love to play. They may battle like big leaguers during the long innings of the contest, only to dismay us, indeed to appear disloyal to us, by the camaraderie they share with each other during pauses or after the game is over for the day.

Jury Selection
Eventually, the bailiff will escort a large number of persons, members of the jury panel from which our jurors will be selected, into the courtroom, seating them in the front rows of the spectator's gallery. The process of choosing the jurors is known as *voir dire*, or "to speak the truth." The court or the attorney conducts *voir dire* with the prospective jurors to ascertain if they harbor unacceptable biases or prejudices that would interfere with being fair and impartial through the often probing and sometimes highly personal questions that citizens accept in a

free society as the price of achieving a measure of justice for litigants. The law does not require a perfect jury, only a fair and impartial one.

A perennial question for those of us who go to trial is, "How can a jury of retired or nonmedical persons or of those less well educated or of different races, creeds, or national origins from us ever be considered our peers? Shouldn't patient care decisions be restricted to physicians?" Our constitution considers every citizen of the United States equal in the eyes of the law so that, as citizens, we all bear the responsibilities associated with our system of justice. Our legal outcome depends on how individuals, no matter how well or poorly educated and regardless of how different their experiences are from our own, judge the care of our patient. Despite our many protests that, given the complex content of our cases, we should receive special or different treatment, we are all subject to this American system of justice.

The judge briefly describes the case and, after reading from a list of those called to jury duty, asks each of them whether they know any of the lawyers, the parties, or the witnesses. A juror may be excused if the relationship is seen as too close for unbiased decision making. The judge asks if anyone has commitments, such as a long-planned trip or a wedding, that will interfere with their jury service. Some, or all, of these individuals may be excused.

Depending on the venue, six or twelve members of the panel will be chosen by lot and seated in the jury box. In some jurisdictions, the judge, relying on questions submitted by the litigants, conducts *voir dire* with these persons himself. Generally, however, both the plaintiff and defense attorney conduct *voir dire*. By carrying it out themselves, experienced lawyers gain and transmit important information, sizing up the jurors, telegraphing key legal concepts, and underscoring difficult factual matters even before the first word of testimony is spoken.

Our lawyer may begin by exploring each juror's general attitude toward physicians. Do they have a personal physician? Have they had good experiences, or have they had problems with their physician? Have either they or members of their families ever experienced unexpected, or less-than-optimal, medical outcomes? How did they feel about that? Did they hold that against their physician? Have they, or any member of their families, ever sued a physician?

If the case involves catastrophic injuries, our lawyer may probe to identify the potential jurors who are unable to discharge their duties dispassionately. For example, the neurologically impaired child may have cerebral palsy, be strapped into a wheelchair, and have no control over his or her speech. Anyone unfamiliar with these problems may be disturbed by seeing and hearing such a child throughout a four- to six-week trial. Such exposure can so move some persons that regardless of the facts of the case, they will vote for a multimillion-dollar award.

The defense also conducts *voir dire* to explore juror attitudes and to educate the jury members on their responsibilities.

Defense counsel may ask:

> Now, Mr. Smith, at the close of the case, the judge will instruct you that you must base your verdict solely on the evidence and that you may not allow sympathy to sway you. Do you think you can follow that instruction?

Or defense counsel may inquire:

> Mrs. Jones, all of our hearts go out to the plaintiff, Camie Wilson (pointing to the child in the wheelchair), her parents, and her brothers and sister. They have already endured much and now face a lifetime of difficulties none of us will ever encounter. As a juror in this case, Mrs. Jones, can you set aside those feelings, listen to the evidence for *both* sides, and render a fair and impartial verdict based on the evidence you hear and the law as given to you by the judge in the instructions to the jury?

Sometimes, wanting the jury to hear less-than-flattering information before the other side presents its interpretation of the facts, counsel will say:

> Mrs. Jones, you will hear testimony and see pictures of the patient's chart indicating that my client made certain entries there shortly after learning the plaintiff had suffered a stroke in the ICU. And the testimony will be that my client did that not to mislead anyone or to cover anything up but because he remembered something important at that time and wanted to make sure that the record contained the entire information relevant to the care of the patient. And, finally, the testimony will show that my client followed the recommendations of the hospital and his specialty society in appending information into the chart. Now, Mrs. Jones, if the evidence shows all of this, will you hold these late entries against my client?

Defense counsel may pursue a similar line of *voir dire* relating to the law of the case:

> Mrs. Jones, I believe the judge will instruct you that you are not to base your decisions about my client's care of the plaintiff's using hindsight. Can you do that?

Or defense counsel may ask:

> I believe the court will also instruct you that my client's care is to be judged by the community standard; that is, what a reasonable physician in the same or similar community in the same or similar circumstances would have done given the same facts as were presented to my client at that time. Will you follow the law if this is what the judge instructs you, Mrs. Jones?

Some plaintiff attorneys like to emphasize the importance of following the law, creating the impression with jurors that the law is on *the plaintiff's* side. They may ask:

> Mrs. Jones, do we have your commitment that you will follow the law no matter where that law will lead you? Will you will follow it no matter what?

Defense counsel may also ask:

> In regard to the standard of care, I believe the judge will also instruct you that you are not to count the number of witnesses on each side but weigh the evidence fairly and impartially in order to render your verdict. This is just a hypothetical but say we only produce one expert who supports my client's care, while the other side produces five experts who say my client violated the standard of care. Would you agree, Mrs. Jones, that, if you decided that our one expert was correct, you could not just count the number of witnesses on each side and say, "Oh, the plaintiff has four more so I will find in their favor"?

A plaintiff attorney may also gauge a juror's attitude toward compensation in a case of severe injury by asking:

> Mrs. Jones, if the judge instructs you that the law allows it and the evidence warrants it, would you agree to vote a verdict in the millions of dollars?

After completing their examinations of the prospective jurors, each side can choose to exercise one or more preemptory challenges. Although the numbers vary by state, each side can use such challenges to dismiss a set number of prospective panel members without stating a reason. The court generally determines whether and how many of these challenges are permitted.

The Art of Jury Selection

Picking juries, long acknowledged as an art, is also becoming a quasi-science. Lawyers sift potential juries carefully to separate the advantageous flecks of gold from the disadvantageous chunks of dross, seeking what they consider the right mix of such factors as race, gender, class, and sexual orientation. Good defense and plaintiff attorneys, however, rely primarily on their own instincts and experience in picking a jury.

Plaintiffs look to rid themselves of jurors who will hurt them and to accept jurors who can be moved by emotion, are sensitive to even the possibility of injustices, and are eager to right any perceived wrongs. Among jury characteristics to be avoided, according to the latest handbook on tort litigation of the American Trial Lawyers Association, is evidence of a "personal responsibility bias."[3] Such individuals, who espouse traditional family values and strong religious beliefs, are biased, we are told, because they expect people to take personal responsibility for their actions, a conviction that may inhibit their developing empathy for many plaintiffs.

For the case of a neurologically impaired infant, for example, the plaintiff attorney may seek male jurors who, because they have young children and earn something close to minimum wage, can understand the burden such injuries impose on young families. Such jurors are likely to be quite sympathetic to the plaintiff, be receptive to the classically effective argument that jurors must send a message that unsafe conditions cannot be tolerated, and, persuaded that all physicians have deep pockets of insurance coverage, will not hesitate to empty them, no harm done, with multimillion dollar verdicts.

The defense, on the other hand, looks for persons who have a stake in the economy, who, in real time, have made decisions affecting the well-being of others, or who have had experiences involving health care similar to those at issue in the trial. The defense, in such a case, may seek management position women with grown children who have first-hand experience with the complexity of childbirth, understand the responsibility of meeting budgets and payrolls, and, tutored in life's often unfair demands, understand that not every tragic event is caused by somebody else's mistake.

Both sides accept the impossibility of empaneling their perfect dream jury. Experienced trial attorneys who exercise their challenges wisely can severely reduce the chances that either the defense or the plaintiff will obtain an ideal jury. Inexperienced lawyers, however, may unknowingly and unwittingly accept enough jurors sympathetic to one or the other side that the trial may be won before the judge gavels the court into order.

Each side tries to identify a potential foreperson, a man or woman who can be elected by the other jurors as a leader to guide and shape the views and decisions of a cohort filled out by a number of sufficiently like-minded individuals. In a high-profile case, lawyers may also use a jury consultant to assist in picking a favorable jury.

Before the trial, we should discuss with our counsel the elements of our ideal jury. This discussion gives us insight into our lawyer's approach to trial strategy in general and how he applies it to our case in particular. Knowing that, as physicians, we have well-honed skills at reading people, they may welcome our input from the *voir dire* to the conclusion of the trial.

Jury selection is complete. These twelve persons, six in federal trials, will, along with their alternates, decide our fate.

The relationship between the jury and the lawyers is critical to the outcome. Dr. Cynthia Davis thought that her attorney related well.

> I don't have any basis to judge my first lawyer. My first attorney looked more like an attorney. He was taller than the other one, slender, and nicely dressed. The one I ended up with is a little shorter, pudgy, and his clothes were kind of baggy. Cook County jurors tend to identify with the underdog and thus, my attorney, being not necessarily attractive, they could identify more easily with him than with the other attorney.[4]

Maureen Anderson felt her attorney never "connected" with the jury.

> I think the insurance lawyer was a better lawyer. I think the case was the last case. The people for the jury were diminished and I have to say it was such a young bunch

of jurors that they were college students that maybe were served with jury duty right after school got out. That was my feeling and that was the feeling of my lawyers. The insurance company's lawyer was very dramatic and very theatrical compared with our lawyer who was more middle aged. The other one was young and flamboyant and our lawyer was subdued and, seemed like, just trying to get the facts. And he kept saying, "What do you want me to say?" And we kept saying, "You have to do what you feel. We don't know." I felt the lawyer was looking to us for direction which struck me as really odd. I think the lawyer for the insurance company had their attention. The people kind of trusted him a little more than our lawyer. It was obvious to me. In retrospect, she felt that the younger jurors identified much more with the young vigorous defense attorney.[5]

The Trial Begins: Things to Watch For

At the conclusion of the testimony and the closing arguments of counsel, the judge instructs the jury on the law to be followed in the case. Jurors swear an oath to follow these instructions, a solemn responsibility that both sides expect the jury to fulfill conscientiously. These instructions contain key concepts with significant value to our successful defense. We should be alert, as the trial unfolds, to the following themes.

The Burden of Proof

Plaintiffs bear the burden of proof in a medical negligence case. They must prove by a preponderance of the evidence, meaning greater than 50 percent, that our care fell below the community standard and resulted in an injury to the plaintiff, for which compensation should be paid. In a familiar symbol, the blindfolded goddess of justice balances two plates. To recover compensation, plaintiffs only need to tip the scale in their favor. Defense counsel can maintain the balance between the two plates by successfully attacking plaintiff's evidence, making clear to the jury that, failing to meet the burden of proof, they also fail to break the tense balance between the scales.

Subject to the same burden, we can plead and prove affirmative defenses, including the argument that the plaintiff's own negligence contributed to the injury. This concept of comparative fault is illustrated by a patient's failures to show up for follow-up appointments or tests, thereby delaying the diagnosis of a malignancy. If we demonstrate that their own negligence contributed more than 50 percent to their injuries, plaintiffs receive no compensation.

The Standard of Care

As the court defines the standard of care, it explains several important limitations on its applicability. Jurors are instructed, as noted earlier, not to base their conclusion on which side called the greater number of expert witnesses. The judge also instructs them that where there is more than one medically acceptable way to treat a condition or perform a procedure, the physician is not negligent if he chooses one or the other.

Credibility of Witnesses

The court may instruct the jury that witnesses found to be false in one part of their testimony may be disregarded in other parts. Both sides use this "impeaching" as they examine each other's witnesses. This illustrates the importance of our thoroughly knowing the documentation, including our own deposition, and of our listening and answering truthfully only to the question that is asked of us.

Case Themes: "The Story"

Nothing about a trial is haphazard for the opposing attorneys. Both sides script events in detail, striving mightily to maintain control of both the atmosphere and the agenda. Their finest plans are frequently disrupted and, like crafty boxers, the opponents may spend as much time measuring and reacting to each other as they do in throwing punches. Each side therefore arrives in court with one or more well-developed case themes in their briefcases.

One theme is *fact based*. The patient presented in the physician's office on a Friday at 5:00 PM with abdominal pain but, at that time, the patient exhibited only two of four common indicators of a ruptured appendix. Based on the then known facts, the patient could have been suffering from one or more other conditions. The physician, therefore, suggested waiting to see whether the discomfort subsided or worsened. For plaintiffs, the fact-based theme is one of misdiagnosis based on an incomplete examination. For defendants, the fact-based theme is one of a correct diagnosis based on the absence of one or more of the symptoms of a ruptured appendix.

Themes can also encompass larger concepts. For example, charges of negligence are brought against both the hospital and the surgeon for failing to discover and remove a sponge from the patient before closing the surgical incision. The fact of the retained sponge is irrefutable. The surgeon's defense is based on the *concept* theme that the scrub nurses alone are responsible for the sponge count and that the jury should not, therefore, find the surgeon negligent.

Themes are important because no trial offers an exact replica of the event that occasioned it. Nor is it a straightforward narrative, but rather a tale interrupted by recesses and delays and witnesses testifying out of the ideal sequence, like a movie in which the film breaks and there are no subtitles for its foreign legal and medical languages. Faced with variously edited versions of events, jurors must use deductive reasoning to arrive at their decision, fitting the facts into a conclusion that favors one side or the other. Armed with a good theme, experienced trial attorneys present or develop a story out of the evidence and cross-examination that is clear, simple, direct, and easily understandable to support a verdict in their favor.

Admitting Liability

On occasion, the defense will admit liability and use the trial to determine how much compensation should be awarded. Admitting liability excises the emotional component from the plaintiff's case, shifting the focus to the less impassioned but still necessary task of determining a fair sum for compensation.

Opening Statements

Plaintiff counsel presents their opening statement first, telling a story that previews the testimony of the fact and expert witnesses and explains the requirements of proof necessary to sustain a damage award. The defense has the option of presenting its own opening statement immediately after that of the plaintiff or doing so only after the plaintiff has presented its case. Although what the plaintiff counsel presents during the opening statement is not evidence, our counsel carefully notes these statements and refers to them during closing arguments if the plaintiff counsel has not produced evidence to support them during the trial.

The Plaintiff's Case

The plaintiff always has the option to call the physician defendant as their first witness. Although our counsel may prepare us technically, we can never be fully prepared emotionally for this possibility. Plaintiff counsel may use this tactic for two reasons: first, of course, is their desire to gain advantage by an ambush of surprise; and second, they want to rivet the jury's attention with the dramatic opening move.

Plaintiffs normally call witnesses in the order that best fits their story line. Because technical medical testimony can wear down even a conscientious lay jury, the plaintiff's attorney prefers that they first hear the human drama from patients or their families. Our counsel cross-examines these fact witnesses to achieve one or more of the following goals: (*1*) to raise significant questions about their credibility, to reduce the adverse impact of their testimony; (*2*) to extract admissions from them that support the defense version of the facts; (*3*) to treat witnesses highly sympathetic to the plaintiff in a kind and courteous fashion, imprinting on jurors an image of the defense as fair, caring, concerned, and empathetic.

The plaintiff calls medical experts to testify that our care was below the community standard and that this failure was a substantial contributing cause of the plaintiff's damages. It can be emotionally jarring to hear professional colleagues fault us for having failed to do this or that and ultimately blame us for the injuries that the plaintiff claims to have suffered as a result of our negligence. Nonetheless, we must not show any emotion whatsoever as their testimony unfolds. Our job is to remain steadfastly impassive—attentive and appropriately concerned but never derisive or in any way disturbed. Observed closely by the jurors, our challenge is to remain what we claim to be: consummate professionals.

Our counsel cross-examines these experts to achieve several goals. Is the expert qualified? Juries not only prefer active over retired clinicians but also favor those who practice in a specialty that is the same or similar to our own. In an effort to raise doubts about their skills in the jurors' minds, our counsel probes the qualifications of the plaintiff's expert witness. What, for example, can we learn of the expert's motivations to testify? Do they fall in the class of professional witnesses who earn their living through testifying on behalf of plaintiffs? Do they believe that, no matter by whose hands or with what skill it is performed, a particular procedure is always wrong? Are they disgruntled because they or some member of their family has been hurt through medical negligence?

How much does the expert really know? Because genuine experts live up to their billing as the very best in their field, they are most damaging when they testify convincingly that we made decisions based on outdated scientific knowledge or that we performed procedures using discredited techniques. They are least effective, however, when they lack real-time, real-world experience in the circumstances we faced or when they refuse to acknowledge the difficulties facing all physicians who, denied the benefits of hindsight, must make real-time critical decisions.

Will the jury "believe" the expert's theories? Our counsel's task, where possible, is to discredit the underlying theme of their presentation by raising doubts about their professional prowess and about the reliability of their testimony.

Can the expert's cross-examination benefit the defense? Rarely, if ever, do plaintiffs' experts admit on the stand that they are totally wrong and that we should be exonerated. Nonetheless, our counsel may attempt to draw the expert into a series of acknowledgments that can be used in final argument to support our case theme. For example, our counsel might ask:

> Doctor, you have the benefit of hindsight when you say my client should have diagnosed the ruptured appendix at the Friday afternoon office visit, isn't that correct? And isn't it also correct that two of the four 'classic' signs, as you call them, were not present during that examination?

The court instructs the jury that negligence is not to be based on what we know from hindsight. Agreement by the expert, however, bolsters our *concept* theme as well as our *factual* theme that, a physician in the same or similar specialty and community would not, in these circumstances, have diagnosed a ruptured appendix.

Motions

Following the presentation of the plaintiff's case, our counsel may make one or more motions aimed at terminating the case. Such an initiative is termed a motion for a directed verdict. If granted, the judge instructs the jury to find for the defendant and to dismiss one or all of the allegations of negligence. Although rarely granted, a successful motion for directed verdict reflects the plaintiff's failure, as a matter of law, to prove one or more essential elements of the claim.

The Defense's Case

The defense presents its case after adverse rulings on its motions for directed verdict. Because both sides enjoy flexibility in presenting their cases, the defense counsel ordinarily presents their witnesses in response to the impact of the plaintiff's case. If, for example, the plaintiff's experts are weak and ours are strong, our counsel may call us to the stand first, to make a strong closing with our experts. Conversely, if we are likely to be the strongest witness in our defense, our counsel may give a strong finish to our case by calling us to testify last.

Although Dr. Laura West never thought that her lawyers would win her case, she wonders, looking back, whether and how some of their strategies affected the outcome.

> The very first day when he called and said, "O.K., we've got the judge and we're going to pick the jury tomorrow," I said, "O.K., I'm coming, I'll be there to do it. But we're going to lose this case." But when I heard his closing arguments it was pathetic. Plus, he made a decision and he asked me my opinion. I have never been in a courtroom. Why would I ask my patient how to do a hysterectomy? So the plaintiff attorney was so furious that I outwitted him, that I had done a good job (in my testimony), that our lawyer thought that the plaintiff's attorney, the next day, when I went back on the stand, was going to eat me alive. So what he decided to do, and he asked my opinion, which I didn't totally understand, he said, "Well, I can put you up on the stand and just go through your CV, then he has nothing to cross-examine and you sit down and that's it and we'll let your partner take all the heat." And I said, "Whatever." And that was a big mistake because nobody knows the case better than the person who's really being sued. My partner was kind of dragged into it. His point was to keep me safe. I looked so good the day before. Don't let the plaintiff attorney get mad and convince the jury that I am a complete, whining, devious doctor. Don't give him the opportunity. Just sit up there and go over my CV and let them see I graduated first in my class and then sit down. But if he had put me up there and used me to do his defense part of the trial, I think we would have done better because my partner said her part, but she didn't read it the way I did.[6]

Presenting a coherent theme in support of our care is essential to our prevailing. We may use some experts to bolster the *factual* theme of our case and others to support our central *concept* theme. We rely on the experts to use language that jurors can readily understand, which is no easy challenge when we are explaining complex medical terms and conditions.

At the conclusion of our testimony, we want each juror to feel, "I wish that was my doctor." Because we are in the best position to present the medicine of the case, as we were the ones who palpated the patient's abdomen or listened to the bowel sounds, our role is to educate the jurors about these facts. We cannot win by simply disputing the plaintiff's version of the events; we must present as our theme a credible alternate explanation of the events in a straightforward and professional manner. No expert can resuscitate our defense if we destroy it by seeming arrogant, vague, or jargon prone or as if we were trying to obscure the truth. In the end, our preparation and our being transparent to the jurors make the decisive difference. As noted, jurors generally like physicians and have a stake in believing that we are competent, caring professionals. Dr. Cynthia Davis says:

> When the doctor testified, something happened that I found really amusing, warmly, I'm not scoffing, warmly amusing. Each time that I'd seen him, I was with him for about five minutes. I was with his assistant who was there the rest of the time. So I don't know whether it was his attorney or my attorney asked, "Now, Doctor, do you remember Dr. Davis?" They always called me Dr. Davis to elevate me for the jury . . . in terms of credibility. "Now, Doctor, do you remember seeing Dr. Davis as a patient?" It was the only time he ever looked over at me. And he looked over at me and said softly, like apologetically, "No." I thought that was eloquent. That was the most human touch in the whole thing. I said it was a game. That was a moment when it wasn't a game. . . . Here we are in this big deal and he can't even remember me? I was rather honored that he had the depth to understand the irony that I held him responsible for the loss of my sight and he couldn't even remember me. And there was pathos in that. So I had more respect for him at that moment. He was being truthful and regretful and . . . it was a human moment in the midst of a big game. It was very powerful and, yet, it may be that he and I were the only ones who realized it.[7]

Motions are offered to the court to allow the plaintiff to put on rebuttal testimony, an option sometimes also open to the defense. The court may, for example, allow testimony to rebut the evidence supporting our defense of comparative fault on the part of the plaintiff.

Closing Arguments

After the allowed rebuttal is completed, the case moves to the argument stage. Because the plaintiff has the burden of proof, their counsel may have two opportunities to address the jury. Argument consists of the plaintiff's *opening*, the defense's *final*, and the plaintiff's *closing*. The court may set time limits on these arguments, which may take several hours.

The judge will instruct the jury thoroughly to understand that what the attorneys say in their arguments is not evidence. Even so, we should never underestimate the importance of their presentations through which, evidence or not, skilled trial attorneys often sway juries to their cause. Plaintiff counsel's opening argument may highlight key facts while also touching on issues of both liability and damage. Our counsel must combine these two issues in their single opportunity to address the jury. Plaintiff counsel conclude by summoning their most compelling arguments in an effort to motivate jurors to award significant damages.

Jury Instructions

Following arguments, the court delivers the jury instructions, which may affect how the jury reaches its decision. The jury is to determine the facts of the case and apply the law as instructed by the judge. Jury instructions tell the jury what law is applicable to the case. Opposing counsel often argue at length outside the presence of the jury, trying to persuade the trial judge to adopt their version of these critical instructions. The side that loses such arguments registers objections to the court's decisions because only objections made on the record are subject to review on appeal. The judge, for example, may instruct the jury: "Your verdict will be for the plaintiff if she was injured and the defendant was negligent and such negligence was a proximate cause of her injury. Your verdict will be for the defendant if the plaintiff was not injured; or the defendant was not negligent; or if negligent, such negligence was not a proximate cause of her injuries." After the judge reads the instructions to the jurors, they retire to deliberate. Jurors first select a foreperson responsible for leading the deliberations and completing the necessary verdict forms. In most cases, the court will allow the jurors to go home at the conclusion of the day's deliberations.

The Verdict

The verdict form prepared by the court may contain questions designed to assist the jury to address all the essential issues in a complex case. In cases with multiple defendants, for example, the jury must determine whether one or more defendants are liable and the percentage of fault, if any, for which they bear responsibility.

Once the jury reaches its verdict, the bailiff notifies the judge, who then summons the parties to the courtroom. The bailiff takes the verdict from the jury foreman and hands it to the judge. After reviewing the form, the judge hands it back to bailiff, who returns it to the foreman, who then reads the verdict. In most jurisdictions, either party may demand that the jury be polled. The judge then asks each juror to state on the record whether they voted for or against the verdict.

Shortly thereafter, the judge thanks the jurors for their service and excuses them.

The Appeal

One or more postverdict motions may be made. In most jurisdictions, the party appealing the verdict must file a notice of appeal within a set period of time, typically thirty days. Appellate courts generally reverse verdicts only when the appealing party brings a mistake of law to the attention of the judge. This is known as "making a record." With rare exception, the appellate court does not substitute its judgment of the facts of the case for that of the jury. If the jury makes an award, the defense must post a bond guaranteeing its payment should the appeal fail. Many states require the bond to cover the full amount of the award. Otherwise, the plaintiff is allowed to execute on the judgment. Interest on this judgment may accumulate at statutory rates that are sometimes as high as 11 percent. Absent the like-lihood of a favorable outcome, the defense, while the appeal is pending, will try to settle for something less than the verdict.

The Emotional Shock of the Trial Experience

Few of us ever go to trial. Of the 184,950 closed claims reported to the Physician Insurers Association of America (PIAA) by its approximately 55 member insur-ance companies between 1985 and 2003, only 6.8 percent (12,640) of the claims have gone to trial. As shown in Figure 11–1, the defendant prevailed in 80 per-cent of the cases.

The word *trial* comes from the Old French word, *trier*, which means "to try." Any one who has ever been on trial can also relate to its family of meanings: "the process of testing" and a test of "faith, patience, or stamina through subjection to suffering or temptation."[8]

Preparing Ourselves for the Trial Experience

Deciding to go to trial, we must also gird ourselves for the battle, for it is no less than a battle on many levels. Each of us prepares in ways that match the demands of our work and the needs of our personalities. Dr. Mary Santos typifies the self-discipline required to deal with a three and one-half–week trial as a sole defendant.

> I totally prepared for the trial. I went through everything. I really sweated. I called the defense attorney frequently. I had an elaborate notebook and timeline and memo-rized everything. I began arising about 4:00 A.M. daily to engage in "mental train-ing," using writing and meditation, which I continue. I was aware of depressed feelings

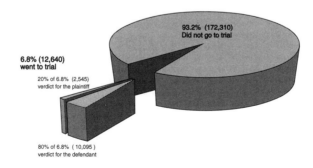

Outcome of 184,950 Closed Claims

Figure 11–1. Outcome of medical malpractice trials. National Data (1985–2003), Physi-cian Insurers Association of America (PIAA), Rockville, MD, with permission.

that came in waves and then as the trial approached, it got worse. I think it was like a battle. You know this inexorable thing, like you're going to land on Omaha Beach and you're going to go to Berlin. And you have to go through it in order to get there.[9]

Getting Our House in Order

While some of us have months, others have only a few weeks before trial to rearrange our schedules. We must commit a great deal of time to study relevant trial testimony and documents, to meet with the lawyers, and to prepare ourselves to testify. Many of us must continue to earn a living and to shoulder our share of the work burden for our group or clinic during the runup to trial.

Most attorneys ask us to be present in the courtroom throughout the trial; our absence tells jurors that we have little interest in their deliberations. Does this subtly suggest that they should decide in favor of the plaintiff who is present and invested in the process?

We need flexible work schedules if we are to devote large segments of our time to the trial itself. Work obligations and coverage options for time away differ for each of us. Psychiatrists, for example, must give their ongoing psychotherapy patients sufficient time to prepare for their absence and give clear instructions regarding coverage during those periods. Other specialists must plan how they will meet their surgical and outpatient obligations. Because trial length is unpredictable, we may need to draw up contingency plans well in advance of the trial and be flexible enough to change them as the case unfolds.

Our individual circumstances determine whether we schedule patient care during trial. Most trial veterans recommend that we maintain only minimal, if any, work obligations during the actual trial. Dr. Laura West recalls:

What my partner did was almost the same thing as what I did. We, weeks in advance, prepared. And some people don't have a chance; they don't have a partner. But in advance we prepared and cut our offices back and set everything up so it wouldn't be an overload for our partners, so they could handle the volume. We didn't take any new patients, any gyns, or annual exams. They could wait a few weeks. We just set up for obstetric patients. We made an effort to make life easier for the people here. Everyone knew we were in court. Patients were told we were out of the office. That's all they knew. They found out later, when they saw the newspaper. There were four of us in the practice, so my two younger associates manned the fort. And it was so upsetting to me everyday so I never came back to the office. I couldn't. I had to go home and read depositions and prepare, keep busy with what was at hand. My partner came back everyday and came in every morning to kind of go over paperwork, sign off on Pap smears, and to keep herself occupied. And also help the partners, so she felt like she was doing her part. She just didn't see patients. So I think we both did the right thing in that I think it is a big mistake to see patients or have anything to do with patient care. It is consuming and distressing and it's just not fair to the patient. You are going to make mistakes, I would think. I can stay up for 36 hours and be sharp as a tack, but this is like nothing I have ever done. To others, I

would recommend: I would not even go to the office. I wouldn't call. I'd have whatever it took. I'd pay whatever kind of money it took to get someone to fill in and not
even think about it.[10]

One of her partners was scheduled for another trial shortly after the completion of
Dr. Mary Santos's trial. Feeling that their practice could not afford such prolonged
absences, she felt financially compelled to continue to see patients periodically.

> Mondays, I operated. Mondays, we don't go to court. I did do a couple of cases in
> the morning on other days before trial but one ended up being more complicated. I
> felt that this is really crazy. So I did not do that. But I did on Mondays and then we
> saw patients in the evening. I had to clear off my desk.[11]

Working with the Attorneys

By the time our trial begins, we will already have spent considerable time with
our attorney reviewing the pertinent case materials, discussing the theories of the
case, giving depositions, and preparing to testify. These activities are merely the
overture to the main act of working intensely with our attorneys during the trial
itself. Meeting with them before and after courtroom sessions is a participatory
rather than a passive experience. Listening to and following their advice does not
mean that we do not make observations or ask questions. The courtroom is to lawyers what the examining room is to physicians. We must let them make the decisions in this environment. We fulfill our role by meeting as closely as possible
their expectations of us. This means that we will do the following.

- *Present ourselves as competent and caring professionals* whether in giving
  testimony, listening to others as they testify for or against us, or, in the sim-
  plest but most difficult of challenges, just waiting for things to happen.
- *Maintain our composure* even under heavy fire from the opposing side.
- *Remember that everything that transpires within the courtroom is directed
  at the jury.* Although counsel asks us questions, we give our answers directly
  to the jury in a friendly, competent manner, using language that helps them
  understand the point at issue. We overcome any temptation to impress them
  with our learning and present ourselves as clinicians well versed in medical
  practice and the care of patients. The plaintiff attorney may attempt to distract us or break our concentration but, if we anticipate these efforts, we can
  handle them.
- *Remember that we answer questions at trial differently than we do in a deposition.* No longer do we give "truthful" but limited responses; we no longer aim
  for the bull's eye but rather for the larger target. At trial, we are permitted to
  take our time and give complete answers so that members of the jury can get
  the information they need to make an informed judgment on the matter at hand.
- *Keep an eye on our own attorney during our testimony.* One or another of
  the attorneys objects many times during the trial. We should never continue

to talk through or over such objections but stop testifying immediately so that the matter can be adjudicated promptly. Sometimes we do not understand the reasons behind the attorneys' objections. The plaintiff attorney, for example, may stop us in mid-sentence during testimony that is strongly in our favor. Naturally, we feel impelled to complete our thought so that the jury will fully understand our point. Instead, we should yield to our attorneys and let them handle these interruptions as they see fit and let the judge rule for or against us. We should never worry about our unfinished point as our lawyers carry out their obligation to see that nothing important to our defense is lost in such exchanges and that all significant material is eventually brought to light.

- *Beware of leading questions.* On the stand, we need to concentrate to avoid being tricked into agreeing to something that is either not true or not in our best interest. The plaintiff attorney may press us to give our opinion about a hypothetical situation, the territory we should never enter unless we are sure of our footing and know exactly the safe path to follow. Our lawyer may interrupt but, if he does not, we should answer the questions as we would in a deposition. If we feel that we cannot respond, we can simply say, "I cannot answer the question in the way it is stated." The rule of thumb is to answer only those questions that relate to actual facts and specific questions.
- *Know our own deposition thoroughly.* The other side will try throughout the trial to impugn our credibility by attempting to impeach us, by getting us to contradict the testimony of our deposition. If we gave a truthful deposition and know it well, we need not fear that we will contradict anything we said before.
- *Make ourselves available to our attorneys throughout the trial.* It is not unusual, at the end of each court session, to meet with our lawyers and associates to review the day, to analyze testimony and evidence or work assigned, and to discuss issues related to the next session or to the overall case. We may well be asked to do some research or obtain materials that respond to the plaintiff expert's testimony. If, during our testimony, we failed to make some points essential to our case, the defense team tells us how and when they will re-introduce these issues. Clearing our calendars of all clinical obligations frees us to participate full-time in these sessions. If, however, we are obliged to see patients between and after court sessions, we not only feel more pressured but we also feel distracted, that we are along as outsiders who are not fully involved in the daily action of the defense team.

After the Trial

A trial is indeed a test. It is, as Dr. Laura West reflects a year after her trial, "like nothing I have ever done."[12] In a study conducted in the late 1980s, 52 percent of physicians who had been on trial felt the entire process was most stressful, while 16 percent said the trial itself was the most stressful aspect of the process. Those who won and those who lost resemble each other, reporting similar symptoms and changes in their behavior as a result of the experience.[13] In a real sense, there are no winners or losers in medical malpractice trials. It is difficult to pin down just how we feel at the end of our long journey.

As winners we may be stunned, exhausted, and pleased but certainly not triumphant. Relieved, yes, but we wonder why we had to go through such a terrible ordeal in the first place. The patient, perhaps, has suffered a tragic injury, but we did not cause it and our care has been judged competent. Why must we go through this painful experience to come to this end? Isn't there a better way to help injured patients?

As losers, we feel overwhelmed, sad, unnerved, and perhaps angry at what passes as justice. We may be exposed to a blitz of damaging publicity as a result of the increasing use by plaintiff attorneys of public relations firms to advertise their successes. Our care may have been judged insufficient, but we know that we are competent and accepted as such by our peers. There may have been extenuating circumstances or questionable legal representation, or the emotionally charged patient's presentation may overwhelm all other factors. Various members of our team or hospital personnel may have made a mistake. Whatever leads to the verdict, we feel singled out as suffering a loss that has consequences for us in its wake. In a study in the 1980s, physicians who lost at trial were more likely than those who won to feel that the patient's case was indeed justified, and they were significantly more likely to feel guilt and lack of social support.[14] The results of the verdict are also reported to the National Practitioner Data Bank and the state medical board. We may need months or years to assess the implications of the verdict and repercussions on our renewal and premium rate.

An appealed verdict involves us further with the lawyers. The defense may appeal the size of the judgment, an issue of utmost concern to us. It may be difficult to remain engaged, especially after a negative outcome, but we must force ourselves to continue to cooperate with the process.

Are we the same persons we were when all this started? Can we take up our lives where we left off, put the event behind us, and go on as if nothing has happened? We may gradually resume our normal routines, but we will be aware of subtle, and not so subtle, changes in our attitudes and in the ways we approach our work.

Listen to some winners and losers: "I plan to discontinue the practice of medicine within five years, as soon as I can arrange to ease into a new profession. I can only hope that liability roulette doesn't strike again in that time" and "For twenty-five years I truly enjoyed seeing patients and trying to help them. The trial has changed that. I wrestle with every decision I make on every patient, knowing how it can be misinterpreted and distorted and manipulated for greed. I don't know how much longer I will continue to practice."[15]

Reflecting on her life a year after losing at trial, Dr. Laura West says,

> The good things are that I'm plugging along. Everything I've done before has got-
> ten me to where I am now. I would have been just completely devastated five years
> ago. So I've been transformed in the sense that I've managed to go on. But I also did
> not decompensate. I went to some departmental dinner, like a week later, and I wasn't
> worried that somebody was going to bug me and ask me all these questions. I went
> and I did everything that I was supposed to do and acted like nothing happened. I've
> come a long way. I have confidence in my abilities, but I do spend too much time
> worrying about who is going to sue me.[16]

Even though Dr. Mary Santos won her trial, she says "I hope I will never have to
go on trial again although I think I probably will. I would say the big thing is that
it's time to turn and fight these charges. But that the bottom line is that it was very
positive. But you really need a good attorney."[17]

As humans, we adjust to the extended effects of trauma. Are we angry? Yes.
Disappointed? Yes. We may even feel a touch of bitterness about the expectations our society places on us, about the law and how lawyers work, and we may
speculate ruefully on the seeming motivation of greed that marks at least some of
them. But we can also feel much stronger emotionally, a bit sadder, perhaps, but
also wiser and still able to take pride in and feel good about ourselves and the
work we do. Our enriched understanding enables us to evaluate accurately the
risks we take in our daily work. We can make realistic plans about our future as
we clarify our life's goals. We appreciate far more our family and friends and take
steps to achieve a better balance between our work and our personal life. Even in
defeat, we have defended our integrity and emerged intact, tested and made more
whole by trial.

Recommendations for Preparing Ourselves Emotionally

A trial tests us in a public setting before people we never saw before and are unlikely ever to see again but who nonetheless hold our destiny in their hands. We
are accused of the professional capital sin, of failing to meet the standard of medical
practice in our care of the patient. Anticipating these and the other stresses of the
trial is our healthiest psychological preparation for sustaining and surviving them
successfully.

THERE WILL BE DIFFERING VIEWS OF THE "TRUTH." During the trial, plaintiff
attorneys and witnesses make statements about our care of the patient that they
believe to be true and that we believe to be blatantly untrue. We are surprised, not
to say startled, and our patience sorely tried when we hear others swear to what,
from our perspective, we know to be false accusations and false testimony. We

are struck with disbelief as we hear experts we once respected dissect our treatment of the patient and charge that we violated the basic standard of care. They must not have reviewed the available documents, we think to ourselves, or they must not have prepared well, or perhaps the plaintiff attorney made them an offer that they could not refuse. Feeling deeply hurt, we are tempted to rise quickly in our own defense. But we must patiently wait our turn, and that usually comes only after the plaintiff attorneys have attacked our integrity and painted what we see as a markedly distorted portrait of us.

THERE ARE ALTERNATING PERIODS OF OPTIMISM AND DESPAIR. We ride a mechanical bull as much as a roller coaster during the alternate case presentations. While being accused, we find ourselves enraged, disappointed, appalled, frustrated, and anxious for our own survival. Can we possibly get through this unscathed? Will our life ever return to normal? As our story is finally told, we feel optimistic and hopeful that we really can win this case. Sometimes our anger is fierce, and it may linger on within us long after the case has been resolved.

Norman Mailer catches the intensity of his rage about his trial in 1980, heard before a circuit judge on Cape Cod, who tried the highly publicized divorce case one day each week. He laughs heartily, self-observant and surprised at the depth of his rage that is easily rekindled:

> I was smoldering. And how manifestly unfair all this was. And we had not had our shot yet. And I thought, Boy, oh boy, when I get my shot, when I get my shot, when I get my shot. I'd wake up in the middle of the night in a murderous rage, which is absolutely the worst. And you can't get back to sleep and there's nothing you can do about it. And you feel all the value of murderous emotions—each value is wasted. Murderous emotions are attached to high ideals, to accomplish wonders. Murderous emotions disconnected from any possibility of being exercised are the most single failing in the entire panoply of people's feelings.[18]

THE UNEXPECTED IS COMMON. Delays materialize, unwelcome, out of the blue as in the true story of the judge at the co-author's own trial, who suddenly called off court for the afternoon to see a visiting congressman, explaining, to our dismay and his unfelt chagrin, that the subject would be pay raises for the judiciary. Or, at the last minute, an expert cannot arrange to give his testimony at the time desired by the plaintiff's side. Witnesses may testify in unanticipated ways that totally surprise us and our attorneys. Issues, sometimes tangential or seemingly easy to settle, suddenly appear that cause the lawyers to research and argue them at length, draining away valuable court time to little relevant purpose. Even before we have had our chance to testify, the plaintiff's side may suddenly raise a settlement flag. That the courtroom, product and symbol of solemn tradition, turns into the stage set for both the unanticipated and the unimaginable makes philosophers of us all.

DIRECT EXAMINATION AND CROSS-EXAMINATION ARE MARKEDLY DIFFERENT EXPERIENCES. We finally take the stand to give our testimony and, with our lawyer's careful encouragement, seize the opportunity to tell our side of the story. We feel quite satisfied and pleased that the jury is finally getting a picture of what really happened. Perhaps for the first time in the process, optimism spreads through us, a welcome feeling that we must guard against revealing to the jury.

The plaintiff attorney may rise to cross-examine us, intent on rattling us, making us slip up, or making us so muddled by anxiety that we present confused and even inaccurate testimony. They want to trip off our frustration and anger so that we overplay or lash out in our response. They may repeat the same question many times, sometimes sarcastically, offering false interpretations that test us mightily. They are not interested in uncovering facts as much as revealing our vulnerability. We quash our temptations to fire back with like anger or sarcasm, remaining as professional as we want to be perceived, calm and in emotional control, persons who maintain their respect for the embroiling process. We meet these difficult challenges by presenting ourselves genuinely, by just being ourselves in that simple way that speaks powerfully to the jury and the court.

> The plaintiff attorney who deposed me in discovery could tell I had a short fuse. So when it came to the trial he expected me to blow my stack. So we prepared and prepared and we were ready. My testimony at trial was an A+. I was so cool, he never got me upset and he pretty much said, "You're a liar, you're this, you're that." And he tried everything. He didn't care if he lied. I fortunately knew the medicine and he didn't and I got to calmly point out the error of his ways and so it went really well, so well that afterwards at a break, he told my lawyer, "You did a great job preparing this witness." Well, most of the preparation was mine but, indeed, my lawyer knew I needed to be a different person than the day I was at the first deposition and I was the person I needed to be at the right time in front of the jury.[19]

WE WILL FEEL ALONE AND VULNERABLE. We seldom feel more alone than when we are publicly accused of incompetent behavior before a random group of fellow humans. Even though we have confidence in our attorneys and feel support from our associates and family, we—especially if we are the only defendant—feel that we are well-defined targets—isolated, exposed, and vulnerable—on the boundless plain of the process. If we are accused in public, only we can defend our honor in public. Many of us have family and associates who stop by, often daily, to lend invaluable support to us in the courtroom. As Mike Wallace reflects, this is a time when "you learn who your friends are."[20]

WE MUST PREPARE FOR THE OUTCOME. Even though, along with our lawyers, we monitor the reactions of the jury members during the trial, we are never sure just how they will judge the case. We enter a strange interlude of expectation after the jury retires to deliberate. While they weigh our fate behind closed doors, we discover a new challenge—managing our anxiety as we prepare to stand in the well of the court and face the jurors as they render their verdict. The verdict usually comes back after a reasonable interlude, but time stretches and bends beyond our control while we wait.

Mike Wallace describes his experience:

> What I used to do occasionally, a couple or three times a week after the morning session was over, I'd go up to my psychiatrist's office, which took a ½ hour trip, then spend an hour with him and then go back down and so forth. He said, "I'll tell you what. We've got to get you ready to do two things: First of all, to testify. You're afraid to testify, and the reason you are is because you've been asking that kind of question, the gotcha question for so long, that, you know, you figure that it's going to happen to you and you're not sure you've got the proper answers and besides which you are obsessing and feeling this way. And then, we've got to get you ready to lose. Because if you lose, you think your life is over. Let me tell you something, you are sick. You're wrong on both scores. There's no question that they can ask you questions that you don't know the answer to. And you're not going to lose in a million years. And even if you were to lose," and he has educated himself by this time about me, he said, "if you lose, you think your credibility is destroyed for all time. Therefore, you won't have a career. Therefore you won't be able to make a living. . . ."[21]

With the help of his psychiatrist, Mike Wallace was able to view his deepest thoughts and fears and to confront them head on, preparing himself for the daily attacks on his integrity and the final outcome of his trial.

12

Case Over: What's Next?

At the end of this long journey, we have mixed feelings that resist easy or quick sorting. Finding closure remains beyond our grasp. Our lives are not the same for we are now intensely aware of the risks as well as the satisfactions of our profession. How did things get to this point?

A Brief History

The Law

The medical and legal professions and the insurance industry have been fit, sometimes forced, together over many centuries into the patchwork quilt of medical malpractice litigation. Mohr dates the definition of *mala praxis*, or "malpractice," to Sir William Blackstone's 1768 volume *Commentaries on the Laws of England*.[1] The goal of malpractice laws is to fix blame and award compensation to the injured party. Although an outbreak of lawsuits erupted in the United States against medical practitioners in the already professionally turbulent mid-nineteenth century, legal action against them was relatively infrequent until another century had passed. In the 1960s, social transformations swept through every American institution, including that of medicine.[2] In the early 1970s, dramatic increases in the number of malpractice claims against physicians and the payouts awarded by juries precipitated a crisis of insurance coverage. We have witnessed cycles with only brief periods of stable predictability and relative calm since then.

Insurance and the Law

Born in nineteenth-century England, liability insurance flourished on its transfer to the highly industrialized and booming American economy. Heralding progress with showers of sparks, locomotives crossed the continent, setting businesses and homes ablaze. Who was responsible, and who would pay for these fires? The law at the time espoused strict liability, as in the *res ipsa loquitur* doctrine—"the thing speaks for itself." It spoke simply: the railroads that caused the fires rather than those who built businesses and homes along the tracks, bore the responsibility for the damage. The widespread application of this doctrine raised a barrier against progress as it threatened American industry with financial ruin. This crisis prompted reflections on, and accommodations to, America's Manifest Destiny, that is, its sense of being called to expand itself beyond all borders. Two parallel responses occurred. Liability insurance became available to industries to manage their risk of financial ruin while legislative changes and new understandings of tort law reinterpreted the very notion of fault, holding that persons who used ordinary care and foresight could not be held liable for an injury or accident in which they were involved.

As the twentieth century dawned, the worlds of health and work were clearly risk-laden. The vulnerability of ordinary people to unemployment and growing old without sufficient resources to support themselves were also clear. A developing social conscience motivated society to become the insurer and the provider of a safety net for its citizens. Legal historian Bernard Schwartz, observing how the social climate always influences changes in law, noted that "the law of torts has steadily moved from a fault to a social insurance basis."[3] The "pro-plaintiff changes in common law doctrine" that abolished the immunity of many charitable entities have also contributed to the increase in malpractice claims.[4]

Medicine, Insurance, and the Law

Medical care relies increasingly on technological developments that demand the exercise of great skill in demanding circumstances by the professionals who use them. Along with pharmacological and diagnostic advances, these developments expand the risk potential for patients. Meanwhile, the ever-expanding medical–industrial complex is viewed as impersonal, a tissue match to big business, increasingly financed by the government, which can absorb the costs of the negative outcomes that go along with increased risks.

Medicine's social contract with the public requires that practitioners and healthcare entities adhere to a high standard of ethics and discipline as they define and follow an accepted standard of care. If as a result of physicians' failures to meet the standard, patients suffer negative outcomes, we are judged responsible for a situation that imposes on patients the costs of all subsequent medical care and other expenses. To safeguard our own assets while meeting the fiduciary obligation to provide compensation for such patients, we pay premiums to purchase liability insurance. Conflicts routinely arise about whether, in fact, we failed to meet the standard of care and whether our actions contributed to the injury of the patient. In civil society, tort law settles such disputes between physicians and patients by determining who is at fault and therefore responsible for providing compensation.

Where Are We? Not Everything Works According to Design

The Law

Physicians and insurers blame lawyers and the legal system for the increase in malpractice suits filed against them. Some critics blame judges who have "abdicated their role as gatekeepers" and "lost sight of the idea that lawsuits concern not only the particular parties to the dispute, but everyone in society."[5] It is relatively easy for patients to file malpractice claims because their lawyers' contingency fee arrangements minimize their personal risk in doing so. As Tocqueville noted of Americans two centuries ago, "this entire independence, which they enjoy continually vis-à-vis their equals and in the practice of private life, disposes them to consider all authority with the eye of a malcontent. . . ."[6] This skepticism about authority often motivates juries to award damages for reasons not necessarily related to a breach of the standard of care. In a prosperous and wealthy country, large jury awards seem equitable because, in this populist vision, the patient "deserves" something.

A recent congressional study recognizes that physicians are not alone in their anger and frustration about lawyers and the legal system they appear to master.

> The medical liability system in the U.S. suffers from several major shortcomings that adversely impact the negligently injured as well as the general population. The system fails to achieve either of its central goals: compensation and deterrence. First, the vast majority of negligent injuries do not lead to a claim. By definition, if injured parties do not file claims, then the tort system provides them no compensation. Second, among those claims that are filed, the vast majority shows no signs of an injury or harmful event. If such claimants receive a payout, then the tort system is providing compensation for the wrong people. Third, when a legitimate claim is filed, the system typically takes years for the injured party to receive anything. Finally, even when legitimately injured parties are able to prove negligence, plaintiffs' lawyers routinely take 33% to 40% (or more) of that for legal fees. On balance, it seems clear that the medical liability tort system broadly fails as a means of compensating the negligently injured.
>
> On the second goal, the deterrence of negligent behavior, the tort system also fails to achieve its mission. Since most acts of medical malpractice do not result in a claim and most claims are not tied to actual negligence, the tort system is unable to

convey to doctors the appropriate signals about the optimal level of care. Moreover, the litigious environment created by the tort system discourages the reporting of mistakes, which impedes efforts to identify and prevent medical errors. In fact, the threat of malpractice litigation induces doctors to practice defensive medicine, subjecting patients to unnecessary treatments and therapy.[7]

State legislatures have responded by addressing the economic repercussions of this system on the insurance industry rather than by any substantive change in tort law itself. A few experiments have offered alternative modes of obtaining compensation for injured patients but, after a generation of tinkering by state legislatures, the basic problems remain if not largely unexamined, at best unreformed.

Insurance

Because of escalating insurance premiums, large jury awards, and unrelenting increases in claims incidence in the 1970s, the insurance business itself became all the things it set out to modulate for its clients: risky, unpredictable, and potentially unprofitable. Insurers then revealed their business natures by withdrawing from the market, leaving many physicians without coverage. Organized medicine responded by forming nonprofit physician-owned companies that offered physicians lower premiums, options about settlements, participation in evaluating the merit of claims, and a focus on service rather than on profit. In 2004, there were approximately 55 physician-owned member companies in the Physician Insurers Association of America (PIAA), a nonprofit trade organization of professional liability insurance companies whose Data Sharing Project is the world's largest database of open and closed claims. It identifies common areas of physician liability with the goal of designing educational programs to prevent further mishaps. The group's strong efforts for tort reform are partially motivated by data revealing that approximately 50 percent of the monies available for compensation to injured patients is disbursed instead to attorneys and to pay for other litigation expenses.[8]

Tort reform, aimed primarily at stabilizing the medical liability insurance market, has been on state and federal legislative agendas since at least the mid-1970s. The model reform is the 1975 California Medical Injury Compensation Reform Act (MICRA), the crown jewel of which is its noneconomic damage (i.e., pain, suffering, and loss of consortium) cap of $250,000. This has enabled California insurers to reinstate some predictability about the amount of compensation they will have to disperse, thereby allowing them to provide more predictable insurance premiums for their doctors. The American Medical Association (AMA)'s Report 32 of the Board of Trustees and its supplements offer an extensive review of tort reform measures and structures for the resolution of medical liability disputes.[9,10] It explores such proposed and enacted alternative liability reforms as the fault-based administrative remedies and the no-fault plans in Virginia and Florida for the compensation of neurologically impaired children. The latter reforms require concessions from all parties, remain underused and, in large part, have proved to be unsatisfactory to both plaintiffs and physicians.

In 2003 in Texas, a state noted for problems associated with runaway litigation and an aggressive plaintiffs' bar, savvy political strategies were used to pass the most sweeping tort reform since MICRA.[11] The Texas Alliance for Patient Access, a nonpartisan, broad-based consortium of over 250 physician groups, hospitals, professional liability carriers, and professional associations led the effort. After the initial legislation was passed by both houses and signed by the governor, the Texas electorate narrowly passed a constitutional amendment guaranteeing the bill's statutory cap on noneconomic damages in civil, not only medical malpractice, lawsuits. This put the reform beyond the reach of any judicial review.

Medical Practitioners

Physicians remain at the center of the medical malpractice crisis even as their work with patients becomes increasingly risky. Managed care and other practice arrangements have introduced changes into the traditional physician–patient relationship that may influence patients' interest in pursuing litigation. Most physicians have to supervise staff, run a business, and ensure the financial stability of their practice despite diminishing reimbursements so they can pay their staff and support their families. Medical liability insurance is a key factor in preserving the financial health of a medical practice.

Insurance premiums, however, change with market conditions and have drifted upward in recent years. Exceptions occur, as when in 2003 the Texas Medical Liability Trust promised a rate reduction if both tort reform and the constitutional amendment passed.[12] In the same year, in states with limited tort reforms such as Illinois, the approximately 35 percent premium rise across all specialties threatened to swamp physicians who were trying hard to keep afloat. Across the country, stories are common of physicians who, unable to afford their insurance premiums, either leave practice or leave town for another location.

To many of us, lawyers seem to use the law as an instrument of intimidation. Lawyers, who file suit to earn a living as well as to represent their clients, view settlement very differently than we do. Obtaining some compensation by settlement, even though no deviation of care is established, achieves their ends. But we protest, "Why should we pay when we are not guilty of negligence?" We bear the scars of settlement long after the wound of the case has been largely forgotten if not completely healed. "He jests at scars," Shakespeare tells us, "that never felt a wound."[13]

Although lawyers claim that their primary interest is the plight of the injured, they are extremely selective about whom they represent. Some become advocates only for severely injured or deceased patients. The whole system strikes us as grossly unfair to us and to our patients.

Particularly threatening and intimidating is the recent trend of attaching settlements and jury awards that are in excess of coverage to our personal assets. In Illinois, for example, at least six physicians have declared bankruptcy in recent years because of the obligation imposed on them to pay for awards that exceed their insurance coverage. Tort reform legislation to shield physicians' assets by limiting the recovery in medical malpractice cases to the amount covered by the physician's insurance was introduced in the Illinois legislature in 2004 but failed to pass. In the past, in the world then governed by gentlemen's agreements, plaintiff attorneys never settled beyond the limits of the policy. Their former strategy of suing a number of defendants to guarantee adequate funding of a large award no longer holds. Their clear message to physicians now is, "Settle, or we'll go after everything you own."

Threatened with potential bankruptcy, physicians have become more hesitant, asking, "Why shouldn't I settle, even if I've done nothing wrong, rather than go to trial and take the chance of losing everything?" The always-adversarial battle between lawyers and physicians is no longer the impersonal: "It's just the cost of doing business in today's world." The news of professional reverberations and possible financial ruin make it even more personal and make more difficult any compromise or search for alternate solutions.

Where Are We Going?

The Law

Tort reform opponents view the medical malpractice climate primarily in economic terms. They dismiss the need for reform since, according to the Congressional Budget Office, the direct cost of insurance premiums and indirect costs associated with defensive medicine constitute only about 2 percent of total health-care expenditures.[14] Proponents of tort reform, exasperated by the slow progress of state-based reform, espouse a federal solution; pending federal legislation, in the form of H.R. 5 (the Help Efficient, Accessible, Low-Cost, Timely Healthcare [HEALTH] Act of 2003), would contribute $12.1 billion to $19.1 billion in budgetary savings each year.[15] Although passed by the House of Representatives in 2003, the Senate has failed to act on this legislation. If passed, federal legislation may deliver economic relief while leaving in place tort law's use of personal fault as a bludgeon that does real damage to physicians.

Medical malpractice litigation, viewed narrowly as an economic problem, will not stimulate significant changes in tort law in the short term. Far more persuasive is the growing and hotly debated problem of patients' access to care that is attributable to the present malpractice system.[16,17] Access has been attenuated because of prohibitive costs of insurance premiums and, less directly, through the noneconomic costs the system extracts from practitioners. Physicians are weary of sitting in courtrooms when they could be in their offices seeing patients or in the operating room performing surgery. They are worn down by the personal assaults on their integrity while they are delivering the best of care, and they are intimidated by the threat of financial ruin after spending their lives in service to the community.

The Texas experience demonstrates that a campaign of public awareness is essential for the success of any reform. Educating the public, especially about access to care, not only prompts the passage of reform legislation but also increases the level of sophistication that jurors bring to the multilayered problems of medical malpractice litigation.

The current medical malpractice system is acceptable "as is," when it is profitable for such interested parties as insurers, plaintiff and defense attorneys, and a subset of the patient population. Substantial reform will not take place as long as the system reinforces itself by rewarding enough people, enough of the time, in enough of the general population.

Because the effort for tort reform is piecemeal at best, it must wait on an integrated consideration of its legal, insurance, and medical themes.[18] In the meantime, it would be prudent to allow genuinely useful tort reform efforts to proceed while developing those alternatives that promote substantive changes in administering compensation in the health care system.

Insurance

Insurance is a business and insurers must remain solvent to deliver their services. They not only support tort reform but also initiate other methods, such as "high-low" contracts, to stabilize their losses. Insurers and the plaintiff attorneys recognize that it is to their mutual advantage to strike agreements in certain circumstances, such as on the eve of trial, in cases in which although no liability appears present, the parties recognize that catastrophic damages remain a possibility because of the possible volatility of juries. Plaintiff attorneys, knowing that most trials result in a defense verdict, stipulate to a settlement process through which the insurer guarantees them a mutually agreed-on payment even if the plaintiff loses the trial. Both sides "bet" that they will win. The agreement's high amount is the insurer's payout limit, a figure that is always within the defendant's policy limits. This agreement is a form of jury nullification—should the jury award the plaintiff $10 million and the contract's high value is $1 million, the latter sum is paid. Should the jury find for the defendant, awarding no damages, the insurer pays the low value, $100,000, for example, as agreed-on in the contract. The contract usually requires the parties to abstain from an appeal and to forego any applicable prejudgment interest.

Insurance companies also invest in risk management education activities to disseminate information about how to address legally problematical areas of medicine through changes in practice. Some insurers conduct site visits that evaluate physicians' offices and provide remedies that lower risk. The Colorado Physicians Insurance Company sponsors an "early offer" program in which physicians who recognize a patient injury, other than death, contact the insurer within seventy-two hours and, together with the risk manager and without attorneys, work to resolve the problem, usually by an offer of compensation.[19] As noted earlier, other insurers also offer a range of services to provide educational and emotional support to sued physicians to help them become better defendants.

Medical Practitioners
If there is little hope for quick and substantive change in tort law and if reforms camouflage the dangers rather than reveal a safe course for the Titanic, what are we, the practitioner passengers, to do?

As in war, there is no substitute for victory, so in medicine, nothing supplants the competence that includes keeping abreast of advances in our field and fostering good communication with our patients. In the cruelest of ironies, we can do all things well and still be sued.

Recommendations

We can use our best energies to adapt to the situation in ways that match and serve our personal and professional circumstances.

A PLAN FOR OUR FINANCIAL HEALTH DEPENDS ON OUR LOCATION, OUR INDIVIDUAL CIRCUMSTANCES, AND OUR EMOTIONAL STAMINA. Asset protection attorneys, a new legal specialty, are gaining credibility as they advise their clients on using such mechanisms as trusts and partnerships to protect their assets. An estimated 20 percent of physicians in Florida's Miami-Dade County follow another scenario by no longer carrying malpractice insurance. Aware that state law protects their homes and annuities from creditors, these physicians are permitted to practice without insurance if they self-insure, informing their patients of this arrangement through which they assume financial responsibility for as much as $250,000 for any judgment against them.[20] In some jurisdictions, physicians are required to post a bond to ensure payment in the event of an award.

Confronted with skyrocketing premiums, many Texas physicians are buying affordable policies with lower limits even though this renders them no longer eligible for privileges at many hospitals. Many hospitals responded to this loss of doctors by lowering staff requirements for minimum malpractice coverage to $100,000. The jury remains out on whether, as a growing conviction among physicians in some states suggests, lawyers will be less likely to sue us if we purchase lower limit policies.

WE CAN PLAY AN ACTIVE ROLE IN REFINING THE CURRENT TORT SYSTEM. Working with our specialty and state medical societies as well as our liability insurers, we can, for example, identify those experts who provide inaccurate or misleading testimony. Medical societies have sanctioned members found guilty of this latter behavior and insurers, such as the Illinois State Medical Inter-insurance Exchange, do not hesitate to report such experts to the state disciplinary board. Founded by two physicians, the Coalition and Center for Ethical Medical Testimony (CCMET) aims to expose dishonest, incompetent, or unethical medical experts.[21]

ONLY WE CAN SHAPE OUR OWN PRACTICE ENVIRONMENT, refusing, for example, to practice outside our sphere of expertise. We can insist that our staff understand their responsibilities and that they implement good risk management principles in our offices. Only we can balance our personal and professional time commitments so that our families do not suffer unnecessarily.

WE CAN STRIVE TO DEVELOP AND MAINTAIN HEALTHY PHYSICAL AND EMOTIONAL LIVES for ourselves and our families by having our personal physician, working out or engaging in regular exercise, taking family vacations, and maintaining a social life that is recreational and supportive.

IN AN IDEAL WORLD, TAKING A WINNABLE CASE TO TRIAL, ALTHOUGH DIFFICULT, IS FAR BETTER THAN SETTLING. Each of us will choose what actions best prepare us for the experience and its aftermath. Dr. Mary Santos sums it up for many of us:

> I do feel the need to get the word out about fighting these suits. I treated it like an adventure. I would not let it interfere with my love of medicine and my patients. I would be a better doctor. I would meet amazing people. It was a terrific challenge. Not allowing the negative distractions associated with the case to interfere with my focus and taking time away from patient care during the trial were important lessons. After my trial, I had one regret, I should have had a week's vacation.[22]

13

Closing Arguments

> In peace there's nothing so becomes a man as modest stillness and humility:
> But when the blast of war blows in our ears, then imitate the action of the
> tiger: Stiffen the sinews. Summon up the blood.
> —Shakespeare, *King Henry V*, Act 3, Scene 1[1]

As long as we work with patients in the high-risk environment of health care, we
will live with the possibility of adverse events. After signing off on difficult cases
of every kind in long careers in medicine, we come upon one for which we will
never gain closure. It began in a moment that grew into years of turmoil as we
were formally accused and had to defend ourselves against medical negligence.
Responsible or not, we wonder, Did I do anything personally that contributed to
the bad outcome?

We understand Saul Bellow's words, "The unexamined life may not be worth
living but the examined life is driving me crazy."[2] Trained to constant self-
examination, we are disquieted by the emotions—doubt and guilt, shame and disappointment, anguish and fear—it stirs within us.

Despite our shell shock, we are still obligated ethically and humanly to talk
with our patients with respect and empathy. But the shadow of the law falls across
us and we worry that if we say, "I made a mistake" or we say nothing at all, we
may be sued for malpractice. Rather than responding in a natural and caring way,
we find ourselves trying awkwardly to keep our balance on the high wire of
impersonal rules and regulations. Self-consciously, we feel compelled to save
ourselves rather than serve our patients self-forgetfully, and thus we find that
protecting ourselves from legal actions may supercede healing our patients of
their ills.

Being sued gives us more rules to follow, of which the most frustrating forbids us to talk to anyone about our case. Litigation is indeed a form of trauma, and we must stir ourselves to take on its main challenges.

- *We must tame this dehumanizing experience by making it as human as we can.*
- *We must integrate, that is, make something whole of an experience that threatens to disintegrate our worlds and our work.*

We are better off in every way if we remain human during this demanding and deeply traumatizing experience. As humans, we must talk with others. We can free ourselves to do this if we avoid detailed discussions that advertise or extend our liability. We are not monks who must take vows of silence but professionals who use prudence as we participate actively in a process whose every detail we should understand thoroughly.

We reject victim status as we aggressively take on two challenges that are really one—informing ourselves about the law and defending our integrity. Despite the emotional and financial cost, we can resist the plaintiff bar's efforts to seduce and intimidate us and take defensible cases to trial. Nothing is more important than the lawyer who represents us and we must demand, and fight for, if necessary, legal representatives who are competent, experienced, and fully committed to our cause. It is *our* reputations and *our* lives on the line and we must demand the best leadership for the battle before us.

Experience teaches us that those of us who take an active role in our defense, no matter at what stage or for how long, are far more satisfied than those who accept passively being overwhelmed and victimized. Nobody is going to fight in our place. We take courage from the fact that taking an active role makes it far more likely that we will win than lose and thereby help shake up and change a system whose biggest secret is that it can be changed by men and women who remain true to themselves and to their highest personal and professional ideals.

Appendix 1

Case Histories

1. Richard Allen, M.D.—Interview with SCC on January 10, 2000

Dr. Allen saw a 60-year-old woman on one occasion in a presurgical consultation and recommended that surgery be delayed until her conditions of hypertension and anemia were stabilized. The orthopedic surgeons decided, in view of her pain and distress, to proceed with an anteroposterior lumbar fusion. Postoperatively, the patient developed a pulmonary embolus and, because Dr. Allen was on vacation, his partner treated her with anticoagulants. She sustained cardiac arrest and died the morning Dr. Allen returned to work. An autopsy showed that she had a large retroperitoneal bleed that apparently led to shock and death. Just before the statutes of limitation expired, the patient's estate sued Dr. Allen, his partner, and the radiologist while not naming the orthopedic group or the orthopedist, who was later found to be a friend of the family. After 2 years of discovery, Dr. Allen settled for $50,000; his partner, for $225,000; and the radiologist, for $500,000.

2. Mrs. Maureen Anderson—Interview with SCC on October 30, 1999

Mrs. Anderson sued the urologist who had operated on her father for benign prostatic hypertrophy, alleging that he failed to diagnose her father's fatal postoperative myocardial infarction. Five years later, after a two-day trial, the jury ruled in favor of the urologist. Ms. Anderson's lawyer offered to appeal the decision, but she felt that she had done what she set out to do and that for her, "it was all over."

3. Saul Bellow—Interview with SCC on September 13, 1999

Mr. Bellow's former wife sued him, contesting the financial arrangements of a divorce settlement. The bench trial progressed over an 8-year period before a few different judges and culminated with a judge's decision that the settlement monies be increased substantially. Mr. Bellow appealed the decision to the Appellate Court, one of whose members was a judge who had presided over the bench trial, and lost.

4. Leonard Cerullo, M.D.

Dr. Cerullo surgically removed, by a trans-sphenoidal approach, a pituitary adenoma from a middle-aged woman. Two or three days after surgery, she developed double vision and a pulsating exophthalmus. He suspected a carotid cavernous sinus fistula, which was confirmed by testing. A specialist in the area agreed to accept the patient, but she died before the transfer could take place. Dr. Cerullo was charged with, among other things, failure to diagnose the condition in a timely manner and failure to perform additional surgery or refer the patient to the appropriate expert. Eleven years after the surgery and after a four-week trial, the jury returned a guilty verdict and assigned damages of $300,000. A posttrial settlement resulted in a $1 million award.

5. Joseph Daley, M.D.—Interview with SCC on June 17, 2003

Dr. Joseph Daley repaired a herniated disc in a middle-aged man. Postoperatively, the patient did well. Some time later, the patient sustained a back injury while shoveling snow, a proscribed activity. Because Dr. Daley was ill, a local university professor operated on the patient and referred the patient back to Dr. Daley. The professor dictated a lengthy note, alleging that the referring physician's (Dr. Daley) original surgery created scar tissue that required him to open another disc space. The patient did not do well and sued Dr. Daley, alleging that his original operation was inadequate. The insurance company judged that the case, supported by expert testimony, was defensible in that the patient's current symptoms were due to the second surgery. At the time, Dr. Daley had, for personal reasons, coverage of only $100,000/$300,000. He hired a private attorney to protect his interests, and the case was eventually settled for $100,000.

6. Cynthia Davis, Ph.D.—Interview with SCC
on September 12, 2000

Dr. Davis became legally blind after a number of episodes of nausea, headache, pain, and right-sided disturbed vision. After consultation with two physicians who diagnosed and treated her for acute conjunctivitis, she consulted with a specialist, who instead gave her a diagnosis of acute glaucoma, which resolved with surgery. She sued one of her previous ophthalmologists for misdiagnosis and, approximately 5 years later after a three-day trial, was awarded over $350,000 in damages.

7. Norman Mailer—Interview with SCC on October 29, 1999

Norman Mailer was a defendant in a highly publicized 1980 divorce case. A judge presided over a bench trial one day each week. At the time, Mr. Mailer lived in New York and, for approximately six months, was required to travel to Massachusetts for the weekly proceedings. His estranged wife charged him with failing to reveal his full economic status, the cause of her alleged unjust divorce settlement. Mr. Mailer eventually paid significant, but less than demanded, monetary damages because evidence supported his claim about his current financial holdings.

8. Mary Santos, M.D.—Interview with SCC on July 25, 2003

Dr. Santos's patient had a previous cesarean section but was committed to having her second child delivered vaginally. Although Dr. Santos and her nurses had talked with the patient about the associated risks, the patient persisted in her desire for a vaginal birth after cesarean (VBAC). Nonetheless, Dr. Santos prepared the operating room and she or one of her assistants was present at all times during the patient's labor, which progressed rapidly. As evidence of variable decelerations occurred, a scalp pH was found to be 7.22 and, within 30 minutes, the patient delivered an essentially dead infant. Dr. Santos had extensive documentation throughout the labor and delivery, including information about the risks and statements of "Do you wish to proceed with this?" to which the patient reaffirmed her commitment to the procedure. Dr. Santos attended the funeral and received a thank-you note from the patient for her care and concern. A year later, she was sued, and after 7 years of pretrial maneuverings and a 3½-week trial, she was found not guilty of negligence.

9. John Schmidt, M.D.—Interview with SCC
on September 19, 2003

A woman in her mid-40s, who was not wearing protective headgear, was catapulted over the handlebars of her bicycle, hitting her head on the sidewalk. Dr. Schmidt saw her in the emergency department, and a CT scan (prior to MRI) confirmed a subarachnoid hemorrhage. She was alert and oriented and had mild nausea but no focal signs. Within 24 hours, she developed signs of delayed traumatic intracerebral hemorrhage and deteriorated rapidly. She was intubated and put on a ventilator. The family insisted that she be moved to a university hospital in another city, where she died. Dr. Schmidt was accused of having missed the diagnosis and failing to administer pain medications appropriately. He settled for less than his $200,000 policy limit.

10. Mike Wallace—Interview with SCC on October 22, 1998

General William Westmoreland, the former U.S. Army commander-in-chief in Vietnam, sued Mike Wallace in 1982, along with CBS and *60 Minutes* staff members, for libel and asked for damages of $120 million. The trial began on October 9, 1984, and continued until February 18, 1985, when General Westmoreland withdrew the case just short of the verdict. He accepted that the CBS statement citing his "long and faithful service to his country" and saying that the network never intended to portray him as "unpatriotic or disloyal" counted as an apology by the network and cleared his name. (E. Randolph, *Washington Post*, February 19, 1985.) CBS denies making any apology and will make no payment (*U.S. News and World Report*, March 4, 1985).

11. Laura West, M.D.—Interview with SCC on June 19, 2003

Case 1: Dr. West saw a patient, whom she judged was an obstetric emergency with an anticipated placenta accreta and who, in retrospect, probably also experienced an amniotic fluid embolism. Before the delivery, Dr.West conducted a well-documented informed consent conference and lined up experienced back-up. After the delivery, the patient developed adult respiratory distress syndrome and was recovering when, on her eighty-fifth day in the intensive care unit, a nurse placed a fatty emulsion tube feeding into her intravenous tube instead of the port. The patient died immediately of a pulmonary fat embolism. Dr. West, in conjunction with the university hospital, was sued for wrongful death. The hospital settled, and after 4 years and just before trial, Dr. West's case was dismissed with prejudice.

Case 2: Dr. West performed a laproscopic tubal ligation on a 39-year-old woman. Shortly after surgery, the patient developed a suspected uroma, requiring a return to the operating room. The surgical team performed a laporatomy and repaired a bladder injury, after which the patient became septic. She then developed adult respiratory distress syndrome and a necrotizing fasciitis and died within ten days. Dr. West was accused of failing to obtain proper informed consent and failing to diagnose and treat properly the necrotizing fasciitis. The hospital settled for $350,000 and, after 4 years, a jury dismissed the informed consent claim but, on the second count, found a $6.5 million judgment against Dr. West and her partner.

12. Thomas White, M.D.—Interview with SCC on July 21, 2003

Dr. White's patient, in her third uncomplicated pregnancy, began to bleed thirteen weeks before her due date and delivered a nonviable baby. A few weeks before the statute of limitations expired, she sued Dr. White for $6 million, alleging that he ignored her complaints of vaginal bleeding for a few weeks before the delivery. His office has a procedure for responding to such complaints, and neither he nor the staff had any memory or record of this complaint. Expert testimony supported the contention that the fetal death was secondary to a thrombophelia. After 2 years of discovery, the case was dismissed just before trial.

Appendix 2

Selections from a Contemporaneous Diary
Plaintiff vs. Cerullo, et al.

Leonard Cerullo, M.D., a Chicago neurosurgeon, experienced the death of a patient after surgery for a pituitary adenoma. Eleven years after the surgery and 9 years after being sued, he dictated extensive notes before and during his trial, from which these selections are taken.

April 1 (50 days before trial)
I talked with my wife for the first time about the possibility of settling out of court, the pros and cons, and at the same time remained extremely ambivalent. I also talked with my partners that night and explained to them that I would really want their input regarding settling the case and how this would affect our practice, and how trying the case would affect our practice as well.

April 3
My partner talked to me this morning, giving me his strong feeling that to go to court would serve no useful purpose and would be disastrous to the practice in terms of patient flow and surgical flow. From the point of view of certain of my friends who would consider this kind of an act of a soldier going to war, willing to sacrifice himself, if need be, for the common good, the common good being, of course, the medical malpractice situation in the country. I'm not sure now, nor was I sure then, that I am willing to sacrifice myself for a system which doesn't

care at all about me. On the other hand, I don't want to have to live with giving up to what I perceive to be an injustice just for the sake of a few dollars or a few days. So, it is this that is now weighing heavily on my mind. The question for me becomes a moral one, rather than a financial one, but the disappointment and dis- illusionment of knowing that if we go to trial and win, the only real winner is the insurance company from a financial point of view, and the real loser is me from my financial point of view, as well as, of course, the plaintiff's lawyer. On the other hand, if we win from a moral point of view, both the insurance company and I have scored victories. If we go to trial and lose, and very likely the award will be in excess of what I am insured for and, therefore, I lose big, being person- ally liable for the remainder.

April 8
The meeting with my defense attorneys ended after about an hour and a half or an hour and three quarters on a very upbeat note. I feel now for the first time, the lawyer has a more comprehensive and accurate picture of the mechanism of both of injury and of death.

April 30
The lawyers are scheduled to take the second half of the deposition of the neuro- pathologist early next week, and he apparently, too, is coming on very strongly in favor of this being a congenital thinning of the artery as a reason for the fistula. He apparently is bolstering our case.

May 6
I called my personal attorney (one of the area's premier plaintiff attorneys) and I can't explain the tremendous feeling of relief I got from talking with him. "Would you like me to become involved?" and I, of course, had a tremendous sigh of re- lief, and said that I would. He understood from the beginning the trauma of the event. I explained to him that it was mainly related to the amount of time that I would be wasting in court and the feeling of abandonment by not really having any true representation of myself. At any rate, he was just marvelously support- ive and very confidant sounding.

May 7
My personal attorney said, "Well, are you afraid of losing the case?" And I stated that I wasn't afraid of the fact but I was concerned about the capriciousness of juries.

May 11
It is somewhat disconcerting to me that here we are less than a week before jury selection and just about a week before the actual trial, and there are still so many

unresolved issues. It is my gut feeling that they are going to try for some sort of a postponement, if not an actual settlement, but again, maybe I'm just being unduly optimistic about this. Maybe we're going to go to trial with a lawyer, who at least to date has not impressed me with his level of preparation or commitment to my innocence regarding the whole matter.

(Having reviewed the plaintiff's expert opinion) I reiterated to my defense attorney my contention that whether or not we injured the carotid at the time of surgery was totally irrelevant, whether or not we diagnosed the carotido-cavernous fistula a day or two later or earlier was irrelevant, and that the only relevant issue from my point of view was how the jury was going to respond to what could be a very graphic demonstration of a very traumatic death. He assuaged my fears in this matter by reading through the nursing notes . . . and really there is very little of a grotesque nature.

He stated that his major fear (in terms of my expert witness) was his arrogance and impatience. Whereas it's apparent that the plaintiff expert has spent many, many hours studying and preparing for this case, I doubt that (my expert) has done more than glance cursorily at the chart, at least that's my defense attorney's allegation.

May 19

My personal attorney called to apprise me of the latest developments, particularly that he had sent a letter to the defense attorney stating that I was his client, and stating that he had reviewed the documents and had suggested settlement within the limits of the policy, that this was basically to protect me in case we should lose in excess of the limits of the policy, the insurance company, and not me, would be liable. I asked him point blank that if I were offered the opportunity to settle, should I take it, and he certainly indicated that I should, the point being why take the chance if it's not needed.

May 20 (day 1 of the trial)

It's May 20 and it's a beautiful day. Today should be a very interesting day in my life. I'm sorry I didn't have a chance to talk with (a friend who has been on trial) prior to this, but I think I'm ready for it.

I started the morning by arriving at the office around 5:30. I came in and cleared my desk and now will go to surgery until 8:00 AM at which time I will meet the defense attorneys at their office. We started a case of medial sphenoid tumor invasive into the cavernous sinus. I then went to the lawyer's office (who) prepared me by discussing some things I should and should not do in the trial and both when I'm on the witness stand and when I am not; specifically, he mentioned for me to keep a calm demeanor, to look interested, to not react, to make eye contact with the jury. He advised me to go very carefully over my depositions so that when I'm on the witness stand I cannot be impeached.

We then went to the courtroom, where, after meeting the judge and the jury, the plaintiff's opening statement was made, extending from 10:00 o'clock to a quarter of 12:00. In the early portions of his statements, it was appalling the number of errors he made in technical terms and descriptions, but in the closing . . . I felt he was quite effective; he overestimated blood loss and overestimated the amount of time this occurred over, and basically painted a very emotional picture. At least in the early part of his discussion, I looked at the jury frequently and found them to be quite bored.

My lawyer gave a nice opening statement, beginning about 1:53 PM and ending just after 3:00 PM. The statement covered most, if not all, of the points: specifically talking about acromegaly as a more important disease than a cosmetic deformity; the lack of evidence that there was puncture of the artery by the laser or by any other instrument; the fact that carotico-cavernous fistulas are very classic in their presentation, and when in the immediate postoperative period her symptoms disappeared, the diagnosis would be highly questionable at best; the fact that an angiogram was performed in a timely fashion when the disease was suspect; and, finally, the appropriateness . . . to transfer this patient to a recognized authority within the city.

May 21

The plaintiff's attorney deposed (presented the testimony of) the brother and then the sister, and then finally the daughter (whose) deposition (examination) was interrupted by her crying, and the judge warned the witness after the jury had been dismissed that the crying witness concept might cause him to throw the case out of court if she couldn't control herself. He was certainly sympathetic to her grief and sorrow, but wanted her to understand that this may be prejudicial to her case.

Immediately after a conversation (with my personal attorney), the judge asked the plaintiff's attorney if he would be willing to settle, giving a $1.75 million figure. (The latter) felt that similar cases had been settled recently in the neighborhood of $12 million, and he would not be at all interested, nor would he recommend that his client settle for this amount.

This afternoon was worse than this morning. The girl turned out to be a fairly decent witness and her brother turned out to be an excellent witness. When I finally got to the stand, there was a very, very brief questioning of me. I was called as an adverse witness, which apparently has a difficult interpretation in terms of Illinois case law. What it basically means is that they probably cannot quiz me from a text, and the fact that they called me early and spent virtually no time indicates: (1) that they had nothing in my deposition to hang their hat on; (2) they recognized that I'm a good witness, and (3) that this would force my lawyer to put me on later.

(The letter Dr. Cerullo's private attorney wrote to the insurer suggested settlement within the limits of the policy and was now in the defense lawyer's hands.)

The court ended early shortly after 3:00 PM, and my lawyer immediately took me back to the conference room. It was obvious that he was pissed (about the personal lawyer's actions). I feel like I'm somewhere between a rock and a hard place and this is not a good feeling. I finally told my lawyer that since I trusted him and that I felt he was doing a good job, at least insofar as I'm capable of ascertaining, that I would continue to follow through but that I was relying on him as a gentleman and as a quasi-friend to inform me if he felt the case were going badly and he felt we ought to settle. He, in turn, promised me that after tomorrow's deposition (testimony) of the plaintiff's expert, if he had that feeling, that he would so notify me and that he would then immediately go and affect a settlement. I think this is a reasonable compromise. It costs me one more day and gives me a chance to demonstrate my faith in a fellow human being. I'm concerned, I'm scared, I'm pissed, but at least I feel good about myself, not just turning around and running away.

May 22

I met with my lawyer just before trial time this morning, and he explained to me that he had talked to my private attorney this morning and was prepared to get me a consent form for me to sign and pull out of the case at this time. We discussed intimidation, and I told him "that, yes, I was intimidated, but, no, that I didn't feel that he necessarily was intimidating me."

At any rate, the plaintiff expert's deposition (direct examination) took the entire morning from about 9:30 AM to 11:45 AM. He really over-extended himself in terms of making points about negligence and failure to live up to the standard of care, etc. to the degree that my lawyer asked, "What does this guy have against you?"

It was a marvelous afternoon. My lawyer was nothing short of theatrical, and the result on the expert was absolutely devastating. We got off to a real slow start and my heart was in my throat. I thought if this was the way it was going to go, I was dead. I was ready to sign the papers; I was ready to cut my throat. But then he picked up speed and dealt with every single issue that had been planned, quoting from the literature and forcing him time after time to either renege on a statement, to impeach himself, or to qualify what he had previously said, so that by the end of the session the defense group practically got up and cheered.

May 26

It's Tuesday morning. The judge called my lawyer back to his chambers and told him that his cross-examination of the defense on Friday was the best he had ever seen. Although he had recommended settlement in the neighborhood of $1.75 million prior to that, now he really in good conscience could not recommend settlement to the lawyers, and he would really have to see how the case proceeded from here before making any kind of recommendations one way or another regarding settlement.

My lawyer then got on for his re-cross and was devastating to the plaintiff's expert in terms of many of the allegations that he had made in terms of many of the inconsistencies, which kept coming up throughout the deposition (testimony).

The plan is to let the plaintiff's attorney finish his experts and then to proceed with me on Friday. Hopefully, I'll be a good witness, and hopefully the jury will have a great deal to think about over this weekend. I don't feel as bad about the trial as I had several days ago, but on the other hand, I don't feel great either. It's been and continues to be a difficult thing. I feel that my testimony is going to be very important in this case, and I think that I'll be able to come across to the jury as being an honest, sincere, and competent caregiver.

May 27
It was a real rough morning. I think eventually I'm going to be forced into demanding settlement and I think that I'm going to be forced into that posture because my defense attorney doesn't seem to be able to take the idea of settling very lightly and without a great deal of ego loss. On the other hand, it is true that I very much want to get on that witness stand, I very much want to tell those people my side of the story. During this time when I know that the plaintiff's attorney is out after my ass and I know that my lawyer's sitting back there and stewing and feeling negatively about the whole thing, I wonder who's worried about me? Obviously, yet once again this impression comes up that there are all these people playing with each other, and the only person who has anything to lose in this whole event is me, and yet I'm the only person who seems to be unprotected, even with my personal attorney, because at least this morning or at least after that meeting in chambers, I felt that he had done more to hurt my defense than to help me. Yet, he was, I know, doing it for good reasons, and I know that my defense attorney shouldn't have responded that way; yet, here I am, still holding the bag, so to speak.

This afternoon was another treat to my lawyer's cross prowess. He had the witness contradicting himself and, in fact, impeaching himself so many times, it was almost too painful to watch. In fact, every time he said, "Do you remember your sworn testimony of blank-blank date?" the man let out a visible and audible groan, as if to say, "Now, what are you going to do to me?"

May 28
I think the posture that I'm going to adopt with regard to the insurance company will be that if they will go to the wall for me, I'll go to the wall for them. That is to say, if they will guarantee my excess liability, I will continue through the case and not recommend settlement within the policy limits, even if that means $5 million. On the other hand, if they are unwilling to go to the wall for me and offer me the coverage, then there is really no reason why I should put myself at risk when I have a policy for this magnitude paid for with good money in good faith.

God smiled on me today. The plaintiff called one of the nurses as their witness. When my attorney got up to cross-examine her, he went over her history and ascertained definitively that she had appreciated no changes in the patient's condition; that bilateral orbital swelling and photophobia and conjunctivitis were routine following this type of surgery; that nasal drainage of blood on the mustache dressing was routine following this type of surgery; that I always responded to nursing questions and queries; and that I always did what I said I was going to do to a patient.

(After the afternoon session, meeting the witness and others in the hallway) The nurse said again, "You know, I just didn't want to hurt you. I think you're the best doctor that I know, and if I ever need any surgery, I want you to operate on me." Well, this was just too much for me. I started to cry, and I turned around and walked back into the courtroom for a few minutes to compose myself, but I then came out. I felt embarrassed, but by the same token I wasn't embarrassed because she had done a marvelous thing, and that's what I told her. I said, "You know, you got up there and told the truth. You know, this has not been a pleasant thing for me. I've never gone through this before, and hopefully I never do again, but after hearing people tell lies and lies and lies for the last four days, to hear somebody tell the truth was just such a breath of fresh air that I was totally, totally grateful."

May 29
(No session was held because of difficulty in scheduling experts so the lawyer and doctor discussed impending testimony.) We specifically discussed in detail the few areas that had been concerning me, namely my recollections as opposed to memory of the exact events, and he seemed to have no problem with me using vague recollections and then becoming fairly specific in terms of what I say. The other issue that concerned me was the difference in dictation of the operative note from the date of surgery to the date of alleged dictation and transcription, and he reminded me that records do get lost, they get misplaced; sometimes they even have to be re-dictated, but in my recollection I dictated the operation on the day of the surgery, and therefore any difference between that recollection and what is typed on the operative note has to be explained by the hospital administration and not by me.

June 1
Last night I met with my defense attorney and discussed the case in detail, particularly from the standpoint of my testimony, going over the program, so to speak. I feel very good about going into court today. The former resident gave his deposition the other night, and was quite supportive. In addition, he discovered on the poly-tomograms evidence of a false floor to the sella turcica. This is different from the lateral sphenoid septum that the plaintiff's expert had described, and I think

very nicely supports all of the contentions in the operating note and dismisses the allegation of the plaintiff's expert that the lateral sphenoid septum was interpreted as being a false floor. My lawyer instructed me on my demeanor in the courtroom, and I should answer his questions and the opposing lawyer's questions with equal candor and equal equanimity.

We then get the former resident on the stand, and he did very, very well with the direct examination. The plaintiff's attorney, however, picked up, because of the answers and the questions that were asked by my lawyer, that he had been coached and demanded a *voir dire* to quiz him on that. So the jury was released, and indeed on Friday evening from 5:30 PM to 7:30 PM he had met with his and another lawyer. He stated that 95 percent of the conversation was spent going over his testimony but that he had been apprised of the testimony of the plaintiff's expert and also that he had seen one of the drawings of the expert. He said this did not change his opinion in any way, and, basically, the judge allowed the trial to go on.

The judge has a friend who died and has a funeral to attend on Wednesday, so there will be no trial on Wednesday, and that's terrible as far as I'm concerned because it puts our defense that much further back and puts the resolution of this whole thing that much further back. Sometimes, it is more frustrating than other times, and today is one of those particularly frustrating days when the only person's time that is not being considered is mine. The jury gets paid, the lawyers get paid, the judges get paid; I don't get paid.

Part of the frustration I was able to vent today, talking to the man from the insurance agency. I said, "If this ever happens again, I am settling. I'm not going to go through this nonsense again. This is ridiculous."

I finally got on the stand and testified for about an hour, only on my credentials. They had a side bar, and at that time the judge dismissed the jury. The point is if the question has not been asked in depth, can it be asked in the court room, and it seems to me ridiculous that the only questions they can ask you are questions they have already asked you, so that if they were too stupid to ask an important question, then I'm not allowed on direct questioning by my attorney to answer that. This is just inconceivable to me. I hope the judge will rule in our favor, but if he doesn't, the plaintiff's expert has already testified to this. The point, though, here is this crazy law that says that they have to know everything ahead of time before going into court and learn nothing in court. It just is inconceivable to me that if you don't look for something and you don't find something, that you should be rewarded for that.

At any rate, I think the jury responded very well to my presence. They looked at me. They had their eyes open. I think we're beginning to relate, which honestly speaking is the first time I can say that. My lawyer chastised me a bit this evening because I had pre-guessed his questions and would answer them before they were asked, and he felt I was moving things along too fast and that I was lacking in foreplay, so tomorrow I'll be a little more laid back and allow him to call the shots. I think the real problem is that he is annoyed that he is not getting to ask as many questions as he would like to ask because once I get started I just continue on to the next answer and the next answer and the next answer without any questions. At any rate, I feel pretty good about the jury, and we'll see what happens tomorrow.

June 3

It's Wednesday morning. I was able to begin the testimony this morning, and I think it went very well, at least my lawyers all thought that it went well.

Following the morning session, I spoke with them for a while outside the courtroom, and basically we talked about hung juries and what that would mean. My lawyer stated that if the jury were to hang, his recommendation to the insurance company would be to settle. He also stated that it was too bad that they didn't sue the corporation, because if they had, then he could offer to the plaintiffs a certain amount of money without having my record besmirched by this event, that is, in case I lose. On the other hand, I told him that really at my stage of career, it doesn't make any difference whether I have this in the National Practitioner Data Bank or don't have this in the National Practitioner Data Bank. Obviously, I would prefer not to but it really doesn't make all that much difference to me. He said not to worry, that we're going to win anyway, but that if it looked like we weren't going to win, he would follow the recommendation that he encourage the plaintiff to re-sue or add another party to the suit, that being the corporation, and he said he would do that. This thing gets more and more complicated all the time but basically the beat goes on.

The shit hit the proverbial fan. (One defense expert was accused of having talked with a lawyer whose client had been dropped from the case.) At any rate, the plaintiff's lawyers are now moving to strike the witness's testimony altogether or to *voir dire* both the lawyers regarding their involvement in this case. And it is, at least, one lawyer's opinion that they may move for mistrial, but I have a strong feeling that even if we win this case, it's going to go on appeal and as my lawyer told me earlier, this will mean that he will recommend settlement.

Reportedly, it's been the law in the state of Illinois, at least for the past 4 or 5 years, that the plaintiff's attorney can speak to any treating physician at any time regarding his opinions in the case but the defense attorneys can only speak to a treating physician at time of deposition, regardless of whether they have anything positive or negative to say. I think this puts the defense at a significant disadvantage, and certainly raises the cost, and I have no idea why this law is allowed to exist, but that's the way it is. It is totally incredible to me how little truth has to do with the running of this case and how vulnerable the defense is in this situation. I am continually amazed and, in fact, overwhelmed that the truth really has very little to do with the case, merely the adversarial relationship between the two sides and the maintenance of equal rights for both to lie; that seems to be the heart of the issue. The final negative effect of this whole afternoon of nonsense is that this case is going to go at least through most of next week, as well, and that's extraordinarily depressing to me.

It's interesting to me that the other day the bailiff, who has been present for most of the proceedings, asked me after my deposition (testimony) whether I was an ophthalmologist. It seems that he has early cataracts and was going to just chat with me about some information. If he, who is used to hearing testimony every day and who is probably smarter than the average juror, thinks I'm an ophthalmologist, and this case is about the eye, I wonder what the rest of the jurors are thinking. Another point is on depositions. It seems that depositions are basically taken prior to trial to discern truth, which then can be gussied up or distorted or obliterated entirely in time for the main event.

I operated on a patient with a brain tumor this morning with Ed. It was a lot of fun, and this afternoon I'll see outpatients.

June 4

It's Thursday morning, June 4th. The morning started off with a bang. I got in very early to do a thoracic laminectomy for rhyzotomy, then Ed came and relieved me, and I came to court.

The plaintiff started off with two written motions. One was to bar my expert's testimony altogether. It seems to me kind of a late hour to make such a motion but that's what they did. The second motion was for a mistrial or, alternatively, to strike and bar certain testimony, namely that of the treating anesthesiologist and to give relief, which I guess means a chance for them to hire an expert anesthesiologist to counter the opinion of the treating anesthesiologist.

My expert then got up and my lawyer beautifully took him through his CV, which is indeed as least as impressive as any that I've heard ever, and more so than most. There were numerous objections when he got into the meat of his discussion regarding the case. There were numerous, numerous requests for a side bar but the judge refused them and said that he would deal with them all later.

Overall, I think that my expert was absolutely superb. I think that while the jury fell asleep during the cross-examination, they certainly woke up for the re-cross. This certainly has been a roller coaster day in terms of my emotions, and I'm sure glad it's coming to a halt pretty soon.

June 5

It's Friday, the 5th of June, and the beat goes on. This morning was kind of nondescript. I did a craniotomy first thing in the morning, and then got to court around 9:30 AM, on time as usual, and, of course, the deposition (testimony) never started until 10:00 AM, again as usual, and also, as usual, the plaintiff's attorney had a few motions to eliminate this or that or bar this or that. As it turns out, the anesthesiologist has been disqualified, and the jury, I think will be told to disregard his testimony.

The afternoon of June 5th was quite memorable for a number of reasons; the first is that my lawyer was really good in terms of the continuing direct examination. We ended up with his asking me about covering and cross covering with my partner and about the last few days of the patient's life. His final piece d'resistance was the death certificate, which was signed by my partner and on which he said that he last saw the deceased on the day before, that is, the Saturday before. We also got into the record that I did not leave town until 8:00 o'clock Monday morning, that is to say, about six hours after she died. There was a tremendous reaction to the death certificate on the part of the plaintiff's attorneys who practically flipped a cork, motioning that this not be allowed as testimony or evidence.

June 8

It's Monday morning, and it's now 10:00 o'clock. We haven't begun yet. The first thing will be the discussion between the attorneys over whether the death certificate can be admitted. Interesting, one defense lawyer met with me and he went over the natural progression, as we anticipated it to be, and that is that I will finish my testimony today, both direct and cross. Tomorrow we'll be off because my lawyer has to leave at 1:00 o'clock this afternoon to go to the funeral for his uncle.

I asked him what the course of action would be if we appealed the case, and he said that if we lost the case and then appealed and won the appeal, that we may have to retry the case, and that's what his bosses like to happen. In fact, when they go back to the office to say, "We won the case," the comment is, "What the hell you mean, you won it?" the idea being the more work that's created for the defense lawyer, the more money they make, and, of course, this is just the opposite for the plaintiff's lawyer; the more they work, the less money they make. The only thing is that nobody really gives a damn how much money I lose, and I told him, "You've got me this year. You won't get me any more this year, so do what you're going to do, but I'm not being back in court this year for any reason at all."

A friend came to court this morning A lot of people have offered to come, but I don't particularly want them to come. I just feel more comfortable doing this thing on my own.

It's now 2:00 PM in the afternoon and the morning went kind of uneventfully. It's disappointing, I guess, one could say, how weak their cross examination has been to date. Unfortunately, they weren't able to finish the cross examination before (my attorney had to leave for a funeral) which means, of course, that I have to go back on Wednesday to continue the cross-examination and hopefully to wind up the testimony.

I feel pretty good and yet, somehow, very let down by the anti-climactic nature of this morning's testimony. I think I was expecting to be hit harder and in a more effective manner and I don't think that I was hit either hard or effectively. Of course, what I think isn't important; it's what the jury thinks that counts. Right now, with these days continuing to add up, it's being more and more costly to me, and I'm not sure that I care what price. I just want to get this thing over with and out of my hair. The letdown of this morning is kind of profound. Right now, I have nothing but disgust, anger, and lack of respect for their whole case and the whole manner in which this has been presented and the fact that we end each day with new motions to try new material and to eliminate people who are contrary to the plaintiff's opinion, the more disgusting the whole thing becomes for me.

At any rate, tomorrow I'll have a normal day, seeing normal outpatients and operating in a normal fashion, and even going to rounds in the morning, and I'm looking forward to that tremendously. There was only one time this morning at which I was even required to go to my deposition, at which time he tried to impeach me, but, in fact, when we did go to the deposition, I think it was pretty clear that I was right and he was wrong.

June 10

(My personal lawyer) had written yet another letter to the insurance company and as yet has received absolutely no response either verbal or written from them. I think this again points out the fact of the matter and that is, that the insurance company is trying to save money for the insurance company and really could care less about the psyche, or for that matter, the excess damages of Leonard Cerullo. This is another sobering truth in the whole case and one that I am sure will continue to embitter me. There's really no reason that this case shouldn't have been settled in the beginning within the limits of my policy and my personal attorney felt that it could have been done for well under $2 million. So the insurance company wins, maybe; the plaintiff's attorney wins, maybe; and I lose for sure. I did, as I mentioned, however, receive a great deal of experience, which, as has been said, is invaluable at any price. At any rate, it's the 10th of June, the beat goes on, and we'll see what happens today.

This thing just keeps dragging out longer and longer, but if any of these (recent motions) are allowed, then certainly it's not going to end on Thursday, and the judge has already said he is already taking off Friday to go to a golfing outing by the Trial Lawyers' Association. This thing is really beginning to wear thin.

As we were preparing to leave, my defense attorney came to me and said, "Well, do you want to settle?" The judge told him that, in his opinion, we had a pretty strong case but not an airtight case, and that there were enough emotional issues and enough emotional jurists that it really could go either way, and, in fact, it was the judge's opinion, that if the jury went out at this minute without any further testimony from anybody that they would probably be a hung jury, which means, of course, that we would be in this whole fiasco over again.

At this stage of the game that suits me just fine. I think that justice has not been done. I think that it's been miscarried but on the other hand I think that the case is just too complicated to expect any reasonable jury of citizens, and maybe even a jury of neurosurgeons, to understand the nuances and come up with the correct answer. So that while in my heart of hearts, I'd certainly like to come out of this thing having won, by the same token I'm not so naive as to recognize that there's at least a significant chance that I will not win, at least this time around, and that means more investment of my time, which I just really cannot do. They said they would contact me this afternoon, and I'm sure I'll hear something one way or another.

It just is amazing to me that we should have gone through this charade for this period of time basically in order to save the insurance company money because if we had started out with the plaintiff's attorney's demand for the limits of the policy and given them that, then everything would be hunky dory, the case would be over, and everyone would have been home a month ago, but in the interim, what we've basically done is save the insurance company between $3 and $3.5 million and managed for Leonard J. Cerullo and CINN Medical Group to lose probably in the neighborhood of $200,000 to $300,000. At any rate, as I told my attorney earlier, I leave it in his hands; I feel confident with him making this decision and I feel that whatever happens, it was a good experience. Also whatever happens I'm not going back to the courthouse this afternoon.

It's Wednesday evening. Things have gone from bad to worse. I got the word that the plaintiff's attorney offered $2 million to settle, and negotiations were about to begin when my lawyer called the insurance company, who now refused to settle at any price. Meanwhile, the judge has heard the various motions from the plaintiff's attorney, who wants to bring in not only a rebuttal neurosurgeon, but also a rebuttal anesthesiologist and a rebuttal radiologist to counter the various testimonies. The judge, according to one of the lawyers, is bending over backwards to accommodate them with all these rebuttal experts and he told me that he wouldn't be surprised if the case went another two weeks. I informed him that I had requested settlement papers and I requested the consent form to sign, and I have never received it. I further told him that I didn't plan to go to court any longer, and if the insurance company wanted to continue to pursue this, they could do it on their own time because I wasn't spending any more time in court, and I am now trying to get in touch with my personal lawyer. This situation has become intolerable, as far as I'm concerned. The emotional roller coaster is unbelievable but more than that is the stupidity of continuing on this travesty while the plaintiff's attorney is allowed to try to rehabilitate a loser case mainly because my insurance company is too stupid to recognize the financial benefits of settling, and meanwhile, as usual, I am still the guy with his ass flopping in the wind. (This lawyer also talked about) if I refuse to go to court, and he informed me that this, of course, would violate my insurance contract, and then I would have no coverage at all. So it looks like I'm the pickle in the middle, and will just have to wait to see how this whole thing unfolds.

Tomorrow, there will be no court, and then on Friday, the judge is at his golf outing, and so there won't be any court on that day either.

That brings us to Monday, and yet another week that I have to reschedule patients and gerrymander things around. In addition, I had planned to be off on Monday to spend a day with the family but it looks like now that it's not going to be in the offing either. This is getting to be more and more distasteful on a daily, in fact on an hourly, basis.

June 11

It's Thursday afternoon, the 11th. Good news finally came in. I got a message from one of the lawyers that the judge is disallowing any further rebuttal experts and that the closing arguments will be given Monday morning, and the jury will go out Monday afternoon. This roller coaster ride is about to end, and it won't happen soon enough for me. I just talked with my lawyer. Apparently, the jury has been given their instructions, and basically there are five points that they are to consider: (1) that I opened the lateral wall of the sphenoid, that means not just the lateral wall of the sella but also the lateral wall of the sphenoid; (2) that I cut or injured the carotid artery; (3) that the diagnosis was not made in a timely fashion; (4) that I did not perform emergency surgery in spite of the fact that there were no case reports of this ever in the literature; and finally (5) that I abandoned the patient. By proving anyone of these things, they then have to prove that this caused or contributed in a substantial way to the cause of her death. It seems to me that the only problem will be the fact or lack thereof of emergency surgery, and even then, given a 40 percent chance of stroke versus a 3 percent chance of complications with Mullen's technique, I think that most people would choose to do exactly what we did. Of course, the question is and remains and always has been, will the jury understand that and will they see it my way. But they should go out probably Monday afternoon or at least Tuesday morning, and then we should have an answer within a day or so. Obviously if I win, I'll be happy, but they will appeal, and if I lose, I'll be unhappy and we will appeal it. I would like most of all to win and then to settle.

June 15

It's Monday morning. I slept poorly last night. It's now 10:15 AM. I've been here since 9:30 AM. In the early minutes, the lawyers were all back in chamber, arguing with the judge over what instructions should be made to the jury and how they were to be presented. You hear now the voice of the plaintiff's attorney in the background, hollering at the judge. The point here is that he wants to show an overlay, rather one of those big tablets on an easel, and the judge may not allow him to present this. What it basically does is to force the jury to look at his point of view and be constantly barraged with this information. My lawyer wants, if the judge allows this to happen, to use overheads of quotes made by their expert, as well as quotes from his book.

The morning's testimony went as expected. It took about two hours to go through the story and basically identified seven areas in which he feels I have been negligent, and I'll dictate them a little later. The interesting thing is that in each case he used half-truths and plays on concepts, as well as words, to prove a point. Now they will talk to the jury about damages.

The jury got about a 40-minute lunch break and had lunch in the jury room in order to save time so that we can get back to the proceedings and wrap this up today and have the jury go out today. I talked with my lawyer, who is quite confident that he has a very good rebuttal prepared, and I think he is right; I think he does have a good rebuttal prepared. We discussed some of the inconsistencies in the plaintiff attorney's closing. Basically, how could I not open the sella and then have the patient bleed out through the surgically absent sellar floor? Likewise, how could I close the sellar floor when I never opened it? One of the key issues is the question of reconstruction of the sellar floor with or without hemorrhage. Obviously, there was no hemorrhage at the time of the closure, but he made a pretty strong argument that would support the necessity for doing so. People are now reviewing different pieces of evidence that my lawyer will be putting up, and we'll go from there.

Well, it's a quarter after 5:00 o'clock and to say this was grueling day would be an understatement. My lawyer gave a very beautiful rebuttal to the plaintiff's closing argument dealing with each of the points I think that needed to be dealt with.

I was a little concerned that he was a little too esoteric in terms of his anatomy and that he didn't really get into, in a very graphic way, why what was alleged could not have happened. At the end of his argument, he got into the awards business, and discussed where the money would go and actually what he said was, "Now, they're asking for $2 million for pain and suffering which he is not sure she had, and then they're asking $2 million a piece for each of the children. Who do you think is going to get the first $2 million?" and he says he was referring to the first $2 million being the $2 million for pain and suffering, but there was immediate objection and a motion for mistrial on the part of the plaintiff's lawyers, stating that he was implying, and the jury was understanding, that this reference of "who do you think is going to get the money" was a reference to the lawyers, and they felt that the jury was laughing about it. The judge said that he didn't hear any laughter. My lawyer, himself, said that he didn't see anybody in the jury laughing, but they discussed the matter in detail, and the judge overruled the motion for a mistrial, but it was kind of a hairy time, and unfortunately gives further ammunition should we win and should they decide to appeal.

The plaintiff's attorney then got up and gave a rebuttal to the rebuttal, and was fairly brutal in terms of implying that I lied; that I abandoned the patient; that I was stupid for not identifying the fistula; etc., etc. On the other hand, it was nothing short of demoralizing. On the other hand, my lawyer's rebuttal was very innervating, so I guess one balances against the other and the net result is that it's been a long, hard day. I'm exhausted and am now going back to see some patients, at least two outpatients, and then probably my patients for surgery tomorrow. I'd hoped to get home early tonight and to begin to enjoy normal evenings with my kids and wife before they go away. I guess that's not going to be the way it's going to be tonight, but that being as it may, I don't have to go in tomorrow morning when the judge reads the instructions to the jury. My lawyer said it would be nice if I were there, but he wasn't going to ask me to be there, and, as far as I'm concerned, I've done enough for this case and what is going to be at this point is what is going to be. The anti-climactic nature, of course, is that no matter what happens tomorrow or whenever the jury eventually comes up with a verdict, it's going to be challenged in one way or another unless—Oh, no. There is no "unless." The only thing that would obviate a challenge would be a hung jury, which, as far as I'm concerned would be a fate worse than death at this stage of the game. At any rate, the next time I dictate anything I think it will be on the verdict and my thoughts at that time on the matter.

June 16

It's Tuesday morning at 8:20 AM, and I'm in the courtroom alone. My spirits are much better, although last night sleeping was somewhat difficult. I really was exhausted at the end of yesterday and didn't realize how tired I was. I think the day took more out of me than I admitted to at first. At any rate, we will observe the instructions to the jury, and I'm doing this because of a phone conversation with my personal attorney last night, who suggested that I attend, so here I am. Sometime today, hopefully, or if not today, tomorrow, we will have an answer from the jury. Obviously, I would love to see a "not guilty," but I have to steel myself against the possibility of the alternate.

I think one of the things that weighs on my mind is that 80 percent of cases, malpractice cases, are decided in favor of the defendant, and if two of my friends both got awards in their behalf, why shouldn't I, and the alternate side of that coin, obviously, is if I don't, does that mean I'm worse, more guilty, etc., etc.? Obviously, the answer is no. These are the things that one thinks about at a time like this.

The jury went out at 9:35 AM, after having been instructed by the judge. It seemed to me that the instructions were very difficult to understand and highly tilted in favor of the plaintiff. I asked my lawyer about this afterward, who said that they were, indeed, just because 70 to 80 percent of the lawmakers who deal with that and the justices who deal with that at all levels are plaintiff's or were plaintiff's lawyers, and he felt that it was a very unfair system, but that's the way it is. He also felt, though that the jury deals out what he calls "rough justice," which seldom is related to the facts, especially the more esoteric facts and more likely related to the gestalt of who they feel is innocent, who they feel is guilty, etc., etc. As we were leaving, one of my lawyers went to interview the alternate juror, and my defense lawyer and I went downstairs. Just before we parted I met one of his associates, and then he pulled this one on me. He said, "You know, really the best thing that could happen is if they came back with a guilty, and then said, 'What the hell, let's give them a million ' and then you'd be done with it." He said, "It sure is better than a hung jury, and it sure is better than a verdict which takes years and then requires a retrial somewhere down the line." It's amazing to me that he should be saying this now and not at the beginning of the trial, but then one has to realize that he just did one month's work and will bill for it one way or another, while he would not intend to lose that opportunity to gain capital. By the same token his interest, I'm sure at this point, has peaked and is now on the wane. At any rate, there are still many slips left between the cup and the lip, when one considers that they can get in touch with each other at this stage of the game, that is, the plaintiff's and defense lawyers can get in touch with each other at this stage of the game and make a settlement before the jury comes out, so now it's in the hands of the gods, and we will see what happens. Actually, although what my lawyer says is true about the guilty verdict and the opportunity to get it over with, I still would like to see a "not guilty."

June 17

It's now Wednesday, the 17th. Last evening, just after 7:00 PM, I got a page and answered the call, but there was no answer on the line, so I kept trying and eventually reached my lawyer. He informed me that they had come out with a verdict against me but only an award of $300,000. He reported that the one area that the jury had decided unanimously for me was on the question of abandonment; they decided that I in no way abandoned the patient. He reported that the men on the jury seemed to be inclined to give only $50,000, but the women managed to knock the figure up to $300,000, which was actually good because if they had come out with the $50,000, this would be very appealable, but with the $300,000 there is less of a chance for an appeal, and obviously they can't appeal the decision. Obviously, also, the insurance company doesn't want to appeal anything, so that the winners are the insurance company and the defense firm, and the losers are the plaintiff's family, as well as the plaintiff's law firm and, of course, the biggest loser is Cerullo because not only have I wasted this time, but I now have this judgment against me.

There's something very unsettling about the whole thing, the finality of it on one hand, and the bitterness of not succeeding juxtaposed with the relief of the finality.

I talked to my defense attorney today, and he, too, was very happy with the outcome but also understood my feeling. He said that in retrospect and in having discussed the issues with the jury, that he should have spent more time explaining how it was impossible to know that a delay in treatment would be fatal since there had never been a reported case of this in the literature and since this was the area in which the jury was most unanimous, though not completely, in deciding my guilt. I have to read the tapes, but it seems to me that in the very beginning this was my concern, and the area that I thought should be emphasized. On the other hand, even though we went into great lengths and had multiple witnesses, including the former resident, the anesthesiologist, and myself, explain how the carotid artery could not have been injured at the time of the operation, several of the jurors felt it had indeed had been and that I was guilty in that regard, as well. This was nowhere near as unanimous, however, as the opinion regarding the delay of treatment. I think that the plaintiff's attorney was very effective in equating blood loss, which at different times in the trial was estimated anywhere between 3,000 and 5,000 mL with a carotid injury, and try as we would to undue this impression on the part of the jury, we were never really successful.

Notes

Chapter 1

1. Linda T. Kohn, Janet M. Corrigan, and Molla S. Donaldson, eds., *To Err Is Human: Building a Safer Health System* (Washington, DC: National Academy Press, 1999), 3–4.

2. Sara C. Charles, Richard B. Warnecke, Amy Nelson, et al., "Appraisal of the Event as a Factor in Coping with Malpractice Litigation," *Behavioral Medicine* 14 (1988): 148–155.

3. Richard I. Cook and David D. Woods, eds., "Ben Kolb Case," in *Assembling the Scientific Basis for Progress on Patient Safety*, Volume I (Chicago: National Patient Safety Foundation, 1997).

4. Linda T. Kohn, Janet M. Corrigan, and Molla S. Donaldson, eds., *To Err Is Human: Building a Safer Health System* (Washington, DC: National Academy Press, 1999) 3–4.

5. Damon Adams, "Grants Spur Medical Groups, Hospitals to Pursue Perfection." *American Medical News* October 8, 2001, 18.

6. Robert J. Blendon, Catherine M. DesRoches, Mollyann Brodie, et al., "Views of Practicing Physicians and the Public on Medical Errors," *New England Journal of Medicine* 347 (2002): 1933–1940.

7. Albert W. Wu, Susan Folkman, Stephen J. McPhee, et al., "Do House Officers Learn from Their Mistakes?" *Journal of the American Medical Association* 265 (1991): 2089–2094.

8. David Hilfiker, *Healing the Wounds: A Physician Looks at His Work* (New York: Pantheon Books, 1985), 85.

9. Linda T. Kohn, Janet M. Corrigan, and Molla S. Donaldson, eds., *To Err Is Human: Building a Safer Health System* (Washington, DC: National Academy Press, 1999) 3–4.

10. Wendy Levinson and Patrick M. Dunn, "Coping with Fallibility," *Journal of the American Medical Association* 261 (1989): 2252.

11. John Lantos, "When Doctors Err," *Chicago Tribune Magazine*, May 4, 1997, 12.

12. James Reason, *Human Error* (Cambridge, England: Cambridge University Press, 1990), 9.

13. James Reason, "Human Error: Models and Management," *British Medical Journal* 320 (2000): 768–770.

14. James Reason, "Human Error: Models and Management," *British Medical Journal* 320 (2000): 769–770.

15. Troyen A. Brennan, Lucian L. Leape, Nan M. Laird, et al., "The Incidence of Adverse Events and Negligence in Hospitalized Patients: Results of the Harvard Medical Practice Study, I," *New England Journal of Medicine* 324 (1991): 370–376.

16. Lucian L. Leape, Troyen A. Brennan, Nan M. Laird, et al., "The Nature of Adverse Events in Hospitalized Patients: Results of the Harvard Medical Practice Study, II," *New England Journal of Medicine* 324 (1991): 377–384.

17. Eric Thomas, David M. Studdert, Joseph P. Newhouse, et al., "Costs of Medical Injuries in Utah and Colorado," *Inquiry* 36 (1999): 255–264.

18. Clement J. McDonald, Michael Weiner, and Siu L. Hui, "Deaths Due to Medical Errors Are Exaggerated in Institute of Medicine Report, *Journal of the American Medical Association* 284 (2000): 93–95.

19. Rodney A. Hayward and Timothy P. Hofer, "Estimating Hospital Deaths Due to Medical Errors," *Journal of the American Medical Association* 286 (2001): 415–420.

20. Robert J. Blendon, Catherine M. DesRoches, Mollyann Brodie, et al., "Views of Practicing Physicians and the Public on Medical Errors," *New England Journal of Medicine* 347 (2002): 1935.

21. James Reason, "Human Error: Models and Management," *British Medical Journal* 320 (2000): 769.

22. Patricia M. Danzon, *Medical Malpractice: Theory, Evidence, and Public Policy,* (Cambridge, MA: Harvard University Press, 1985), 90.

23. Steven A. Schroeder and Andrea I. Kabcenell, "Do Bad Outcomes Mean Substandard Care?" *Journal of the American Medical Association* 265 (1991): 1995.

24. Robert A. Caplan, Karen L. Posner, and Frederick W. Cheney, "Effect of Outcome on Physician Judgments of Appropriateness of Care." *Journal of the American Medical Association* 265 (1991): 1957–1960.

25. Troyen A. Brennan, "The Institute of Medicine Report on Medical Errors—Could It Do Harm? *New England Journal of Medicine* 342 (2000): 1123–1125.

26. Ruth M. Parker and Joanne G. Schwartzberg, "What Patients Do—and Don't—Understand," *Postgraduate Medicine* 109 (2001): 13–16.

27. Louis P. Halamek, David M. Kaegi, David M. Gaba, et al., "Time for a New Paradigm in Pediatric Medical Education: Teaching Neonatal Resuscitation in a Simulated Delivery Room Environment," *Pediatrics* 106 (2000): (4) e45.

28. David Gaba, "Anesthesiology as a Model for Patient Safety in Health Care," *British Medical Journal* 320 (2000): 785–788.

29. Martin Reznek, Rebecca Smith-Coggins, Steven Howard, et al., "Emergency Medicine Crisis Resource Management (EMCRM): Pilot Study of a Simulation-Based Management Crisis Management Course for Emergency Medicine," *Academic Emergency Medicine* 10 (2003): 386–389.

30. Anesthesia Patient Safety Foundation, "ASA/ASPF Safety Video Library" [Online]. Available at: http://www.apsf.org/references /video_library.php [August 24, 2004].

31. National Patient Safety Foundation, "Let's Talk: Disclosure After an Adverse Event," [Online] *National Patient Safety Foundation*. Available at: http://www.npsf.org/html/publications.html [August 24, 2004].

32. "Perspective on Disclosure of Unanticipated Outcome Information," (Chicago: American Society for Health Care Risk Management, April, 2001) [Online] Available at: http//www.hospitalconnect.com/ASHRM/resources/files/disclosure.2001.pdf [August 28, 2004].

33. Joint Commission on Accreditation of Healthcare Organizations, "Revisions to Joint Commission Standards in Support of Patient Safety and Medical/Health Care Error Reduction, Rev. July 2001 [Online]. Available at: http// www.utmb.edu/patientsafety/ JCAHOStandardsRev.pdf [August 28, 2004].

34. "Policy for Disclosing Medical Errors to Patients," Reviewed by Board of Trustees, Boston, MA, Dana-Farber Cancer Institute, July 17, 2001.

Chapter 2

1. Dr. Laura West, Interview with author (SCC), June 19, 2003 [Appendix 1].

2. Albert W. Wu, "Medical Error: The Second Victim," *British Medical Journal* 320 (2000): 726–727.

3. John F. Christensen, Wendy Levinson, and Patrick M. Dunn, "The Heart of Darkness," *Journal of General Internal Medicine* 7 (1992): 424–431.

4. Marc C. Newman, "The Emotional Impact of Mistakes on Family Physicians," *Archives of Family Medicine* 5 (1996): 71–75.

5. Albert W. Wu, Susan Folkman, Stephan J. McPhee et al., "Do House Officers Learn From Their Mistakes?" *Journal of the American Medical Association* 265 (1991): 2092.

6. John W. Ely, Wendy Levinson, Nancy C. Elder, et al., "Perceived Causes of Family Physicians' Errors," *Journal of Family Practice* 40 (1995): 337–344.

7. Nathan P. Couch, Nicholas L. Tilney, Anthony A. Rayner, et al., "The High Cost of Low-Frequency Events," *New England Journal of Medicine* 304 (1981): 634–637.

8. Robert J. Blendon, Catherine M. DesRoches, Mollyann Brodie, et al., "Views of Practicing Physicians and the Public on Medical Error," *New England Journal of Medicine* 347 (2002): 1937.

9. James Reason, "Human Error: Models and Management." *British Medical Journal* 320 (2000): 770.

10. American Psychiatric Association, *Diagnostic and Statistical Manual of Mental Disorders, 4th Edition, Text Revision (DSMIV-TR)* (Washington, DC: American Psychiatric Association, 2000) 463.

11. Carol S. North, "Psychiatric Epidemiology of Disaster Response" in *Trauma and Disaster: Responses and Management,* Review of Psychiatry, Volume 22, ed. Robert Ursano and Ann E. Norwood (Washington, DC: American Psychiatric Press, 2003), 38.

12. Anonymous, "Personal View: Looking Back . . . ," *British Medical Journal* 320 (2000): 3: 812.

13. D. Jeffrey Newport and Charles B. Nemeroff, "Neurobiology of Posttraumatic Stress Disorder," *Current Opinion in Neurobiology* 10 (2000): 211–218.

14. Dennis S. Charney, "Neuroanatomical Circuits Modulating Fear and Anxiety Behaviors," *Acta Psychiatrica Scandinavica: Supplementum.* 417 (2003): 38–50.

15. Bruce S. McEwen, "The Neurobiology and Neuroendocrinology of Stress. Implications for Post-Traumatic Stress Disorder from a Basic Science Perspective." *Psychiatric Clinics of North America* 25 (2002) 2: 469–494.

16. Joseph E. LeDoux, "Emotion Circuits in the Brain," *Annual Review of Neuroscience* 23 (2000): 155–184.

17. Mardi J. Horowitz, *Treatment of Stress Response Syndromes* (Washington, DC: American Psychiatric Publishing, 2003) 16.

18. Carol S. North, "Psychiatric Epidemiology of Disaster Response," in *Trauma and Disaster: Responses and Management*, Review of Psychiatry, Volume 22, ed. Robert Ursano and Ann E. Norwood (Washington, DC: American Psychiatric Press, 2003) 55.

19. James L. McGaugh, "Memory—A Century of Consolidation," *Science* 287 (2000): 248–251.

20. James L. McGaugh and Benno Roozendaal, "Role of Adrenal Stress Hormones in Forming Lasting Memories in the Brain," *Current Opinions in Neurobiology* 12 (2002): 205–210.

21. American Psychiatric Association, *Diagnostic and Statistical Manual of Mental Disorders, 4th Edition, Text Revision (DSM-IV-TR)* (Washington, DC: American Psychiatric Press, 2003) 463.

22. Carol S. North, "Psychiatric Epidemiology of Disaster Response," in *Trauma and Disaster: Responses and Management*, Review of Psychiatry, Volume 22, ed. Robert Ursano and Ann E. Norwood (Washington, DC: American Psychiatric Press, 2003) 40, 41, 55.

23. Carol S. North, Sara J. Nixon, Sheryll Shariat, et al., "Psychiatric Disorders Among Survivors of the Oklahoma City Bombing, *Journal of the American Medical Association* 282 (1999): 755–762.

24. Paul T. Bartone, Robert J. Ursano, Kathleen M. Wright, et al., "The Impact of a Military Air Disaster on the Health of Assistance Workers: A Prospective Study," *Journal of Nervous and Mental Disease* 177 (1989): 317–328.

25. Carol S. North, "Psychiatric Epidemiology of Disaster Response," in *Trauma and Disaster: Responses and Management*, Review of Psychiatry, Volume 22, ed. Robert Ursano and Ann E. Norwood (Washington, DC: American Psychiatric Press, 2003) 54.

26. Patricia J. Watson, Matthew J. Friedman, Laura E. Gibson, et al., "Early Intervention for Trauma-related Problems," in *Trauma and Disaster: Responses and Management*, Review of Psychiatry, Volume 22, ed. Robert Ursano and Ann E. Norwood (Washington, DC: American Psychiatric Press, 2003), 105.

27. Justin A. Kenardy and Vaughan J. Carr, "Debriefing Post Disaster: Follow-up After Major Earthquake," in *Psychological Debriefing: Theory, Practice and Evidence*, ed. B. Raphael and J. P. Wilson (Cambridge, England: Cambridge University Press, 2000), 174–181.

Chapter 3

1. Council on Ethical and Judicial Affairs, *Code of Medical Ethics: Current Opinions with Annotations* (Chicago: American Medical Association, 2002–2003 ed.) Opinion 8.12, 217–218.

2. *Merriam-Webster's Collegiate Dictionary*, 11th edition (Springfield, MA: Merriam-Webster, 2003), 356.

3. *Merriam-Webster's Collegiate Dictionary*, 11th edition (Springfield, MA: Merriam-Webster, 2003), 11.

4. *Merriam-Webster's Collegiate Dictionary,* 11th edition (Springfield, MA: Merriam-Webster, 2003), 58.

5. California (West's Annotated California Evidence Code § 1160), "Admissibility of expressions of sympathy or benevolence." Other states that have a current (2003) law

protecting expressions of beneficence are Washington (Chapter 5.66.010 RCW), Massachusetts (Mass. Ann. Laws ch. 233, § 23D), Texas (Vernon's Tex. Stat. & Code Ann., Civ. Prac. & Remedies Code § 18.061), Florida (Section 90.4026) and Tennessee (Evidence Rule 409.1).

6. Bruce N. Barge and Kristofer J. Fenelson, "Dealing Effectively with Malpractice Litigation," (St. Paul MN, St. Paul Fire and Marine Insurance Company, 1994).

7. AMA/Specialty Society Medical Liability Project, *Risk Management Principles and Commentaries,* 2nd edition (Chicago: American Medical Association, 1995).

8. National Patient Safety Foundation, "Talking to Patients about Health Care Injury: Statement of Principle," *Focus Patient Safety* 4 (2001) 3 [Online] Available at: http//www.npsf.org/download/FOCUS2001vol1no1.pdf [September 2, 2004].

9. Joint Commission on Accreditation of Healthcare Organizations, "Revisions to Joint Commission Standards in Support of Patient Safety and Medical/Health Care Error Reduction," Intent of RI.1.2.2.

10. Kathleen M. Mazor, Steven R. Simon, Robert A. Yood et al., "Health Plan Members' Views about Disclosure of Medical Errors," *Annals of Internal Medicine* 140 (2004): 409–418.

11. Council on Ethical and Judicial Affairs, *Code of Medical Ethics: Current Opinions with Annotations*, Opinion 8.12, 217–218.

12. Lucian L. Leape, "Error in Medicine," *New England Journal of Medicine* 272 (1994): 1851–1857.

13. John Lantos, "When Doctors Err," *Chicago Tribune Magazine*, May 4, 1997, 13–14.

14. A. Russell Localio, Ann G. Lawthers, Troyen A. Brennan, et al., "Relation Between Malpractice Claims and Adverse Events Due to Negligence," *New England Journal of Medicine* 325 (1991): 245–251.

15. Gerald B. Hickson, Ellen Wright Clayton, Penny B. Githens, et al., "Factors That Prompted Families to File Medical Malpractice Claims Following Perinatal Injuries," *Journal of the American Medical Association* 267 (1992): 1359–1363.

16. Charles Vincent, Magi Young, and Angela Phillips, "Why Do People Sue Doctors? A Study of Patients and Relatives Taking Legal Action," *Lancet* 343 (1994): 1609–1613.

17. Steve S. Kraman and Ginny Hamm, "Risk Management: Extreme Honesty May Be the Best Policy," *Annals of Internal Medicine* 131 (1999): 963–967.

18. Mark Crane, "What to Say If You've Made a Mistake," *Medical Economics* August 20, 2001, 28.

19. Kathleen M. Mazor, Steven R. Simon, Robert A. Yood et al., "Health Plan Members' Views about Disclosure of Medical Errors," *Annals of Internal Medicine* 140 (2004): 409–418.

20. Robyn Shapiro, Deborah Simpson, Steven L. Lawrence, et al., "A Survey of Sued and Nonsued Physicians and Suing Patients," *Archives of Internal Medicine* 149 (1989): 2190–2196.

21. Martha S. Gerrity, Robert F. DeVellis, and Jo Anne Earp. "Physicians' Reactions to Uncertainty in Patient Care," *Medical Care 28* (1990): 724–736.

22. Jochanan Benbasset, Dina Pilpel, and Razia Schor, "Physicians' Attitudes Toward Litigation and Defensive Practice: Development of a Scale," *Behavioral Medicine* 27 (2001): 52–60.

23. Aaron Lazare, "Shame and Humiliation in the Medical Encounter," *Archives of Internal Medicine* 147 (1987): 1653–1658.

24. As of 2003, twenty-one states have legislation related to legal protections against disclosure of reported data. See Table 1 in Mimi Marchev, "Medical Malpractice and Medical Error Disclosure: Balancing Facts and Fears," *National Academy for State Health Policy*, [Online] December 2003. Available at: http//www.nashp.org/files/medicalmalpracticeandmedicalerrordisclosure.pdf [August 27, 2004].

25. Dr. Joseph Daley, Interview with author (SCC), June 16, 2003 [Appendix 1].

26. Bryan A. Liang, "Promoting Patient Safety Through Reducing Medical Error: A Paradigm of Cooperation between Patient, Physician, and Attorney," Dr. Arthur Grayson Distinguished Lecture in Law and Medicine, 24 *Southern Illinois University Law Journal* 541 (2000): 541–568.

27. According to a 1998 survey by the American Health Lawyers Association, just three states (and the Department of Defense) appear to specifically protect disclosure of sensitive information to the Joint Commission: Iowa, Georgia, and Maine, with Maine's laws possibly applying to root cause analysis. The rest are either limited or no protection at all [Online]. Available at: http://www.sentinel-event.com/disclosure.htm [September 2, 2004].

28. Carol B. Golin, ed., "Reporting Medical Errors Give Lawyers Tools to Sue, While Doctors May Lose Liability Cover," *Medical Liability Monitor* 26 (2001): 5.

29. *Oregon Revised Statutes* 41.675.

30. Linda O. Prager, "New Laws Let Doctors Say 'I'm Sorry,'" *American Medical News*, August 21, 2001, 1–12.

31. California (West's Ann. Cal. Evid. Code § 1160), "Admissibility of expressions of sympathy or benevolence."

32. Troyen A. Brennan, Colin M. Sox, and Helen R. Burstein, "Relation Between Negligent Adverse Events and the Outcomes of Malpractice Litigation," *New England Journal of Medicine* 335 (1996): 1963–1967.

33. Michelle J. White, "The Value of Liability in Medical Malpractice," *Health Affairs Milwood* (1994): 75–87.

34. Mark I. Taragin, Laura R. Willett, Adam P. Wilczek, et al., "The Influence of Standard of Care and Severity of Injury on the Resolution of Medical Malpractice Claims," *Annals of Internal Medicine* 117 (1992): 780–784.

35. Steven D. Edbril and Robert S. Lagasse, "The Relationship Between Malpractice Litigation and Human Errors," *Anesthesiology* 91(1999): 848–855.

36. Bryan A. Liang and David J. Cullen, "The Legal System and Patient Safety: Charting a Divergent Course," *Anesthesiology* 91 (1999): 609–611.

37. Dan Miller, "Liability for Medical Malpractice: Issues and Evidence," A Joint Economic Committee Study, Jim Saxton, Vice-Chairman, United States Congress, May 2003.

38. A. Russell Localio, Ann G. Lawthers, Troyen A. Brennan et al., "Relation Between Malpractice Claims and Adverse Events Due to Negligence," *New England Journal of Medicine* 325 (1991): 245–251.

39. Ann G. Lawthers, A. Russell Localio, Nan M. Laird, et al., "Physicians' Perceptions of the Risk of Being Sued," *Journal of Health Politics, Policy and Law* 17 (1992): 463–482.

40. Bryan A. Liang, "Error in Medicine: Impediments to U.S. Reform," *Journal of Health Politics, Policy and Law* 24 (1999): 27–58.

41. Amy B. Witman, Deric M. Park, and Steven B. Hardin, "How Do Patients Want Physicians to Handle Mistakes?" *Archives of Internal Medicine* 156 (1996): 2565–2569.

42. John W. Ely, Wendy Levinson, Nancy C. Elder, et al., "Perceived Causes of Family Physicians' Errors," *Journal of Family Practice* 40 (1995): 337.

43. Wendy Levinson and Patrick M. Dunn, "Coping With Fallibility," *Journal of the American Medical Association* 261 (1989): 2252.

44. Daniel O'Connell, "We Made a Mistake," *Presentation at the 4th Annenberg Conference*, Minneapolis, MN, May 2001.

45. Frank Davidoff, "Shame: The Elephant in the Room," *Quality and Safety in Health Care* 11 (2002): 2–3.

46. *Oregon Revised Statutes* 41.675.

47. David A. Alexander, Susan Klein, Nicola M. Gray, et al., "Suicide by Patients: Questionnaire Study of Its Effect on Consultant Psychiatrists," *British Medical Journal* 320 (2000): 1571–1574.

48. Steve S. Kraman and Ginny Hamm, "Risk Management: Extreme Honesty May Be the Best Policy," *Annals of Internal Medicine* 131 (1991): 963–967.

49. Bryan A. Liang, "A System of Medical Error Disclosure," *Quality and Safety in Health Care* 11 (2002): 64–68.

50. Michael D. Cantor, "Telling Patients the Truth: A Systems Approach to Disclosing Adverse Events," *Quality and Safety in Health Care* 11 (2002): 7–8.

51. Albert W. Wu, Thomas A. Cavanaugh, Stephen J. McPhee, et al., "To Tell the Truth—Ethical and Practical Issues in Disclosing Medical Mistakes to Patients," *Journal of General Internal Medicine* 12 (1997): 770–775.

52. Timothy Quill and Penelope Townsend, "Bad News: Delivery, Dialogue, and Dilemmas," *Archives of Internal Medicine* 151 (1991): 463–468.

53. Robert Buckman, *How to Break Bad News: A Guide for Health Care Professionals* (Baltimore, MD: Johns Hopkins University Press, 1992) 65–97.

54. Amy B. Witman, Deric M. Park, and Steven B. Hardin, "How Do Patients Want Physicians to Handle Mistakes?" *Archives of Internal Medicine* 156 (1996): 2566.

55. Robert L. Lowes, "Made a Bonehead Mistake? Apologize," *Medical Economics* May 12, 1997, 104.

56. Mark Crane, "What to Say If You've Made a Mistake," *Medical Economics* August 20, 2001, 28.

57. Bayer Institute for Health Care Communication. Available at: http//www.bayerinstitute.org [August 24, 2004].

Chapter 4

1. Emily Morison Beck, ed., *Familiar Quotations by John Bartlett*, 14th ed. (Boston: Little, Brown and Company, 1968), 453a.

2. Dr. Laura West, Interview with author (SCC), June 19, 2003 [Appendix 1].

3. Dr. Joseph Daley, Interview with author (SCC), June 16, 2003 [Appendix 1].

4. Dr. Richard Allen, Interview with author (SCC), January 10, 2000 [Appendix 1].

5. Mike Wallace, Interview with author (SCC), October 22, 1998 [Appendix 1].

6. Steven H. Miles, "A Challenge to Licensing Boards: The Stigma of Mental Illness," *Journal of the American Medical Association* 280 (1998): 865.

7. Thomas E. Hansen, Rupert R. Goetz, Joseph D. Bloom, et al., "Changes in Questions About Psychiatric Illness on Medical Licensure Applications Between 1993 and 1996," *Psychiatric Services* 49 (1998): 202–206.

8. "Licensed Physician Renewal Form," *State of Illinois* (Springfield, IL: Department of Professional Regulation, 2002).

9. Claudia Center, Miriam Davis, Thomas Detre, et al., "Confronting Depression and Suicide in Physicians," *Journal of the American Medical Association* 289 (2003): 3161–3166.

10. Jonathan R.T. Davidson, "Effective Management Strategies for Posttraumatic Stress Disorder," in *Focus: The Journal of Lifelong Learning in Psychiatry*, Volume 1, ed. Deborah J. Hales and Mark H. Rapaport (Arlington, VA: American Psychiatric Press, 2003), 241.

Chapter 5

1. Dr. Richard Allen, Interview with author (SCC), January 10, 2000 [Appendix 1].

2. Troyen A. Brennan, Lucien L. Leape, Nan M. Laird, et al., "The Incidence of Adverse Events and Negligence in Hospitalized Patients: Results of the Harvard Medical Practice Study, I," *New England Journal of Medicine* 324 (1991): 370–376.

3. Lucien L. Leape, Troyen A. Brennan, Nan M. Laird, et al., "The Nature of Adverse Events in Hospitalized Patients: Results of the Harvard Medical Practice Study, II," *New England Journal of Medicine* 324 (1991): 377–384.

4. Eric Thomas, David M. Studdert, Joseph P. Newhouse, et al., "Costs of Medical Injuries in Utah and Colorado," *Inquiry* 36 (1999): 255–264.

5. A. Russell Localio, Ann G. Lawthers, Troyen A. Brennan, et al., "Relation Between Malpractice Claims and Adverse Events Due to Negligence," *New England Journal of Medicine* 325 (1991): 247.

6. Troyen A. Brennan, Colin M. Sox, and Helen R. Burstin, "Relation Between Negligent Adverse Events and the Outcomes of Medical Malpractice Litigation," *New England Journal of Medicine* 335 (1996): 1967.

7. Patricia A. Danzon and L.A. Lillard, *The Resolution of Medical Malpractice Claims: Modeling the Bargaining Process* (Santa Monica, CA: The Rand Corporation, The Institute of Civil Justice, 1982) vi.

8. Frank A. Sloan, Paula M. Mergenhagen, Bradley Burfield, et al., "Medical Malpractice Experience of Physicians: Predictable or Haphazard?" *Journal of the American Medical Association* 262 (1989): 3291–3297.

9. Randall R. Bovberg and Kenneth R. Petronis, "The Relationship Between Physicians' Malpractice Claims History and Later Claim: Does the Past Predict the Future?" *Journal of the American Medical Association* 272 (1994): 1421–1426.

10. Gerald B. Hickson, Ellen Wright Clayton, Penny B. Githens, et al., "Factors That Prompted Families to File Malpractice Claims Following Perinatal Injuries," *Journal of the American Medical Association* 267 (1992): 1359–1363.

11. Charles Vincent, Magi Young, and Angela Phillips, "Why Do People Sue Doctors? A Study of Patients and Relatives Taking Legal Action," *Lancet* 343 (1994): 1690–1613.

12. Dr. Richard Allen, Interview with author (SCC), January 10, 2000 [Appendix 1].

13. Audrey Vanagunas, Vice President of Risk Management, ISMIE Mutual Insurance Company, Interview with author (SCC), July 9, 2003.

14. Michael J. Gitlin, "A Psychiatrist's Reaction to a Patient's Suicide," *American Journal of Psychiatry* 156 (1999): 1630–1634.

15. Herbert M. Perr, "Suicide and the Doctor-Patient Relationship," *American Journal of Psychoanalysis* 18 (1968): 177–188.

16. "Medical Liability Reform—Now!" June 14, 2004 edition. American Medical Association. Available at: http//www.ama-assn.org/ama1/pub/upload/mm/450/mlrnow June112004.pdf [September 4, 2004].

17. Renée C. Fox, *The Human Condition of Health Professions* (Durham, NH: University of New Hampshire, November 19, 1979) 15–16.

18. Albert W. Wu, Susan Folkman, Stephan J. McPhee et al., "Do House Officers Learn From Their Mistakes?" *Journal of the American Medical Association* 265 (1991): 2089–2094.

19. Cary P. Gross, Lucy A. Mead, Daniel E. Ford, et al., "Physician, Heal Thyself? Regular Source of Care and Use of Preventive Health Services Among Physicians," *Archives of Internal Medicine* 160 (2000): 3209–3214.

20. Jason D. Christie, Ilene M. Rosen, Lisa M. Bellini, et al. "Prescription Drug Use and Self-prescription Among Resident Physicians," *Journal of the American Medical Association* 280 (1998): 1253–1255.

21. Hans Selye, *Stress without Distress* (Philadelphia: J.B. Lippincott, 1974) 32.

22. Susan Folkman and Richard S. Lazarus, "An Analysis of Coping in a Middle-aged Community Sample, *Journal of Health and Social Behavior* 21 (1980): 219–239.

23. Richard S. Lazarus and Susan Folkman, *Stress, Appraisal and Coping* (New York: Springer, 1984), 21

24. Sara C. Charles, Richard B. Warnecke, Amy Nelson, et al., "Appraisal of the Event as a Factor in Coping with Malpractice Litigation," *Behavioral Medicine* 14 (1988): 149.

25. Jack D. McCue, "The Effects of Stress on Physicians and Their Medical Practice," *New England Journal of Medicine* 306 (1982): 458–463.

Chapter 6

1. Mike Wallace, Interview with author (SCC), October 22, 1998 [Appendix 1].

2. Tom Shales, "TV Journalists Pleased but Wary of Impact; Opinions Differ Over 'Chilling' Effect," *Washington Post,* February 19, 1985, A11.

3. Roni Pressler, Assistant Vice President, ISMIE Mutual Insurance Company, Interview with author (SCC), July 15, 2003.

4. Dominic Pellegrino, "Issues That Plaintiffs' Attorneys Consider Before Instituting Suit," in *Professional Liability and Risk Management in a Changing Health Care Environment,* (Chicago: Postgraduate Course #2, 85th Clinical Congress, American College of Surgeons, 1999), 20–21.

5. Gerald B. Hickson, Ellen Wright Clayton, Penny B. Githens, et al., "Factors That Prompted Families to File Medical Malpractice Claims Following Perinatal Injuries," *Journal of the American Medical Association* 267 (1992): 1359–1363.

6. Charles Vincent, Magi Young, and Angela Phillips, "Why Do People Sue Doctors? A Study of Patients and Relatives Taking Legal Action," *Lancet* 343 (1994): 1609–1613.

7. Maureen Anderson, Interview with author (SCC), October 30, 1999 [Appendix 1].

8. Dr. Cynthia Davis, Interview with author (SCC), September 12, 2000 [Appendix 1].

9. See note 8 above.

10. "Privacy of Health Information/ HIPAA" [Online] Effective April 13, 2003. Available at: http//www.hhs.gov [September 8, 2004].

11. Dr. Laura West, Interview with author (SCC), June 19, 2003 [Appendix 1].

12. Information compiled from CNA and Northwest Physicians Mutual Insurance Companies, Oregon Medical Association, Portland OR, 2003.

13. Sara C. Charles and Eugene C. Kennedy, *Defendant: A Psychiatrist on Trial for Medical Malpractice* (New York: Vintage Books, Random House, 1986), xvii.

14. Dr. Richard Allen, Interview with author (SCC), January 10, 2000 [Appendix 1].

15. See note 11 above.

16. Jeremy Gerard, "Callers Besiege CBS over Andy Rooney," *The New York Times,* February 10, 1990.

Chapter 7

1. Dr. Laura West, Interview with author (SCC), June 19, 2003 [Appendix 1].

2. Martindale-Hubbell [Online] Available at: http://www.martindale.com/xp/Martindale/home.xml [August 28, 2004].

3. American College of Trial Lawyers [Online] Available at: http://www.actl.com [August 28, 2004].

4. International Association of Defense Counsel [Online] Available at: http://www.iadclaw.org/StaticContent/pdfs/overview.pdf [August 28, 2004].

5. Dr. Joseph Daley, Interview with author (SCC), June 16, 2003 [Appendix 1].

6. *Merriam-Webster's Collegiate Dictionary*, 11th edition (Springfield, IL: Merriam-Webster, 2003) 679.

7. Barry Werth, *Damages* (New York: Simon and Schuster, 1998), 181.

8. Dr. Richard Allen, Interview with author (SCC), January 10, 2000 [Appendix 1].

Chapter 8

1. Norman Mailer, Interview with author (SCC), October 29, 1999 [Appendix 1].

2. Leon Salzman, *The Obsessive Personality*, (New York: Science House, 1968), ii.

3. Glen O. Gabbard, "The Role of Compulsiveness in the Normal Physician," *Journal of the American Medical Association* 254 (1985): 2926–2929.

4. Dr. Richard Allen, Interview with author (SCC), January 10, 2000 [Appendix 1].

5. Mike Wallace, Interview with author (SCC), October 22, 1998 [Appendix 1].

6. Richard B. Ferrell and Trevor R. P. Price, "Effects of Malpractice Suits on Physicians," in *Beyond Transference*, ed. Judith H. Gold and John C. Nemiah. (Washington, DC: American Psychiatric Press, 1993) 141–158.

7. See note 5 above.

8. See note 4 above.

9. Dr. Mary Santos, Interview with author (SCC) , July 25, 2003 [Appendix 1].

10. Dr. Joseph Daley, Interview with author (SCC), June 16, 2003 [Appendix 1].

11. David Berreby, "Exploring combat and the psyche, beginning with Homer," *The New York Times*, March 11, 2003.

12. See note 10 above.

13. Lori Bartholomew, Physician Insurers Association of America, Personal Communication, April 8, 2003.

14. See note 4 above.

15. Richard S. Lazarus and Susan Folkman, *Stress, Appraisal and Coping* (New York: Springer, 1984) 22–25.

16. Jeremy Gerard, "Callers Besiege CBS over Rooney," *The New York Times*, February 10, 1990.

17. See note 4 above.

18. Sara C. Charles, Richard B. Warnecke, Amy Nelson, et al., "Appraisal of the Event as a Factor in Coping with Malpractice Litigation," *Behavioral Medicine* 14 (1988): 151–152.

19. Sara C. Charles, Charlene E. Pyskoty and Amy Nelson, "Physicians on Trial: Self-Reported Reactions to Malpractice Trials," *Western Journal of Medicine* 148 (1988): 358–360.

20. Renée C. Fox, *The Human Condition of Health Professions* (Durham, NH: University of New Hampshire, November 19, 1979) 35.

21. Paul R. Frisch, Sara C. Charles, Robert D. Gibbons et al. "Role of Previous Claims and Specialty on the Effectiveness of Risk-Management Education for Office-Based Physicians," *Western Journal of Medicine* 163 (1995): 346–350.

22. See note 9 above.

23. Patricia J. Watson, Matthew J. Friedman, Lauren E. Gibson, et al., "Early Intervention for Trauma-Related Problems," in *Trauma and Disaster: Responses and*

Management Review of Psychiatry, Volume 22, Ed. Robert Ursano and Ann E. Norwood (Washington, DC: American Psychiatric Press, 2003) 100.

24. See note 23 above.

25. Sara C. Charles, Charlene E. Pyskoty and Amy Nelson, "Physicians on Trial: Self-Reported Reactions to Malpractice Trials," *Western Journal of Medicine* 148 (1988): 360.

26. See note 23 above.

27. AMA/Specialty Society Liability Project, *Risk Management Principles and Commentaries for the Medical Office*, 2nd Edition (Chicago: American Medical Association (1995).

28. Paul R. Frisch, Sara C. Charles, Robert D. Gibbons, et al., "Role of Previous Claims and Specialty on the Effectiveness of Risk-Management Education for Office-Based Physicians," *Western Journal of Medicine* 163 (1995): 346–350.

29. See note 9 above.

30. Rachel E. Silverman, "Litigation Boom Spurs Efforts to Shield Assets," *Wall Street Journal*, Tuesday, October 14, 2003.

31. Dr. Thomas White, Interview with author (SCC), July 21, 2003 [Appendix 1].

32. Lisa Kelly-Wilson, Jennifer Parsons, and Sara C. Charles, "Physicians and Medical Malpractice Litigation," Report to the Council of Medical Specialty Societies (Chicago, IL: Survey Research Laboratory, University of Illinois, 2003).

33. Dr. Cynthia Davis, Interview with author (SCC), September 12, 2000 [Appendix 1].

34. See note 10 above.

35. See note 33 above.

36. Dr. Laura West, Interview with author (SCC), June 19, 2003 [Appendix 1].

37. Peter M. Marzuk, "When the Patient Is a Physician," *New England Journal of Medicine*, 317 (1987): 1409–1411.

38. George E. Valliant, Nancy C. Sobowale, and Charles McArthur, "Some Psychological Vulnerabilities of Physicians, *New England Journal of Medicine* 287 (1972) 372–375.

39. See note 5 above.

40. See note 5 above.

41. Horowitz, *Treatment of Stress Response Syndromes* (Washington, DC: American Psychiatric Publishing, 2003) 60–68.

42. Saul Bellow, Interview with author (SCC), September 13, 1999 [Appendix 1].

Chapter 9

1. *The Jerusalem Bible* (Garden City, NY: Doubleday, 1966), 764.
2. Dr. Laura West, Interview with author (SCC), June 19, 2003 [Appendix 1].
3. Dr. John Schmidt, Interview with author (SCC), September 19, 2003. [Appendix 1]
4. See note 3 above.

Chapter 10

1. Dr. Mary Santos, Interview with author (SCC), July 25, 2003 [Appendix 1].
2. See note 1 above.
3. Dr. Cynthia Davis, Interview with author (SCC), September 12, 2000 [Appendix 1].
4. Dr. John Schmidt, Interview with author (SCC), September 19, 2003 [Appendix 1].
5. See note 1 above.
6. Dr. Laura West, Interview with author (SCC), June 19, 2003 [Appendix 1].
7. See note 1 above.
8. See note 4 above.

9. National Practitioner Data Bank for Adverse Information on Physicians and Other Health Care Practitioners; Final Regulations. 45CFR, Part 60, *Federal Register, Rules and Regulations*, vol. 54, no. 199 (Washington, DC: Department of Health and Human Services, Tuesday, October 17, 1989).

10. *National Practitioner Data Bank, Data by Profession and State Summary* [Online]. Data as of October 9, 2004. Available at: http//www.npdb-hipdb.com/ [November 28, 2004].

11. "Reporting Medical Malpractice Payments, (d) Interpretation of Information," *Federal Register, Rules and Regulations*, vol. 54, no. 199, Tuesday, October 17, 1989, Section 60.7, 42732.

12. Dr. Richard Allen, Interview with author (SCC), January 10, 2000 [Appendix 1].

13. Dr. Joseph Daley, Interview with author (SCC), June 16, 2003 [Appendix 1].

Chapter 11

1. Mike Wallace, Interview with author (SCC), October 22, 1998 [Appendix 1].

2. Dr. Cynthia Davis, Interview with author (SCC), September 12, 2000 [Appendix 1].

3. Editorial, "Personal Responsibility Bias," *Wall Street Journal*, January 12, 2004.

4. See note 2 above.

5. Maureen Anderson, Interview with author (SCC), October 30, 1999 [Appendix 1].

6. Dr. Laura West, Interview with author (SCC), June 19, 2003 [Appendix 1].

7. See note 2 above.

8. *Merriam-Webster's Collegiate Dictionary*, 11th edition (Springfield, MA: Merriam-Webster, 2003) 1334.

9. Dr. Mary Santos, Interview with author (SCC), July 25, 2003 [Appendix 1].

10. See note 6 above.

11. See note 9 above.

12. See note 6 above.

13. Sara C. Charles, Charlene E. Pyskoty and Amy Nelson, "Physicians on Trial: Self-Reported Reactions to Malpractice Trials," *Western Journal of Medicine* 148 (1988): 359.

14. Sara C. Charles, Charlene E. Pyskoty and Amy Nelson, "Physicians on Trial: Self-Reported Reactions to Malpractice Trials," *Western Journal of Medicine* 148 (1988): 360.

15. Results from Closed Claims Handling Surveys, Oregon Medical Association Portland, Oregon.

16. See note 6 above.

17. See note 9 above.

18. Norman Mailer, Interview with author (SCC), October 29, 1999 [Appendix 1].

19. See note 6 above.

20. See note 1 above.

21. See note 1 above.

Chapter 12

1. James C. Mohr, "American Medical Malpractice Litigation in Historical Perspective," *Journal of the American Medical Association* 283 (2000): 1731–1737.

2. Paul Starr, *The Social Transformation of American Medicine: The Rise of a Sovereign Profession* (New York: Basic Books, 1982).

3. Bernard Schwartz, *The Law in America* (New York: McGraw-Hill, 1974), 242.

4. Patricia Danzon, *The Frequency and Severity of Medical Malpractice Claims*, *R-2870* (Santa Monica, CA: Rand Corporation, 1982) 6.

5. Phillip K. Howard, "When Judges Won't Judge," *Wall Street Journal*, October 22, 2004.

6. Alexis de Tocqueville, *Democracy in America*, translated and edited by Harvey C. Mansfield and Delba Winthrop (Chicago, IL: University of Chicago Press, 2000) 639.

7. Dan Miller, "Liability for Medical Malpractice: Issues and Evidence," A Joint Economic Committee Study, Jim Saxton, Vice-Chairman, United States Congress, May 2003, 24.

8. Physician Insurers Association of America, *Medical Professional Liability Insurance: A practitioner's primer* (Rockville, MD: Physician Insurers Association of America, 2002) ii.

9. Board of Trustees, *Medical Liability Reform: Report on MICRA Enhancements, Report 32 (A-03)* (Chicago, IL: American Medical Association, 2003) [Online]. Available at: http://www.ama-assn.org/AMA/pub/category/10296.html [August 28, 2004].

10. Board of Trustees, *Medical Liability Reform: Report on MICRA Enhancements, Report 13 (I-03)* (Chicago, IL: American Medical Association, 2003) [Online]. Available at: http://www.ama-assn.org/AMA/pub/category/11611.html [August 28, 2004].

11. Howard Marcus, "The Rocky Road to Texas Tort Reform," *Physician Insurer* 18 (2004): 6–10.

12. Howard Marcus, "The Rocky Road to Texas Tort Reform," 8.

13. William Shakespeare, *Romeo and Juliet,* Act ii, Scene 2.4. [Online] Available at: http//bartleby.com/100/138.28html [August 28, 2004].

14. Chris Grier, "Feds/Medical Liability Cap Would Have Little Effect on Health Care Costs," BestWeek: BestWire Services [Online] Rev. January 14, 2004. Available at: Chris.Grier@ambest.com [January 29, 2004].

15. Dan Miller, "Liability for Medical Malpractice: Issues and Evidence," A Joint Economic Committee Study, Jim Saxton, Vice-Chairman, United States Congress, May 2003, 22

16. United States General Accounting Office, "Medical Malpractice: Implications of Rising Premiums on Access to Health Care, GAO-03-836" [Online], Rev. August 8, 2003. Available at: http//www.gao.gov/cgi-bin/getrpt?GAO-03-836 [August 28, 2004].

17. "GAO: Crisis Localized?" *Illinois Medical Express* 4 (2003): 11: 4.

18. James C. Mohr, "American Medical Malpractice Litigation in Historical Perspective," *Journal of the American Medical Association* 283 (2000): 1731.

19. Board of Trustees, *Medical Liability Reform: Report on MICRA Enhancements, Report 32 (A-03)* (Chicago, IL: American Medical Association, 2003) [Online]. Available at: http://www.ama-assn.org/AMA/pub/category/10296.html [August 28, 2004].

20. Rachel E. Silverman, "So Sue Me: Doctors Without Insurance," *Wall Street Journal* January 28, 2004, D1.

21. "Eyeing the Experts" *Illinois Medical Express*, 4 (2003): 8: 2.

22. Dr. Mary Santos, Interview with author (SCC), July 25, 2003 [Appendix 1].

Chapter 13
1. William Shakespeare, *King Henry V*, Act 3, Scene 1 [Online]. Available at: http//bartleby.com/ [February 14, 2004].

2. Saul Bellow, Interview with author (SCC), September 13, 1999 [Appendix 1].

Glossary

ALLEGATION: Assertion, declaration, or statement that is made in a pleading by one of the parties to the action and that tells what that party intends to prove.

ADR (ALTERNATIVE DISPUTE RESOLUTION): Formal malpractice case resolution process outside the jury trial system.

ANSWER: Written response in a civil case; in it, the defendant admits or denies the allegations contained in the plaintiff's complaint.

APPELLATE COURT: Review court above the trial court; appellate courts decide whether there were errors of law committed in the trial court.

ARBITRATION: Process for deciding a legal dispute out of court; a substitute for an ordinary trial.

CASE LAW: Law based on previous decisions of appellate courts.

CASE RESERVE: Money set aside and invested by an insurance company to pay estimated future losses. A company's claim department typically specifies a reserve amount for every claim filed, which may be modified as the claim proceeds in the courts.

CAUSATION: Causal relationship between the alleged act of negligence and the alleged damages. The chain of causation can be broken by a new intervening cause that interrupts the initial sequence of events and produces a result that would not otherwise have occurred from the original act or omission.

CLAIM: Actual demand for compensation (formal claim) in which the patient (or his or her representative) has indicated an intent to pursue the demand. Notice may be made orally or in writing. A claim does not always become a lawsuit.

CLAIM PROFESSIONAL: Insurance company representative who coordinates the activities of the defense team.

CLAIM SEVERITY: Amount of financial liability resulting from settling a claim. A claim that is settled with no payment for damages is generally considered to have a "small" claim severity, whereas a claim in which the carrier pays the full limits of a policy is a "large" severity claim. Trends in claims severity on a specialty-by-specialty basis are important factors in setting rates each year.

CLAIMS-MADE COVERAGE: Most common type of professional liability coverage available. It provides protection for claims that occur and are reported while the policy is in effect (coverage period). Within the conditions of a claims-made policy, a claim must be reported to the carrier in writing by the insured. Tail coverage, or a reporting endorsement, provides coverage for claims that occur during the coverage period but are reported after the policy terminates.

CLOSING ARGUMENT: At the end of the trial, the attorneys are permitted to summarize their case for the jury before the jurors begin their deliberations.

COLLATERAL SOURCE: Worker's compensation benefits, sick pay, and health insurance benefits are collateral sources and may not be deducted from what the defendant owes the plaintiff. In some instances, this allows the plaintiff double recovery; however, many collateral sources have payback provisions that require the plaintiff to reimburse the carrier for benefits paid previously.

COMMON LAW: Court-made law.

COMPARATIVE NEGLIGENCE: Doctrine of comparing degrees of fault among the responsible parties.

COMPLAINT: Document(s) filed with the court to institute a civil action (lawsuit). The complaint must give fair notice to a defendant regarding the alleged basis for the lawsuit and the relief sought. The complaint must be "served" on the defendant, along with a summons.

CONTINGENCY FEE: Fee arrangement frequently entered into by the plaintiff's attorney where, if there is recovery, the client pays the lawyer a percentage, but the plaintiff pays nothing if there is no recovery. Defense attorneys are customarily engaged on an hourly basis.

CONTINUANCE: Adjournment or delay of a scheduled session of a court.

CONTRIBUTION: Right among defendants allowing them to share responsibility for a judgment and pay according to their degree of fault. Contribution is sharing of the loss according to fault. (See also Indemnity.)

COURT COSTS: Awarded to the winning party in a lawsuit. In general, court costs are very minimal. Attorneys's fees are not included.

COURT TRIAL: Trial without a jury; the judge sits as the jury.

CROSS-EXAMINATION: Questioning of a witness of one party by the opposing party during a trial, hearing, or deposition.

DAMAGES: Monetary compensation claimed by a person who has sustained a loss or an injury to his or her person, property, or rights as a result of the negligence or unlawful conduct of another.

DATE OF INCIDENT: Date on which an alleged incident of malpractice occurred.

DATE OF REPORTING: Date on which an incident is reported to an insurance company.

DEFAULT: Failure of either party to file required documents or appear in a civil case within a certain period of time.

DEFENDANT: Person or party sued in a civil case.

DEFENSE ATTORNEY: Attorney who defends the person who is sued (defendant).

DEFENSE COSTS: Expenses directly attributable to specific claims. Includes payments for defense attorneys, medical evaluation of patients, expert medical reviews and witnesses, investigation, and record copying.

DEPOSITION: Question-and-answer period under oath taken by lawyers before the trial, either to find out the witnesses' knowledge of the incident or to preserve their testimony to use at the time of trial instead of a personal appearance.

DIRECT EXAMINATION: Questioning of a witness by the party who calls the witness.

DIRECTED VERDICT: In a trial, a judgment entered by the judge without allowing the jury to participate.

DISCOVERY: Pretrial process, such as a deposition, by which one party discovers the evidence that will be relied upon at trial by the opposing party.

DISMISSAL WITH PREJUDICE: Order to dismiss a case in which the court bars the plaintiff from suing again on the same cause of action.

DISMISSAL WITHOUT PREJUDICE: Order to dismiss a case in which the court preserves the plaintiff's right to sue again on the same cause of action.

DUTY: To prove negligence, the plaintiff must show that the named healthcare provider had an obligation to the patient who was (allegedly) harmed. This duty is usually proved by demonstrating that a provider–patient relationship existed at the time of the event in question.

ECONOMIC DAMAGES: Monetary losses such as medical expenses and loss of income.

EVIDENCE: Fact presented in court through the testimony of a witness, an object, or written documents. For example, exhibit A can be a document or an object that is offered into evidence during a trial or hearing.

EXCESS LIABILITY: Liability insurance designed to provide an extra layer of coverage above the primary layer. The excess insurance does not respond, however, until the limits of liability in the primary layer have been exhausted. The excess layer provides not only higher limits but also catastrophic protection for very large losses.

FEDERAL COURT: Another system of courts similar to state courts, but federal court may accept only certain types of cases. Malpractice cases are generally not filed in federal courts unless a patient from another state sues a physician from another state.

FRIVOLOUS LAWSUITS: Lawsuit that clearly lacks substance or is clearly insufficient as a matter of law. Court may order the plaintiff and/or the plaintiff's attorney to pay the defendant's legal fees if the plaintiff pursues a frivolous lawsuit.

GENERAL AND SPECIAL DAMAGES: In compensating an injured person for the damages that he or she has sustained, the jury will typically assess two basic categories of damages. One category concerns losses that can be determined with some degree of precision—loss of earnings, loss of future earning capacity, medical bills in the past and future, and the like. These are called *special damages*. *General damages*, on the other hand, are less "mathematical" in nature, but often they constitute the most significant loss sustained by the injured person. General damages include physical pain and suffering; emotional pain and suffering; loss of enjoyment of life, and loss of care, comfort, and society when a loved one dies.

INCIDENT: Event or happening that causes unanticipated harm to a patient.

INFORMED CONSENT: Agreement obtained voluntarily from a patient for the performance of specific medical, surgical, or research procedures after the material risks and benefits of these procedures and their alternatives have been fully explained in nontechnical terms.

INSURANCE GAP: When a physician has professional liability insurance under a claims-made policy, once the coverage period has expired without renewal, claims that have not yet been made and reported to the carrier (insurance company) during the "active" policy period are not covered. In such cases, a physician is said to be "bare" (uninsured), unless he or she has purchased an extended reporting endorsement (tail coverage) from the former carrier or has obtained *prior acts* (nose coverage) from a new carrier.

INSURANCE POLICY: Contract between an insurance company and its insured. The policy defines what the company agrees to cover for what period of time and describes the obligations and responsibilities of the insured.

INSURANCE POLICY LIMIT: Maximum amount paid under the terms of a policy. A professional liability insurance policy usually has two limits: a per-claim limit and an annual aggregate limit.

INSURANCE POLICY TERM: Length of time for which a policy is written.

INSURANCE PREMIUM: Amount of money an insured pays for an insurance policy. Rates are calculated by the insurance company's underwriters to bring in enough money to establish reserves for future losses; pay current losses; cover the company's operating expenses, including the cost of defending claims; and, If the company is organized as a profit-making business, generate a profit.

INTERROGATORIES: Series of written questions from one party in the case to the other side to be answered under oath (i.e., the answering party signs a sworn statement that the answers are true). Interrogatories are part of the discovery process.

JOINT AND SEVERAL LIABILITY: A potential exists where one or more defendants cannot pay their liability share of losses. These unpaid amounts are re-apportioned among remaining solvent defendants. Among multiple defendants, a minimally responsible defendant can be held responsible (jointly liable) for all the plaintiff's damages when the other defendants are unable to pay their share of the award—commonly referred to as the "deep pocket." Because of tort reforms, in some states multiple defendants are now only individually responsible (severally liable) for the plaintiff's damages. In other words, the defendants pay according to the percentage of their fault.

JUDGMENT: Official decision by a court regarding the rights and claims of the parties to a civil or criminal lawsuit.

JUDGMENT NOTWITHSTANDING THE VERDICT: Motion for judgment not withstanding the verdict, *non obstante veredicto*, asks the court to reverse the jury's verdict on the grounds that the jury could not reasonably have reached such a verdict. If granted, the court enters a new verdict.

JURY DELIBERATIONS: At the conclusion of a trial—after *voir dire*, opening statements, trial witnesses, closing arguments, and jury instructions—the jurors are given the case to decide. They discuss the case in a separate room— (jury deliberations) and then summarize the result of their discussions on the verdict form.

JURY INSTRUCTIONS: Jurors decide cases based on their review of the evidence presented during the trial. The jurors receive direction from the judge regarding any legal principles they must consider in arriving at their verdict. The judge provides that direction by reading from written "instructions"; this is done at the end of the case, although some instruction may be read to the jury at the outset of the trial. Attorneys for the plaintiff and defendant are given an opportunity to submit their recommended instructions to the judge.

JURY TRIAL: Many state constitutions guarantee the right to a jury trial in most cases, such as malpractice and automobile cases. An exception exists for those cases subject to an arbitration agreement or mandatory arbitration.

JURY VERDICT: After the jury has heard all the evidence and received the judge's jury instructions, the jurors meet and arrive at their decision. The foreman of the jury summarizes the decision on the verdict form that the judge, with input from both sides of attorneys, has given them. The verdict will indicate who has won and who has lost and, if damages are awarded, the amount of the damages.

LAWSUIT: Filing of the necessary legal documents in court (summons and complaint) to recover damages.

LIMITS OF LIABILITY: Maximum amount an insurer will pay out under the terms of a policy. Professional liability policies typically specify both a per-occurrence limit and an aggregate limit for all claims incurred during the term of a contract, such as $1 million (per occurrence)/$3 million (aggregate).

LOSS RESERVES: Amount set aside to pay for reported and unreported claims. For an individual claim, a case reserve or an estimate of the expected loss is set aside.

MALPRACTICE: Professional negligence or failure to exercise that degree of care as is used by reasonably careful physicians in the same or similar community. This failure must be a substantial contributing cause of the injury. In a medical malpractice trial, the plaintiff's attorney must show that the physician's violation of the standard of practice caused the patient's injury. The attorney can prove the violation any one of three ways: (*1*) by medical testimony establishing that the ordinary standards of the medical community were violated and contributed to the patient's bad result, (*2*) *res ipsa loquitur*, or (*3*) lack of informed consent.

MEDIATION: Form of alternate dispute resolution, in lieu of a formal court trial. In mediation, both sides agree on a third party to help them reconcile differences or negotiate a resolution of the matter in dispute. In mediation, the decision-making power lies in the hands of the disputing parties rather than in that of the mediator.

MEDICAL EXPERT: Qualified individual providing evidence based on inference after reviewing available medical information, not personal knowledge of the situation being considered. To be considered an expert, the individual must be qualified (by virtue of knowledge, skill, experience, training, or education) to offer an opinion on the topic.

MICRA (MEDICAL INJURY COMPENSATION REFORM ACT OF 1975) Legislation passed by the California legislature in an emergency session in response to a medical liability insurance crisis that resulted in proposed skyrocketing increases in physician medical liability insurance premiums of between 300% and 500%. MICRA places a $250,000 cap on noneconomic damages (pain and suffering), limits attorney contingency fees, and allows periodic payments of future damages in excess of $50,000. MICRA created the Board of Medical Quality Assurance (now the Medical Board of California).

MISTRIAL: Erroneous invalid trial that cannot stand in law.

NATIONAL PRACTITIONER DATA BANK (NPDB): Federally established repository of information regarding malpractice payments and disciplinary actions against health-care providers.

NEGLIGENCE: Failure to exercise that degree of care that a reasonable person would exercise under the same circumstances. When that failure causes another person to sustain an injury or a financial loss, that person may be entitled to just compensation through our civil justice system.

NONECONOMIC DAMAGES: Pain, suffering, inconvenience, loss of consortium, physical impairment, disfigurement, and other nonpecuniary damages.

NONRENEWAL When an insurer chooses not to offer renewal coverage on a policy for cause such as higher-than-expected hazards or losses or lack of compliance with safety recommendations or because the insurer is withdrawing from a territory or from offering a type of coverage. When an insurer nonrenews coverage, it must be done within the applicable state law as far as the reasons permitted, type of notice that is sent to the insured, and the amount of time the insurer must give the insured before policy expiration.

NOSE COVERAGE: Nose coverage covers claims first made against the physician after the effective date of coverage on the policy. To be covered, such claims must arise out of the physician's acts or omissions before the policy's effective date and after its retroactive date. A policy may have an effective date of January 1, 2004, for example, but its retroactive date may be January 1, 1998. (Both dates are shown on the declarations page of the policy.) Nose coverage is also known as *retroactive coverage* or *prior acts coverage*.

OCCURRENCE INSURANCE: Type of policy in which the insured is covered for any incident that occurs (or occurred) while the policy is (or was) in force, regardless of when the incident is reported or when it becomes a claim. Occurrence insurance for medical liability coverage is rarely offered today because of the difficulty in projecting long-term claims costs under this type of policy.

OPENING STATEMENT: Before the jury begins to hear from witnesses and review exhibits in a trial, the attorneys are permitted to summarize the case and to explain the evidence they believe will be presented during the trial.

PEER REVIEW: Discussions, analyses, and recommendations of a physician's diagnosis, care, and treatment of patients conducted by colleagues with similar training and background in the same practice setting. Upper-level peer review committees may comprise a cross section of many specialties. Peer review is conducted for purposes of employment, appointment, reappointment, privileging, quality improvement, or corrective action. Peer review discussions and notes are protected from discovery by plaintiffs in medical malpractice litigation.

PLAINTIFF: Party who initiates a legal action—in a personal injury lawsuit, the person who alleges that he or she has suffered monetary damages due the negligence of another party.

PLEADINGS: Written documents stating the allegations and claims of the opposing parties in a legal dispute.

PREPONDERANCE OF EVIDENCE: The relative weight, credit, and value of the evidence presented by adversaries in a trial. In a civil trial, the jury is charged with reaching a verdict based on this standard.

PRIVILEGED COMMUNICATIONS: Communications made to a physician, lawyer, minister, etc., by a patient, client, or penitent that are intended to be confidential. These communications may not be disclosed by the physician, lawyer, or minister without the permission of the patient, client, or penitent. Permission may be written or oral. Unless the patient waives the privilege, it exists until he or she takes the stand and testifies in court about the privileged matter. Medical records are generally privileged.

PUNITIVE DAMAGES: This category of damages is not designed to provide compensation for injuries. Instead, compensation is obtained through a jury's award of general damages and special damages. Punitive and exemplary damages, on the other hand, are awarded in circumstances in which the defendant's misconduct should be punished by a specific and separate damage award.

REBUTTAL: Opportunity to present rebuttal evidence after one's evidence has been subject to cross-examination.

RE-DIRECT EXAMINATION: Evidence that attempts to explain, counteract, or disprove facts given in evidence by the other party.

REINSURANCE: Agreement between insurance companies under which one accepts all or part of the risk or loss of the other. Most primary companies insure only part of the risk on any given policy; the amount varies among carriers. The remainder of the policy limits are covered by reinsurance entities. The less primary risk that the company insures, the more premium it has to pay to the reinsurer to cover the remaining policy limits. In general, smaller companies are able to cover only a relatively small proportion of the liability limit. This results in large premium payments to reinsurers. Larger com-panies can cover a large proportion safely, thus reducing the payments they must cede to reinsurers, which indirectly reduces the cost of insurance to their policyholders.

RES IPSA LOQUITUR: Legal doctrine that, when applicable, allows a patient to forego the necessity of an expert witness to testify that the defendant physician violated the standards of practice. Generally it is applicable only in those instances where negligence is clear and obvious, even to a layman, such as foreign object cases where a physician testifies against himself or herself.

RESERVATION OF RIGHTS: Insurance term that refers to the situation arising when there is a question as to whether an incident is covered. Typically, an insurer is obligated to defend a claim during the time the coverage issue between insurer and policyholder is being resolved.

RETROACTIVE DATE: Earliest date for which coverage is afforded under a claims-made form, usually the effective date of the first year of such policy provided to the insured.

SETTLEMENT: Resolution of a formal claim or lawsuit by the parties involved without judicial intervention or proceedings. Settlement is not an admission of negligence but rather a formal agreement that ends the legal dispute and usually includes a negotiated monetary exchange. A settlement can occur at any point in the life of the claim or suit before the actual payment of a monetary judgment imposed by a court against a defendant.

STANDARD OF PRACTICE: Term used in the legal definition of medical malpractice. A physician is liable only if the treatment, or the lack thereof, violates the standards of practice of reasonably competent physicians in the same or similar circumstances, in the same or similar community. The standard is therefore set by what reasonably careful physicians do or do not do, when treating a given condition. There may be more than one medically acceptable method of treating; consequently, several acceptable standards may exist.

STATUTE OF LIMITATIONS: Time period in which a lawsuit alleging malpractice must be brought. It varies by state and patient age.

STATUTORY LAW: Law enacted by the legislature or congress.

STIPULATION: Agreement, admission, or concession made in a judicial proceeding by the parties or their attorneys, thus relieving a party of its obligation to produce evidence in support of an argument or allegation.

STRUCTURED SETTLEMENT: Legal agreement to pay a designated person, usually someone who has been injured, a specified sum of money in periodic payments, usually for his or her lifetime, instead of in a single lump sum payment.

SUBPOENA: Official order requiring a person to appear at a certain place and time to give testimony on a particular matter or to present certain documents in his or her possession.

SUMMONS: Legal document commanding the person sued to appear and answer the claims in the complaint within a prescribed time.

TAIL COVERAGE: In claims-made liability policies, only those claims that occur after the retroactive date and are reported or filed against the insured during the policy period are covered by the policy. The ERP, or tail, is an endorsement available to extend the reporting period for the filing of a claim to give additional time to be considered covered.

TORT: Wrongful act to a person or property for which the law allows money damages (assault and battery, malpractice, libel and slander, etc.). The person committing the wrongful act is called a *tort-feasor*.

TORT REFORM: Legislation designed to reduce liability costs through limits on various kinds of damages and through modification of liability rules.

TRANSCRIPT: Official verbatim record of court proceedings.

TRIAL COURT: Court where all of the testimony is taken and the witnesses appear.

UNDERWRITING RESULTS: Profit or loss of the insurance company, computed by subtracting from earned premium those amounts paid out and reserved for losses and expenses. Any residual amount is called an *underwriting profit*. If those deductions exceed the earned premium, this is called an *underwriting loss*. Underwriting results do not include investment income.

VICARIOUS LIABILITY: Liability that a person may have for the acts of someone else; for instance, in the employer–employee relationship, the physician may be vicariously liable for the acts of the nurses in the physician's office.

VOIR DIRE: This phrase is derived from the French words "to see" and "to say or tell." At the beginning of a jury trial, the court will have summoned a number of people as potential jurors. Most judges permit the attorneys to question potential jurors before the final group of jurors is selected. This process—known as *voir dire*—allows the attorneys to learn more about the jurors, but it also allows the potential jurors to learn about the case. If the discussion between the attorneys and potential jurors demonstrates that it would be difficult for a particular person to serve as a fair and unbiased juror for the trial, then that person can be excused from jury service.

WRONGFUL DEATH: Term given for the money damage claim that exists in favor of a surviving spouse, children, parents, or estate when a person dies due to the wrongful acts of another.

Bibliography

Board of Trustees. *Medical Liability Reform: Report on MICRA Enhancements, Report 32 (A-03)* (Chicago, IL: American Medical Association, 2003) [Online]. Available at: http://www.ama-assn.org/AMA/pub/category/10296.html [August 28, 2004].

Board of Trustees. *Medical Liability Reform: Report on MICRA Enhancements, Report 13 (I-03)*, (Chicago, IL: American Medical Association, 2003) [Online]. Available at: http://www.ama-assn.org/AMA/pub/category/11611.html [August 28, 2004].

Brennan, Troyen A., Lucian L. Leape, Nan M. Laird, et al. "The Incidence of Adverse Events and Negligence in Hospitalized Patients: Results of the Harvard Medical Practice Study, I," *New England Journal of Medicine* 324 (1991): 370–376.

Charles, Sara C. "Coping with a Medical Malpractice Suit," *Western Journal of Medicine* 174 (2001): 55–58.

Charles, Sara C. and Eugene C. Kennedy. *Defendant: A Psychiatrist on Trial for Medical Malpractice* (New York: Vintage Books, Random House, 1986).

Council on Ethical and Judicial Affairs. *Code of Medical Ethics: Current Opinions with Annotations* (Chicago, IL: American Medical Association, 2002–2003 ed.) Opinion 8.12, 217–218.

Danzon, Patricia M. *Medical Malpractice: Theory, Evidence, and Public Policy* (Cambridge, MA: Harvard University Press, 1985).

Fox, Renée C. *The Human Condition of Health Professions* (Durham, NH: University of New Hampshire, November 19, 1979).

Gabbard, Glen O. "The Role of Compulsiveness in the Normal Physician," *Journal of the American Medical Association* 254 (1985): 2926–2929.

Hilfiker, David. *Healing the Wounds: A Physician Looks at His Work* (New York: Pantheon Books, 1985).

Horowitz, Mardi J. *Treatment of Stress Response Syndromes* (Washington, DC: American Psychiatric Publishing, 2003).

Kelly-Wilson, Lisa, Jennifer Parsons, and Sara C. Charles. "Physicians and Medical Malpractice Litigation," *Report to the Council of Medical Specialty Societies* (Chicago, IL: Survey Research Laboratory, University of Illinois, 2003).

Kohn, Linda T., Janet M. Corrigan, and Molla S. Donaldson, eds. *To Err Is Human: Building a Safer Health System* (Washington, DC: National Academy Press, 1999).

Leape, Lucian L., Troyen A. Brennan, Nan M. Laird, et al. "The Nature of Adverse Events in Hospitalized Patients: Results of the Harvard Medical Practice Study, II," *New England Journal of Medicine* 324 (1991): 377–384).

Liang, Bryan A. "A System of Medical Error Disclosure." *Quality and Safety in Health Care* 11 (2002): 64–68).

"Medical Liability Reform—Now!" June 14, 2004 edition. American Medical Association. Available at: http/www.ama-assn.org/ama1/pub/upload/mm/450/mlrnowJune112004.pdf [Septermber 4, 2004].

Miller, Dan. "Liability for Medical Malpractice: Issues and Evidence," *A Joint Economic Committee Study*, Jim Saxton, Vice-Chairman, United States Congress, May 2003).

Mohr, James C. "American Medical Malpractice Litigation in Historical Perspective," *Journal of the American Medical Association* 283 (2000): 1731–1737.

Reason, James. *Human Error* (Cambridge, England: Cambridge University Press, 1990).

Reason, James. "Human Error: Models and Management," *British Medical Journal* 320 (2000): 768–770.

Starr, Paul. *The Social Transformation of American Medicine: The Rise of a Sovereign Profession* (New York: Basic Books, 1982).

Wu, Albert W., Susan Folkman, Stephen J. McPhee, et al. "Do House Officers Learn from Their Mistakes?" *Journal of the American Medical Association* 265 (1991): 2089–2094.

Wu, Albert W. "Medical Error: The Second Victim," *British Medical Journal* 320 (2000): 726–727.

Ursano, Robert and Ann E. Norwood, eds. *Trauma and Disaster: Responses and Management,* Review of Psychiatry, Volume 22 (Washington, DC: American Psychiatric Press, 2003).

United States General Accounting Office. "Medical Malpractice: Implications of Rising Premiums on Access to Health Care, GAO-03-836" [Online], Rev. August 8, 2003. Available at: http//www.gao.gov/cgi-bin/getrpt? GAO-03-836 [August 28, 2004].

Index